Small Animal Anesthesia & Analgesia

Diane McKelvey, B.Sc., D.V.M.

Kamloops Veterinary Clinic
Kamloops, British Columbia, Canada

K. Wayne Hollingshead, B.Sc., M.Sc., D.V.M.

Assistant Professor
Animal Health Technology
University College of the Cariboo
Kamloops, British Columbia, Canada

Second Edition

with 72 illustrations

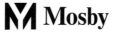 Mosby

An Affiliate of Elsevier Science

St. Louis   London   Philadelphia   Sydney   Toronto

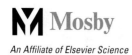

An Affiliate of Elsevier Science

Cover Art: Right center, "© TSM/Ariel S. Kelley, 1999"; left top and bottom, courtesy Dr. Eleanor Hawkins. From Nelson RW et al: *Small animal internal medicine,* ed 2, St Louis, 1998, Mosby.

Second Edition

Copyright © 2000 by Mosby, Inc.

Previous edition copyrighted 1994

NOTICE

Pharmacology is an ever-changing field. Standard safety precautions must be followed, but as new research and clinical experience broaden our knowledge, changes in treatment and drug therapy may become necessary or appropriate. Readers are advised to check the most current product information provided by the manufacturer of each drug to be administered to verify the recommended dose, the method and duration of administration, and contraindications. It is the responsibility of the treating physician, relying on experience and knowledge of the patient, to determine dosages and the best treatment for each individual patient. Neither the publisher nor the editor assume any liability for any injury and/or damage to persons or property arising from this publication.

Mosby, Inc.
An Affiliate of Elsevier Science
11830 Westline Industrial Drive
St. Louis, Missouri 63146

Printed in United States of America

ISBN 0-323-00273-0

02   03   /   9   8   7   6   5

TO OUR FAMILIES

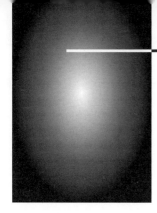

Preface

S mall animal anesthesia has undergone significant change in the 6 years since the publication of the first edition. New preanesthetic and anesthetic drugs have been approved, and sophisticated monitoring devices such as pulse oximeters have become widely available. In preparing this edition, we have included updated information on anesthetic agents and monitoring procedures that may be encountered in current veterinary small animal practice.

There has also been a long overdue surge of interest in detecting, preventing, and managing pain in veterinary patients, and we have included a new chapter on analgesia to reflect these concerns. We have changed the title of this book to recognize the important role of veterinary anesthetists in providing appropriate analgesia for small animal patients.

In the majority of small animal practices in the United States and Canada, veterinarians and veterinary technicians work together as a team to provide anesthesia for their patients. Recognizing the important and expanding role of veterinary technicians in anesthesia, the Veterinary Technician Anesthetist Society (VTAS) and the Academy of Veterinary Technician Anesthetists (AVTA) have been established in order to bring together veterinary technicians and others who share a common interest in the field of veterinary anesthesiology. Testing and certification of technicians in the specialty of anesthesia will soon be a reality. It is our hope that this book will stimulate an increased awareness of the vital role that veterinary technicians play in small animal anesthesia.

Diane McKelvey
K. Wayne Hollingshead

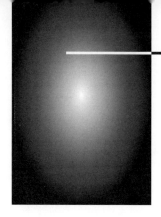

Acknowledgments

In preparing the second edition of *Small Animal Anesthesia and Analgesia* we were fortunate to have the assistance of many veterinarians and veterinary technicians. These include Dr. Tanya Duke, who reviewed the manuscript and gave many valuable suggestions; Dr. Samuel Longiaru; Ms. Wendy Stankevich; Ms. Delli Dreger; Ms. Robina Kay; Dr. Karol Mathews; Dr. Margie Scherk; Dr. Ralph Harvey; Dr. Jeff Ko; Dr. Allan Klide; Ms. Paige Jones; and Mr. Chuck Bishop. We gratefully acknowledge the assistance of Ed Alderman, Teri Merchant, Linda Duncan, and the staff of Mosby, Inc.

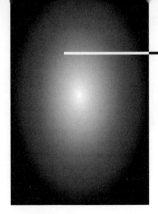

Contents

1 The Preanesthetic Period, 1

Patient Evaluation, 2
  Patient History, 2
  Physical Examination, 5
  Diagnostic Tests, 11
  Classification of Patient
    Status, 14
Selection of the Anesthetic
    Protocol, 14
  Factors That Influence
    Selection, 14
Preanesthetic Patient Care, 16
  Withholding Food Before
    Anesthesia, 16
  Correction of Preexisting
    Problems, 17
  Intravenous
    Catheterization, 17
  Other Preanesthetic Patient
    Care, 21
Preanesthetic Agents, 21
  Reasons for the Use of
    Preanesthetic Agents, 21
  Anticholinergics
    (Parasympatholytics), 23
  Tranquilizers and
    Sedatives, 28
  Phenothiazines, 28
  Benzodiazepines, 30
  Thiazine Derivatives, 32
  Opioids (Narcotics), 35

2 General Anesthesia, 46

Definition of General
    Anesthesia, 47
Components of General
    Anesthesia, 47
  Preanesthesia, 48
  Induction, 48
  Maintenance, 48
  Recovery, 48
Safety of General Anesthesia, 49
Classical Stages and Planes of
    Anesthesia, 50
  Stage I, 51
  Stage II, 51
  Stage III, 51
  Stage IV, 54
  Overview of Anesthetic Stages
    and Planes, 54
Induction Techniques and
    Agents, 55
  Induction Using Injectable
    Agents, 55
  Induction Using Inhalation
    Agents, 56
  Monitoring During the
    Induction Period, 60
Endotracheal Intubation, 61
  Advantages of Endotracheal
    Intubation, 61
  Problems Associated with
    Endotracheal Intubation, 62

Maintenance of Anesthesia, 71
  Monitoring Vital Signs, 72
  Use of Instruments to
    Monitor Vital Signs, 78
  Reflexes and Other Indicators
    of Anesthetic Depth, 88
  Judging Anesthetic
    Depth, 94
  Recording Information
    During Anesthesia, 95
Patient Positioning and Comfort
  During Anesthesia, 99
Recovery from General
  Anesthesia, 100
  Stages of Recovery, 101
  Anesthetist's Role in the
    Recovery Period, 101

3 **Anesthetic Agents and
   Techniques, 109**

Comparison of Inhalation and
  Injectable Anesthesia, 110
Injectable Anesthetics, 111
  Barbiturates, 111
  Cyclohexamines, 120
  Neuroleptanalgesia, 125
  Propofol, 126
  Etomidate, 128
Inhalation Anesthetics, 128
  Characteristics of an Ideal
    Agent, 128
  Classes of Inhalation
    Anesthetic, 129
  Mechanism of Action of
    Inhalation Agents, 132
  Distribution and Elimination
    of Inhalation Agents, 132
  Properties of Inhalation
    Agents, 132
  Halothane, 134
  Isoflurane, 136
  Methoxyflurane, 137
  Other Chlorofluorocarbon
    Agents, 138
  Nitrous Oxide, 139

Agents Used in the Postanesthetic
  Period, 140
Doxapram, 141

4 **Anesthetic Equipment, 147**

Equipment Needed for
  Anesthesia, 148
  Endotracheal Tubes, 148
  Anesthetic Machines, 151
  Vaporizers, 165
Operation of the Anesthetic
  Machine, 172
  Rebreathing Systems, 173
  Nonrebreathing Systems, 173
  Choice of Rebreathing Versus
    Nonrebreathing, 177
  Carrier Gas Flow Rates, 178
  Safety Concerns When Using
    a Total Rebreathing
    System, 180
Care and Use of Anesthetic
  Equipment, 183
  Setting Up Anesthetic
    Equipment, 183
  Maintenance of Anesthetic
    Equipment, 183

5 **Workplace Safety, 191**

Hazards of Waste Anesthetic
  Gas, 191
  Short-term Problems, 192
  Long-term Effects, 192
  Assessment of Risk, 194
  Reducing Exposure to Waste
    Anesthetic Gas, 196
  Monitoring Waste Gas
    Levels, 204
Safe Handling of Compressed
  Gases, 205
  Fire Safety Precautions, 205
  Use and Storage of
    Compressed Gas
    Cylinders, 205

6   *Anesthetic Problems and Emergencies,   210*

Reasons Why Anesthetic Problems
    and Emergencies
    Arise,   211
    Human Error,   211
    Equipment Failure,   213
    Anesthetic Agents,   215
    Patient Factors,   216
Response to Anesthetic Problems
    and Emergencies,   225
    Role of the Veterinary
    Technician in Emergency
    Care,   225
    General Approach to
    Emergencies,   226
    Problems That May Arise in
    the Recovery Period,   242

7   *Special Techniques,   252*

Local Analgesia,   253
    Agents Used in Veterinary
    Anesthesia,   253
    Characteristics of Local
    Analgesia,   253
    Mechanism of Action,   254
    Route of Administration,   255
    Toxicity,   262
Controlled Ventilation,   264
    Types of Assisted or
    Controlled
    Ventilation,   264
    Ventilation in the Awake
    Animal,   264
    Ventilation in the
    Anesthetized Animal,   265
    Manual Ventilation,   266
    Mechanical Ventilation,   268
    Risks of Controlled
    Ventilation,   270

Neuromuscular Blocking
    Agents,   270

8   *Analgesia,   277*

Introduction,   277
    What is Analgesia?,   277
    Why Treat Pain?,   278
General Principles of
    Analgesia,   279
    Physiology of Pain,   279
    Monitoring Signs of
    Pain,   279
    Methods of Pain
    Control,   282
Pharmacologic Analgesia,   284
    Delivery of Analgesic
    Drugs,   285
    Classes of Analgesic
    Drugs,   286
    Opioid Agents,   286
    Nonsteroidal
    Antiinflammatory
    Drugs,   295
    Combination Therapy,   300
    Other Agents,   300

Appendix A
    Standard Values and
    Equivalents,   307

Appendix B
    Catheter Comparison
    Scale,   310

Appendix C
    Equipment and Drugs for
    Use in an Emergency
    Crash Kit,   311

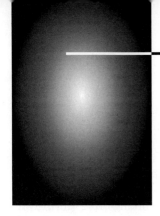

CHAPTER 1

The Preanesthetic Period

PERFORMANCE OBJECTIVES

After completion of this chapter, the reader will be able to:

- Define the term *preanesthetic period.*
- Understand the reasons for patient evaluation.
- Understand the need for obtaining a proper history, know how to take a complete history, and know what pitfalls may be encountered when taking a history.
- List the information that makes up the minimum data base for a patient.
- Understand the rationale for obtaining the owner's consent for anesthesia.
- State the parameters of a proper physical examination.
- Understand the importance of species, breed, weight, and obesity as they relate to the use and choice of anesthetic drugs.
- List the five physical classifications for patients as specified by the American Society of Anesthesiologists.
- Describe the various aspects of preanesthetic preparation, including choice of protocol, fasting, rationale for IV catheterization, and types of IV solutions that can be used and why they might be chosen.
- State which preanesthetic agents are commonly used, the rationale for their use, their mode of action and effects on the body, and their associated adverse side effects.

Preanesthesia is a term that describes the period immediately preceding the induction of anesthesia. Throughout the preanesthetic period and the anesthetic period that follows, the goal of the technician is to work with the veterinarian to achieve efficient, safe, and effective anesthesia with minimal stress to the patient. This chapter describes the responsibilities of the technician during the preanesthetic period.

One of the most important duties of the technician is to help obtain patient information through history, physical examination, and diagnostic tests. This information is useful not only to the technician/anesthetist but also to the veterinarian, who must determine the patient's physical condition and select the anesthetic protocol. The technician also may be responsible for preanesthetic care of the patient, including fasting, intravenous catheterization, and other procedures ordered by the veterinarian. To prepare for anesthesia, the technician must also ensure that the necessary equipment and supplies are available and in good working order (further described in Chapter 4). Finally, the technician is usually responsible for administering preanesthetic drugs to the patient, as requested by the veterinarian, and must have a thorough knowledge of the actions and adverse side effects associated with these drugs.

■ PATIENT EVALUATION

Technicians working as anesthetists in small animal practice soon become accustomed to the variety of patients they see. Animals vary in age, in temperament, and in physical appearance. Some are healthy, and some are critically ill or injured. Some are brought in for minor procedures; others are to undergo lengthy, more complicated surgery. Given this diversity, it is unrealistic to assume that the same anesthetic techniques should be used for all patients. Furthermore, it would be dangerous to expect all patients to react to a given anesthetic agent in the same way. It is therefore vital that, before initiating anesthesia, the veterinarian and technician gather as much information as possible on each patient to discover any factor that might lead to anesthetic complications. Accordingly, it is recommended that a *minimum patient data base* be obtained for each patient. If the information obtained on a given animal reveals a potential problem, the veterinarian may choose to alter the planned anesthetic procedure or postpone (or even cancel) the anesthesia.

The minimum patient data base should include the following (at the discretion of the veterinarian):
1. Patient history
2. The nature of the procedure to be performed under anesthesia
3. A complete physical examination
4. Diagnostic tests requested by the supervising veterinarian, which may include radiography, electrocardiography, urinalysis, hematology, and clinical chemistry
5. In consultation with the veterinarian, determination of the patient's physical status and anesthetic risk

Patient History

No examination of an animal is complete without an adequate history. Obtaining a good history requires skill and care. Like all arts, it must be continually practiced and refined. If the technician asks questions that require only a "yes or no" answer, the history may be incomplete or misleading. Thus asking "Does your dog drink much water?" would not encourage the client to provide specific information. Asking "How much water does your dog drink?" is the preferred option because it requires the owner to describe the amount of water consumed but not judge whether he or she believes the amount to be abnormal. If, for example, the client replied

"About 4 liters," the questioner would then be able to evaluate the information, perhaps deciding that 4 liters of water per day is excessive for a 2-kg Chihuahua despite the owner's belief that this is normal.

Another common error is to ask leading questions of the owner. In this example, asking the question "Your dog doesn't drink much water, does she?" would suggest to the owner that the appropriate response should be "No, I guess not." A technician asking such a question would fail to obtain an accurate patient history.

To obtain a complete history for any patient requiring anesthesia, the following questions should be asked:

1. What is the procedure to be performed on the animal (for example, surgery, dentistry, or diagnostic procedure)?
2. How old is the pet?
3. Has the animal had any previous illnesses, and if so, what was the medical or surgical treatment? Obviously, the patient's record may supplement the owner's information. A history that includes diseases of the heart and circulatory system, respiratory system, kidneys, liver, blood, nervous system, endocrine organs, or gastrointestinal tract may be of significance to the anesthetist and surgeon and should be brought to the attention of the veterinarian.
4. Has the animal exhibited any signs of illness in the past 24 hours, including lack of appetite, coughing, sneezing, vomiting, diarrhea, or any other condition that is of concern to the owner? When was the animal last sick or ill, and has the animal recovered from this disease as far as the owner knows? A report of recent illness should alert the veterinarian or technician to focus particular attention on the physical examination of that organ system. Animals suffering from disease may be at increased risk of anesthetic complications because of dehydration, fever, or electrolyte abnormalities. Sick animals also may introduce pathogens into the hospital, posing a risk to other patients unless they are placed in isolation.
5. How well does the animal tolerate exercise? The owner may be able to describe the type and amount of daily exercise or play that is normal for the animal. Dyspnea or fatigue after mild exercise, such as walking up a flight of stairs, may indicate the presence of cardiovascular or respiratory disease, which should be of concern to the anesthetist.
6. Has the animal undergone recent treatment with drugs or insecticides? Many medications, including corticosteroids, insulin, anticonvulsants, antibiotics, antidepressants, and flea control products, may alter the effect of anesthetics.
7. Is there any history of allergies or drug reactions? The owner may be able to recall the animal's reaction to anesthetic agents used in the past. This information is particularly important if the animal experienced prolonged recovery or personality changes after a previous anesthesia. In addition, if the animal has exhibited signs of an anaphylactic or other allergic reaction to any medication, this should be noted on the record and the information conveyed to the veterinarian.
8. When was the animal last vaccinated, and against what diseases was it vaccinated? Many veterinary clinics require current vaccinations for all healthy patients entering the clinic to prevent the spread of contagious diseases between patients.

9. What is the reproductive status of the animal? Has the animal been spayed or castrated? In the case of an intact female, has the owner observed any recent estrous cycle activity? Is it possible that the animal is pregnant? These questions are of particular importance if the animal is scheduled for an ovariohysterectomy because the animal's reproductive status may affect the length and difficulty of the surgery. Animals in heat also may have increased blood-clotting times because of the effect of estrogen on the clotting cascade. This may result in excessive bleeding during surgery.

10. Has the owner observed any of the following in the animal: abnormal bleeding or bruising, fainting, seizures, unexplained weakness, excessive thirst, or difficulty in passing stool or urine? If the owner answers yes to any of these, the veterinarian should be consulted because a serious illness may be present.

At the same time the patient history is obtained, it is customary to obtain a signed release authorizing anesthesia and surgery. It is illegal in most jurisdictions to undertake surgery or anesthesia on an animal without the owner's written consent. Such consent must be "informed," meaning that the owner is warned beforehand of any unusual risks associated with the anesthesia or surgery. Standard consent forms are available from practice management consultants and from state and provincial veterinary associations. Owners should be asked to provide a telephone number at which they may be reached during the day, in case an emergency or unforeseen complication should arise. It is also advisable that a written estimate of fees be presented to the owner before initiating the procedure.

Obviously, a great deal of information must be obtained for each patient before initiating anesthesia. Ideally, the history is obtained in person by the veterinarian or technician. A trained receptionist may be able to assist, particularly when a young, healthy animal is scheduled for an elective surgery such as castration or ovariohysterectomy. It is important to ensure that any hospital employee who admits a patient and speaks to the owner not only obtains a history but also relays that information to the anesthetist by means of a written record or oral report.

In some cases it may be difficult to obtain the history in person. Some clinics prefer to have the owner fill out a prepared history form, particularly if the clinic has a high volume of patients. In any practice, difficulties may arise when an animal's owner is in a hurry and reluctant to stop and answer questions; however, it is usually possible to obtain a telephone number and call for more information at a prearranged time. Occasionally the person bringing the animal into the clinic is not the owner and is unfamiliar with the pet. In this case, every effort should be made to contact the owner by telephone to obtain a more complete history.

In a busy practice, it is often difficult to set aside adequate time to obtain a good history, and the technician may be tempted to take shortcuts or omit one or more questions. **The importance of obtaining a complete history on each animal cannot be overemphasized.** The experienced anesthetist knows that a thorough history will help avoid unpleasant surprises during anesthesia and surgery. A dog that has been coughing regularly and that tires easily when chasing a ball may have a cardiac problem unknown to the owner. If this problem is not described in the animal's history, the technician may be surprised by having to deal with an anesthetized patient suffering from pulmonary edema, circulatory failure, and, ultimately, cardiac arrest.

Physical Examination

A complete physical examination should be conducted on every animal scheduled for anesthesia. Although the examination is usually carried out by a veterinarian, the technician should be familiar with the procedure. In some jurisdictions, veterinary technicians are authorized to perform basic physical examinations provided they are acting under the direct supervision of a licensed veterinarian.

The physical examination is important because it may reveal the following:

1. The presence of respiratory or cardiovascular disease. These can increase the risk of anesthetic complications and even lead to death.
2. The presence of a disorder such as an enlarged liver or abnormally small kidneys. Either of these may indicate a reduced ability to detoxify or excrete anesthetic agents.
3. The patient's inability to adequately control its state of hydration. A dehydrated patient has increased risk of problems during anesthesia.
4. Conditions requiring veterinary attention. Some of the more common disorders that are easily detected by physical examination include ear mite infestation, otitis externa, dental disease, overgrown nails, the presence of fleas, and anal sac impaction. The owner is often unaware that these disorders are present and, once informed of them, will authorize the veterinarian to treat the animal while it is anesthetized.
5. Physical factors that may affect the procedure to be performed. One surprisingly common example is the discovery that a cat brought in for an ovariohysterectomy is actually a male. It is far better to discover this mistake before undertaking anesthesia than to become aware of the problem during surgery! Another common example is the presentation of a cryptorchid animal for castration. The owner should be informed that the animal is a cryptorchid and that an increased fee may be charged for the surgery.

It is often helpful to have the owner present during the physical examination to give pertinent history regarding any physical abnormalities that are found. Any unusual findings should be brought to the attention of the veterinarian for confirmation. It is the veterinarian's responsibility to formulate an appropriate treatment plan and advise the technician accordingly.

Some veterinary clinics routinely recommend that animals scheduled for elective surgeries be brought into the clinic for an appointment before the day of surgery. Procedures that can be done at this time include obtaining a complete history, performing a physical examination in the presence of the owner, administering necessary vaccinations, undertaking routine preanesthetic screening such as heartworm testing and other blood tests, giving information on preanesthetic fasting of the animal, obtaining signed consent forms, and giving the owner an estimate of surgery and anesthesia fees. If such an appointment is scheduled several days before the planned surgery, unforeseen problems can be discovered and addressed well in advance of surgery.

The complete physical examination should include the signalment, disposition, and activity level of the animal and an examination of the organ systems.

Signalment.   The signalment includes the species, breed, weight, age, sex, and whether the patient is neutered. Some of this information is best obtained as part of the animal's history, but as previously mentioned, it is wise to double-check the owner's opinion on issues such as the animal's gender and age.

Species and breed.   Each species has a characteristic response to specific drugs. The metabolism of many drugs differs significantly between cats and dogs, and the recommended dose of many drugs reflects this fact (for example, the dose of morphine recommended for cats is much less than that recommended for dogs).

The technician or veterinarian may occasionally encounter an unfamiliar species, such as a rabbit, iguana, or parrot, and should consult specialty references and the veterinarian before undertaking anesthesia.

Differences in anatomy and physiology among the various breeds also may affect the response to an anesthetic agent or procedure. For example, endotracheal intubation may be difficult in a brachycephalic dog such as a bulldog. Brachycephalic dogs also are more likely to have breathing difficulties during anesthetic recovery because of airway obstruction from excess soft tissue in the oropharyngeal area. Sighthounds such as the greyhound or saluki may experience a prolonged recovery from thiobarbiturate anesthesia because of their relative absence of body fat and slow metabolism of barbiturates compared to other breeds of dogs.

Weight.   It is important to weigh each animal accurately before anesthesia because anesthetic dosages and intravenous fluid drip rates are calculated according to body weight. Estimating an animal's weight may lead to incorrect dosages, particularly in smaller patients. Animals lighter than 15 kg should be weighed on a pediatric scale or electronic scale; the chance of errors is greater if a less sensitive scale is used. The patient's weight should be compared to previous weights (as noted on the patient record) to determine whether weight gain or loss has occurred. Changes in weight may reflect changes in the patient's nutritional intake or in the overall state of health.

Age.   The age of the patient can be an important consideration when deciding the anesthetic protocol or types of drugs used. The neonate (up to 2 weeks of age) or pediatric animal (2 to 8 weeks of age) is much less capable of metabolizing any injectable drug than is the adult animal because the necessary liver metabolic pathways are not fully developed. At the other end of the scale, a geriatric animal may be unable to tolerate normal doses of some drugs because of poor hepatic or renal function. The net result in either case may be a slow recovery from anesthesia, particularly when injectable agents are used.

Disposition and activity level.   Before initiating anesthesia, the veterinary technician should observe the animal's temperament and activity level, both of which will affect the selection of anesthetic agent and the route of administration. For example, an animal that is anxious or aggressive may not become adequately sedated if a phenothiazine tranquilizer is used. In this case, combining a phenothiazine tranquilizer with an opioid may be preferable. On the other hand, animals that are calm and easily handled may be adequately sedated with phenothiazine tranquilizers alone, or the veterinarian may elect to omit sedation.

Aggressive or fearful animals are occasionally scheduled for anesthesia and surgery. Special handling techniques such as anesthetic chamber inductions, oral administration of ketamine, or the use of intramuscular or oral tiletamine/zolazepam, may be necessary to restrain such patients without endangering hospital staff. Orally administered anesthetics are slow to take effect (a range of 30 to 90 minutes has been reported). Some agents appear to have a narrow safety margin when given orally. Oral use of anesthetics generally constitutes off-label use and requires the owner's consent.

Examination of organ systems.   There are probably as many ways to perform a thorough physical examination as there are veterinarians and technicians. The main criterion is that the examination be done in a systematic manner (for example, from head to tail). Ideally, the examination should include all of the following:

1. *Notation of overall body condition* (for example, dehydrated, emaciated, obese, weak, or pregnant). All patients should be routinely evaluated for hydration status, which indicates if the amount of body water is normal. Table 1-1 outlines the parameters used to determine whether or not a patient is dehydrated, including the appearance of the skin, eyes, and oral cavity. Clinical chemistry and hematology tests may also give clues about the hydration status of an animal.

   Obesity is commonly observed in companion animals scheduled for anesthesia, and this condition poses some difficulties for the anesthetist. Obese animals often have reduced exercise tolerance and may show signs of dyspnea at rest, indicating inadequate cardiovascular and respiratory function. Venipuncture and auscultation may be difficult in these animals. When anesthetizing obese animals, drug dosages should be calculated based on the animal's *ideal weight* (however difficult this is to imagine) rather than the actual weight. Although the animal's size is indeed increased by the deposition of fat stores, the size of the target organ of anesthesia (that is, the brain) is unaffected.

TABLE 1-1

Evaluation of State of Hydration Using Clinical Signs

Physical Feature	Mild (5%) Dehydration	Moderate (6%-9%) Dehydration	Profound (10%-12%) Dehydration
Eyelid pinch	Mild tenting, pinch slowly relaxes	Severe tenting; pinch persists	Severe tenting; pinch persists
Cornea	Cornea moist, tearing still possible	Cornea drier and tearing is infrequent	Dry cornea and no tearing
Position of eyeball in orbit	Minimal (1-2 mm) space between medial canthus and globe	Pronounced space (2-4 mm) between medial canthus and globe	A space of more than 4 mm between medial canthus and globe
Skin of neck	Decreased pliability	Tented skin persists 3-5 seconds	Tented skin persists more than 5 seconds
Oral mucous membranes	Moist, warm and pink	Warm, sticky, and pale	Dry mucous membranes; cold, cyanotic or very pale; poor capillary perfusion
General condition	Standing; extremities are warm	Often recumbent	Often comatose, extremities are cold

Modified from *Veterinary Teaching Hospital Manual*, Guelph, Ontario, Canada, 1992, Ontario Veterinary College.

Excessive thinness is also of concern to the anesthetist because it may indicate the presence of an underlying disorder such as renal failure or chronic parasitism. Animals with little body fat may be unusually sensitive to the effects of some anesthetics and also are prone to hypothermia.

Pregnant animals present unique challenges to the anesthetist. Patients in early gestation or mid-gestation may be at risk if given drugs that can cause abortion (such as xylazine). Animals brought in for cesarean surgery also merit special consideration: the patient must be sufficiently anesthetized to allow the procedure to be performed humanely, yet the level of anesthesia should be as light as possible because some anesthetics may adversely affect the newborn puppies or kittens.

2. *Notation of body temperature.* The normal temperature range in the cat is 37.8° to 39.2° C (100.0° to 102.5° F). The normal range in the dog is 37.5° to 39.2° C (99.5° to 102.5° F). The veterinarian should be informed if the patient's temperature is outside the normal range.

3. *Examination of the head, including eyes, oral cavity, pharynx, ears, and nose.* The technician should examine the animal for wheezing or stertor (snoring), which indicates that an airway obstruction may be present. Any disorder that could impede endotracheal intubation, such as the presence of redundant tissue in the oropharynx or difficulty in opening the mouth, should be noted. The gingivae should be observed for mucous membrane color and capillary refill time (CRT), which indicate whether cardiovascular function is adequate. If the gingivae are pigmented, mucous membrane color and CRT may be observed at other sites, such as the conjunctiva of the lower eyelid, the entrance to the vulva, or the tip of the prepuce.

4. *Observation of the pupillary light reflex and consensual light reflex* (Fig. 1-1). The pupillary light reflex is elicited by shining a beam of light (usually from a penlight or other portable light source) into one eye and noting whether the pupil of that eye constricts in response (direct reflex). Pupil constriction (miosis) is the normal response; dilation of the pupil (mydriasis) in the presence of light is abnormal. At the same time, change in pupil size should be observed in the other eye (consensual reflex). Again, miosis is the expected response. Normal animals will demonstrate both a direct and a consensual light reflex in each eye, although this reflex may be altered in excited animals or after the administration of some preanesthetic and anesthetic drugs.

5. Auscultation of the heart and lungs. Auscultation of the chest is performed to determine the heart rate and rhythm and to check for the presence of abnormal heart or lung sounds. Auscultation of the lungs is best performed by listening to at least four different areas of the chest, including the right and left anteroventral lung fields and the right and left dorsal lung fields. Auscultation of the heart should also be performed on both the left and right sides of the chest. It is important to evaluate each of the four valves of the heart: the pulmonic, aortic, and mitral valves on the left side of the chest and the tricuspid valve on the right side of the chest. It is possible for the animal to have a heart murmur that will go undetected unless each valve is ausculted independently.

The normal range of heart rates for dogs is 60 to 180 beats per minute (bpm), with pediatric patients and smaller breeds tending to have rates more

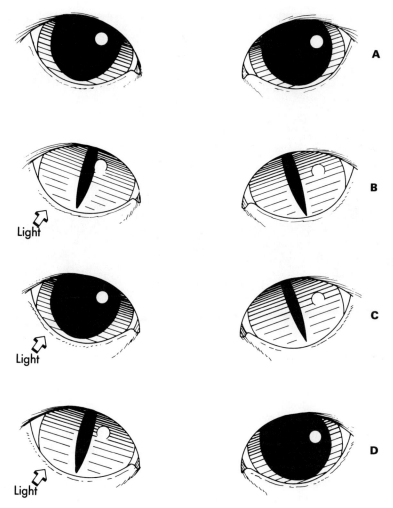

FIG. 1-1 Pupillary light reflex. **A,** Normal pupils. **B,** Direct and consensual light reflex (normal). **C,** Consensual but no direct light reflex (abnormal). **D,** Direct but no consensual light reflex (abnormal).

rapid than those of larger breeds. The heart rate in giant breeds should be less than 100 bpm. The normal range of heart rates for cats is 110 to 220 bpm. The rhythm in both dogs and cats should be reasonably regular, although it is common for the heart rate to increase slightly during inspiration (that is, sinus arrhythmia). Sinus arrhythmia is more commonly found in the dog than in the cat.

Exercise or the stress of handling may cause the heart rate to increase. The heart rate should be measured on a calm animal and, if possible, not immediately after inserting a rectal thermometer or collecting a blood sample.

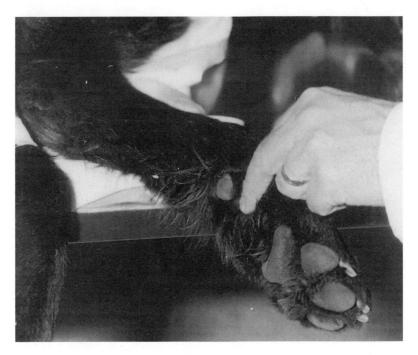

FIG. 1-2 Palpation of the metatarsal/metacarpal artery.

6. *Palpation of pulse and comparison of pulse rate and heart rate.* For the dog and cat, the pulse is most easily palpated at the femoral artery, on the medial side of the rear leg. Other sites that may be palpated include the metatarsal and metacarpal arteries (Fig. 1-2). Palpation of the pulse gives some indication of systolic blood pressure: a weak or absent pulse may indicate hypotension (low blood pressure). It is also important to compare the heart rate with the pulse rate. If the two are not the same (for example, if the heart rate exceeds the pulse rate), a pulse deficit exists. This may indicate the presence of cardiovascular disease.

7. *Determination of respiratory rate and observation for dyspnea.* The normal respiratory rate for dogs is 10 to 30 breaths per minute and for cats is 25 to 40 breaths per minute. Animals experiencing *dyspnea* (that is, difficult or labored breathing) may exhibit signs such as mouth breathing, flared nostrils, excessive panting, exaggerated chest or abdominal movements on inspiration, wheezing, and reluctance to lie down. In extreme cases, an animal with breathing difficulty may exhibit *cyanosis* (that is, mucous membranes that appear purple or blue). Any animal showing signs of dyspnea should be brought to the veterinarian's attention immediately. Dyspnea must be differentiated from normal rapid breathing and from panting.

8. *Examination of the thorax, abdomen, and limbs to note the condition of hair coat and presence of parasites or any cutaneous lesions.* Although examination of the skin is seldom relevant to the anesthesia itself, it may indicate the presence of a disorder requiring treatment.

9. *Observation for lameness or localized pain in the extremities.*
10. *Palpation of superficial lymph nodes.* Enlarged lymph nodes may indicate the presence of a local or systemic infection, allergy, or neoplastic disease (cancer), all of which would be of concern to the anesthetist and surgeon.
11. *Abdominal palpation for pain, organ size and location, and the presence of fluid, gas, fetuses, or feces.*
12. *Observation of mammary glands for signs of lactation (in the case of intact females), particularly if the animal is pregnant or postpartum.* The vulva should also be observed for indications of estrous activity or the presence of a discharge.

Diagnostic Tests

In a small animal practice, it is normally the responsibility of the veterinarian to decide which diagnostic tests are recommended for a given patient. The technician's responsibilities usually include obtaining blood and urine samples and either performing the tests or forwarding the samples to a diagnostic laboratory. All test results should be reviewed by the veterinarian.

There are no universal guidelines for preanesthetic diagnostic tests. Depending on the clinic policy, certain tests may be routinely performed on every animal scheduled for anesthesia. The veterinarian may request additional tests, based on the patient's age, history, and the results of the physical examination. Economic considerations may, in some cases, limit the number and type of tests approved by the client.

Diagnostic tests and procedures that provide information of particular interest to the anesthetist and supervising veterinarian include the complete blood count, urinalysis, blood chemistries, blood clotting tests, blood gases, electrocardiogram, and radiographs.

Complete blood count.   One commonly requested preanesthetic test is a complete blood count (CBC). The CBC includes the determination of packed cell volume (PCV), hemoglobin (Hb), total plasma protein (TPP, sometimes referred to as total solids and protein or TsP), and evaluation of a blood smear for white blood cell, red blood cell, and platelet abnormalities. Normal values for these parameters in the dog and cat are given in Table 1-2. Some variation may be expected depending on age, breed, and geographic location.

The information obtained from the PCV and Hb indicates the ability of the blood to deliver oxygen to the tissues. A PCV above normal limits suggests that the relative amount of red blood cells has increased. This is most often a result of fluid loss leading to dehydration. An elevated PCV is of concern to the anesthetist because hemoconcentration and increased blood viscosity will be present. These, in turn, lead to poor tissue perfusion and a reduction in cardiac output. On the other hand, a PCV below the normal range may indicate anemia caused by blood loss, hemolysis, or the failure to produce adequate numbers of red blood cells. The net result in each case is a decreased capacity to supply oxygen to the tissues.

The total plasma protein value is also of interest to the anesthetist. An increase in TPP, similar to an increase in PCV, may indicate dehydration. A decreased TPP usually indicates hypoproteinemia, which may be a result of renal, hepatic, or gastrointestinal disease. Alterations in TPP are particularly significant to the anesthetist because they indicate that the patient's response to anesthetic drugs may be altered. Many anesthetic agents are distributed in the blood in such a way that a

TABLE 1-2

Normal Values for Selected Parameters in Dogs and Cats

Parameter	Canine	Feline
HEART RATE (bpm)	60-180	110-220
TEMPERATURE	99.5°-102.5° F	100.0°-102.5° F
	37.5°-39.2° C	37.8°-39.2° C
RESPIRATORY RATE (bpm)	10-30	25-40
HB (g/dl)	14-18	9-16
TPP (g/dl)	5.7-7.8	6.3-8.3
PCV (%)	35-54	25-45
TOTAL LEUCOCYTE ($\times 10^9$/L)	6.0-18	6.0-20
Pao_2 (mm Hg)	91-97	91-115
$Paco_2$ (mm Hg)	30-43	28-43
ARTERIAL pH	7.36-7.46	7.34-7.43

Modified from Muir WW III, Hubbell JAE: *Handbook of veterinary anesthesia*, St Louis, 1989, Mosby.

portion circulates freely and another portion is bound to plasma proteins. Only the portion of the drug that is free and unbound to plasma proteins can affect the drug receptors. In the hypoproteinemic patient, a decreased proportion of drug is bound to plasma proteins. This results in an increased proportion of unbound drug and, consequently, increased drug potency for that particular patient.

The CBC should also include a differential count and an examination of white blood cells, which may indicate whether the animal is undergoing severe infection or stress. Such conditions may be exacerbated by anesthesia and surgery and also increase anesthetic risk.

Urinalysis.   The results of a urinalysis (particularly the urine specific gravity) provide information about the ability of the kidneys to excrete many anesthetic agents. Any animal with a urine specific gravity of less than 1.025 should be brought to the veterinarian's attention because further tests may be needed to assess renal and endocrine function. Urine dipstick results are also useful, allowing rapid screening for conditions such as diabetes mellitus and urinary tract infection. The interpretation of urinalysis results may be aided by microscopic examination of urine and by blood chemistry results such as blood urea nitrogen (BUN).

Blood chemistry.   Some patients scheduled for anesthesia may be known or suspected to suffer from renal, hepatic, endocrine, or other disease. In many cases the degree of organ dysfunction can be determined through appropriate biochemical tests. The most common of these include tests for alanine aminotransferase (ALT), alkaline phosphatase (AP), BUN, creatinine, blood glucose, and serum electrolytes (such as sodium and potassium). Normal values for these parameters vary with the instrumentation used and should be obtained from the laboratory doing the tests. Interpretation of test results requires specialized knowledge of disease and is therefore the responsibility of the veterinarian.

Blood clotting tests.   Blood clotting tests usually are performed only on animals with suspected coagulation disorders or animals of breeds known to be commonly affected by von Willebrand's disease (such as the Doberman pinscher and Scottish terrier). A toenail cuticle or buccal bleeding time gives a rough estimate of blood clotting ability and can be easily performed on any anesthetized animal. To perform a toenail cuticle bleeding time, the nail is cut slightly short using a pair of nail trimmers, such that the quick is entered and a small amount of bleeding results. The nail is allowed to bleed without any effort to wipe away accumulated blood. In a normal animal, bleeding should stop within 4 minutes. The buccal bleeding time is performed by nicking the tissue on the inside of the cheek using a small lancet. As with the toenail bleeding time, bleeding should stop within 4 minutes. More precise evaluation of hemostasis can be obtained through the use of more sophisticated tests such as partial prothrombin time (PPT) and platelet counts. A patient with reduced ability to clot blood will require special handling by the anesthetist and the surgeon because hemorrhage during surgery may result in prolonged recovery, shock, or death.

Blood gases.   Determination of blood gases (that is, the partial pressure of arterial blood carbon dioxide [$PaCO_2$], arterial blood oxygen [PaO_2], and blood pH) is not routinely done in general practice, and in any case is seldom necessary before the patient is anesthetized. Further details on blood gas determination are in Chapter 2 under monitoring techniques.

Electrocardiogram.   The electrocardiogram (ECG) monitors the electrical activity of the heart muscle, allowing the veterinarian to assess the pattern and rhythm of the myocardial contractions. Abnormalities in the size, duration, shape, and rhythm of the ECG tracing provide useful information about cardiac function. An ECG is not routinely done on every patient before anesthesia; it is usually reserved for those patients with known or suspected heart disease, chest trauma, or electrolyte disturbances such as hyperkalemia (abnormally high potassium concentration in the blood). The ECG also can be used to screen for cardiac disease before anesthetics are given to higher-risk animals, such as geriatrics. The ECG may allow the veterinarian to determine what type of dysfunction, if any, is present; and to evaluate the risk of anesthesia for a particular patient. Electrocardiograms are discussed in Chapter 2.

Radiography.   Because of economic considerations, chest radiographs are not routinely obtained for every patient scheduled to receive a general anesthetic. Radiography may be warranted in animals that show signs of dyspnea or those in which abnormal heart or lung sounds are detected during the physical examination. It is also advisable that animals that have had major trauma (such as being hit by a car) undergo chest radiographs before any surgery, including fracture repair. This will alert the veterinarian to the presence of pneumothorax, pleural effusion, or pulmonary trauma before making the decision to anesthetize the patient. Patients must not be stressed during radiography procedures, particularly if dyspnea is present. In some cases the patient should be radiographed in the standing position, instead of being placed in lateral or dorsal recumbency, to minimize patient discomfort and anxiety. Oxygen delivery by mask or nasal cannula will often reduce dyspnea and increase safety during radiography and other procedures.

Miscellaneous tests.   Depending on the geographic location of the practice, other diagnostic tests may be routinely performed before anesthesia. For example, veterinary practices in some areas require a heartworm test for all canine patients before anesthesia.

Classification of Patient Status

The veterinarian should evaluate the patient's minimum data base (that is, physical examination, history, and results of diagnostic tests) and assign a status to the patient before the anesthetic protocol is chosen and the anesthesia is initiated. The most widely accepted classification system is the one proposed by the American Society of Anesthesiologists (ASA). It is summarized in Table 1-3. Classification of risk is subject to personal interpretation. Two anesthetists might disagree, for example, on whether a particular animal should be assigned to class II (slight risk) or class III (moderate risk). Whatever the preoperative status assigned to an animal, it should be recorded in the animal's hospital record and in the anesthetic logbook. The anesthetist should recognize that a patient's ASA status may change. For example, patients that receive appropriate therapy such as IV fluids before surgery may have their ASA classification changed to a lower-risk category. On the other hand, a patient whose condition is deteriorating may be changed to a higher-risk category.

The technician acting as anesthetist should not hesitate to discuss abnormal findings from the minimum data base with the veterinarian because such information may lead to changes in the planned anesthetic protocol. The presence of organ dysfunction in an animal does not necessarily require that anesthesia be postponed or cancelled, although this may be necessary in some situations. Often anesthesia may be successfully achieved by selecting the agents that are least likely to have adverse effects on the animal. For example, if the physical examination and diagnostic tests suggest that heart disease is present in a 13-year-old dog scheduled for surgery, the veterinarian may choose to use isoflurane instead of halothane because isoflurane is less likely to induce potentially dangerous cardiac arrhythmias. If the patient is severely ill, the veterinarian may decide that the animal's condition must be stabilized before an anesthetic is administered. Patients that are severely dehydrated, acidotic, anemic, or suffering from a serious systemic disease or electrolyte imbalance are poor anesthetic risks, and every attempt should be made to correct the condition before anesthesia, if time allows. If the planned procedure is not immediately necessary to save the patient's life, and the patient's condition may be improved by nursing care, it is likely that anesthesia can be safely postponed.

■ SELECTION OF THE ANESTHETIC PROTOCOL
Factors That Influence Selection

In all jurisdictions in the United States and Canada, it is the veterinarian, rather than the veterinary technician, who chooses (that is, prescribes) the anesthetic drugs for a given patient. The veterinarian also chooses the dose and the route of administration of each agent. In most hospitals the veterinarian establishes one or two standard anesthetic protocols to be used for routine surgeries on healthy patients. However, the standard protocol must be evaluated for its suitability for each individual patient, and changes should be made to the protocol when necessary for the safety of the patient. The technician who has a good understanding of anesthetic principles and who demonstrates sincere interest in patient care and monitoring can communicate valuable observations and suggestions to the veterinarian. Nevertheless, the supervising

TABLE 1-3

Classification of Patient Physical Status

Category	Physical Condition	Examples of Clinical Situations
CLASS I Minimal risk	Normal healthy animal No underlying disease	Ovariohysterectomy, castration, declawing operation, hip dysplasia radiograph
CLASS II Slight risk, minor disease is present	Animals with slight to mild systemic disturbances Animal able to compensate	Neonate or geriatric animals, obesity, skin tumor, uncomplicated hernia, local infection
CLASS III Moderate risk, obvious disease is present	Animals with moderate systemic disease or disturbances Mild clinical signs	Anemia, moderate dehydration, fever, low-grade heart murmur or cardiac disease
CLASS IV High risk, significantly compromised by disease	Animals with preexisting systemic disease or disturbances of a severe nature	Severe dehydration, shock, uremia or toxemia, high fever, uncompensated heart disease, diabetes, pulmonary disease, emaciation
CLASS V Grave risk, moribund	Surgery often performed in desperation on animals with life-threatening systemic disease or disturbances not often correctable by an operation; includes all moribund animals not expected to survive 24 hours	Advanced cases of heart, kidney, liver, lung, or endocrine disease; profound shock; major head injury; severe trauma; pulmonary embolus; terminal malignancy

veterinarian has the ultimate responsibility for the patient's safety and must make the final decision regarding the anesthetic protocol.

The patient's physical status is not the only factor that determines the anesthetic protocol to be used. Other factors that affect the veterinarian's decision include the following:

Availability of facilities and equipment. Some anesthetic techniques require the use of specialized equipment. For example, halothane and isoflurane anesthesia require the use of a precision vaporizer designed for use with a volatile liquid anesthetic.

Familiarity with the agent. In all procedures, familiarity and skill with the chosen anesthetic and preanesthetic agent are desirable. For most patients, any one of several anesthetic procedures is likely to result in successful and safe anesthesia, and it is reasonable to use the method with which the anesthetist is most familiar, provided patient safety is ensured. It is seldom beneficial to anesthetize a critically ill patient with a new combination of drugs that the anesthetist may have heard or read about but never tried before.

Nature of the procedure requiring anesthesia.   Procedures vary in their anticipated duration and in the amount of analgesia and restraint required. For example, local analgesia may be suitable for short procedures in which the patient requires only minimal restraint. On the other hand, patients that are to undergo thoracic or abdominal surgery usually require general anesthesia.

Special patient circumstances.   Anesthetics that may be appropriate for animals undergoing a routine surgery (such as ovariohysterectomy or castration) may not be the first choice for every surgical procedure. For example, the choice of anesthetic for a cesarean section is partially determined by the need to avoid agents that may cause respiratory depression in the newborn puppy or kitten.

Cost.   Anesthetic agents vary in cost, and in a situation in which two agents are of equal value from the standpoint of patient safety, the less expensive may be preferable.

Speed.   Critically injured animals may require rapid induction of anesthesia to initiate emergency therapy. For example, a patient that has an obvious hypovolemia because of blood loss cannot wait for a premedication given intramuscularly that needs 15 to 20 minutes to take effect. Rapid induction using a combination of preanesthetic and induction agents given intravenously may be preferable in this case.

■ PREANESTHETIC PATIENT CARE

During the preanesthetic period the technician should ensure that the patient receives appropriate nursing care, including fasting, intravenous catheterization, and any other procedures requested by the veterinarian. The technician also must ensure that each patient is clearly identified, usually by means of a card attached to its cage or an identification band placed around the animal's neck.

Withholding Food Before Anesthesia

Animals that are anesthetized without prior fasting may vomit or regurgitate stomach contents during anesthesia or during the recovery period. As anesthetized animals lack the ability to swallow, vomitus in the airway may be aspirated into the trachea, bronchi, and lung alveoli. If the vomitus blocks the airways, immediate respiratory arrest may result. An animal that survives the episode may develop aspiration pneumonia several days after the incident.

To prevent vomiting during the anesthetic period, it is generally accepted that food should be withheld from adult dogs and cats for 12 hours before anesthesia and that water should be withheld for 2 hours before anesthesia. These times are based on research that indicates that complete emptying of food from the stomach requires an average of 10 hours in the dog. Birds, "pocket pets" such as hamsters and guinea pigs, and dogs and cats younger than 3 months of age should be fasted for a shorter period or not at all because of their tendency to develop hypoglycemia. The technician must ensure that dehydrated animals receive adequate intravenous fluids to prevent further dehydration when water is withheld.

Despite every precaution, vomiting may occur during the preanesthetic, anesthetic, or recovery periods. Fortunately, the animal is most often well into the recovery period when vomiting occurs, and at this time the swallowing reflex is present and aspiration is unlikely. Possible explanations for vomiting in an animal that was supposedly fasted include individual patient variation and owner noncompliance.

Some protection against vomiting may be offered by the use of preanesthetic drugs with antiemetic properties (for example, acepromazine). Also, the use of cuffed endotracheal tubes helps prevent aspiration of regurgitated or vomited stomach contents, provided the endotracheal tube remains in place until the animal regains the swallowing reflex during recovery. In the case of animals known to have ingested food within a few hours of anesthesia, it may be best to postpone the anesthetic procedure. It is also possible to give a preanesthetic with emetic properties (for example, morphine in dogs) to ensure that the stomach is empty.

Animals undergoing gastrointestinal procedures may require special feeding and care to minimize the amount of digestive material within the gastrointestinal tract at the time of surgery. If a surgical procedure involving the stomach or intestine is planned, food is generally withheld for 24 hours and water is withheld for 8 to 12 hours before anesthesia. If surgery of the colon is planned, it may be advisable to administer one or more enemas within the 12 hours before the procedure.

The anesthetist should be aware that although preanesthetic fasting is recommended, prolonged fasting might be detrimental to the animal. Many seriously ill animals are anorexic and, in fact, may refuse to eat for several days before and after anesthesia. For example, a dog that has been hit by a car may arrive at the veterinary clinic with a fractured femur and pneumothorax. The veterinarian may elect to postpone fracture repair for several days to allow the pneumothorax to resolve. The animal may be in too much pain, too frightened, or too weak to eat throughout this period. By the time the surgery is performed, the animal may have gone without eating for more than 4 days. Lack of nutrition impedes the healing process and prolongs recovery. Efforts should be made to reestablish caloric intake in the anorexic animal, whether by hand-feeding palatable foods, syringe bolus feeding, the use of feeding tubes, or intravenous nutrition.

Correction of Preexisting Problems

Animals scheduled for anesthesia are sometimes found to be suffering from systemic disorders such as dehydration, anemia, respiratory distress, shock, and hypothermia. As already mentioned, these patients are at increased anesthetic risk, and in the interest of patient safety, it may be best to postpone anesthesia to allow time for appropriate nursing care. In some cases (for example, a patient with a gastric tortion or uncontrolled internal bleeding) the veterinarian may decide that the risk of delaying surgery outweighs the increased anesthetic risk and will elect to proceed with anesthesia. These patients, perhaps, pose the greatest challenge to the technician's skills as an anesthetist and as an intensive care nurse.

Intravenous Catheterization

Reasons for catheterization.   Not all animals are catheterized before anesthesia. However, the presence of an intravenous (IV) catheter is of potential benefit to both the patient and the anesthetist. Reasons for catheterization include the following:

1. Intravenous catheters are a convenient way to administer anesthetic agents that can be irritating if injected perivascularly (such as thiopental).

2. Intravenous catheters allow concurrent injection of incompatible drugs (such as diazepam and oxymorphone) by the use of separate syringes and a catheter adapter.

3. Intravenous catheters allow the rapid administration of emergency drugs (such as epinephrine and prednisone sodium succinate) and for this reason are particularly recommended for high-risk patients. They are useful not only during the anesthetic period itself, but also during the recovery period, when treatment of complications such as bleeding, respiratory obstruction, or seizures may require intravenous access.

4. Intravenous catheterization allows the administration of balanced electrolyte solutions or saline during surgery. Fluid administration is not mandatory for routine surgeries in healthy animals, but it is highly recommended for some patients, including the following:
   ▪ Animals that are in shock
   ▪ Animals undergoing any surgery that may result in significant blood loss, including cesarean sections
   ▪ Animals that are debilitated or dehydrated because of renal, gastrointestinal, or other systemic diseases
   ▪ Animals undergoing lengthy surgery. Many anesthesiologists advise that a secure IV access (by indwelling catheter or butterfly) be established for any animal undergoing a surgical procedure lasting over 1 hour. This allows administration of fluids or drugs if the need arises. The incidence of anesthetic complications is greater in animals undergoing lengthy anesthesia (over 2 hours) than for animals undergoing routine, short procedures, and fluid administration is therefore advisable in these patients.

5. Some animals require a constant infusion of electrolytes or drugs (such as insulin) during anesthesia. These animals are usually catheterized, and the drug is mixed with the IV fluids for convenient administration.

6. Some types of anesthetic agents (in particular, propofol and pentobarbital) are given "to effect," meaning that the drug is given intravenously in small amounts adequate to maintain unconsciousness. In these animals, use of an intravenous catheter is preferable to needle and syringe because the accidental dislodgement of the needle within the vein can lead to perivascular drug administration and the development of a hematoma. Accidental manipulation of the needle and syringe also may lead to inadvertent administration of excessive amounts of the drug.

Risks of catheterization.   The administration of fluids and drugs through an IV catheter is not without risk of complications. These include the following:
   ▪ The introduction of air. This should be avoided, although significant air embolism is unlikely if a peripheral vein is used.
   ▪ Broken catheter tip. Care should be exercised when placing the catheter to avoid breaking off the tip and creating a catheter embolus.
   ▪ Accidental overhydration. This occurs when fluid administration is too rapid. Animals weighing under 5 kg and those with cardiac disease are at greatest risk.
   ▪ Catheter-induced sepsis. Careful antiseptic technique helps reduce the risk of bacteria colonizing the catheter site, but it is generally recommended that a

catheter in a peripheral vein should be removed after 72 hours to reduce the chance of phlebitis and sepsis.

- Blood clot formation. While the catheter is in place, it may be beneficial to infuse heparin to reduce the chances of blood clot formation.

Fluid administration rates.   The rate of fluid administration varies depending on the patient and the procedure. The following guidelines may be useful:

- *Maintenance fluids:* Daily maintenance fluids are commonly given to hospitalized patients at a rate of 2 ml/kg/hr (large dogs) to 4 ml/kg/hr (small dogs/cats).
- *Fluids given during anesthesia:* A fluid infusion rate of 10 ml/kg/hr is the standard fluid administration rate during routine anesthesia and surgery and is safe for almost all patients. Animals suffering from cardiovascular, respiratory, or renal disease are at increased risk of overhydration and may benefit from a slower infusion rate during surgery (for example, 5 ml/kg/hr). Fluids can be given more rapidly, particularly if bleeding or decreased blood pressure is encountered during surgery (20 ml/kg in the first 15 minutes is recommended). If excessive blood loss occurs, the anesthetist should ensure that 3 ml of fluids are given for every 1 ml of blood lost. If blood transfusion therapy is used, the amount of blood given should approximately equal the amount of blood lost.
- *Rapid rehydration:* Fluids can be given more rapidly than the maintenance and surgery rates just discussed. Healthy dogs may tolerate up to 40 ml/kg for 1 hour. Cats are more prone to overhydration than dogs, and for this reason the fluid infusion rate should not exceed 20 ml/kg/hr unless the animal is in shock.
- *Shock therapy:* Fluids are given at very rapid flow rates when treating shock (for example, up to 90 ml/kg/hr for dogs and 50 ml/kg/hr for cats).

When in doubt, the technician should consult with the veterinarian regarding the optimum fluid administration rate and should carefully monitor the amount of fluids being given to the patient during surgery. The use of a burette (Fig. 1-3) decreases the risk of accidental volume overload by allowing the accurate measurement and administration of small volumes of fluids rather than direct administration from a bag or bottle.

When monitoring any anesthetized patient that is receiving IV fluids, the anesthetist should be alert for signs of overhydration. These include ocular and nasal discharge, chemosis (edema and swelling of the conjunctiva), restlessness, increased lung sounds, increased respiratory rate, and dyspnea.

Types of IV fluids.   The choice of intravenous (IV) fluids is governed by the animal's condition and the veterinarian's preference. *Crystalloid* solutions, which are aqueous (dissolved in water), are the most commonly administered type of fluid. There are three types of crystalloid solutions. (See Table 1-4 for composition of fluids.)

1. *Balanced electrolyte solutions.* As the term implies, these solutions contain several electrolytes (most often sodium, potassium, chlorine, magnesium, and calcium) in concentrations that reflect the electrolyte composition of blood. Lactated Ringer's solution is one of the most commonly used balanced electrolyte solutions.

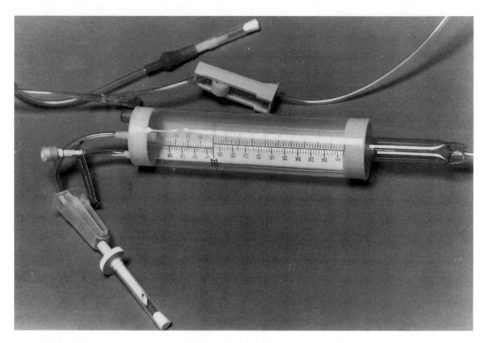

FIG. 1-3 Burette.

TABLE 1-4

Composition of Intravenous Fluids and Plasma

					mEq /liter		
Solution	pH	Carbohydrate	Na^+	K+	Ca^+	Mg^{+2}	Cl^-
PLASMA	7.5	5.6% dextrose	144	5	5	1.5	107
0.99% NaCl	5.4	None	154	0	0	0	154
5% DEXTROSE	5.0	5% dextrose	0	0	0	0	0
LACTATED RINGER'S	6.5	None	130	4	3	0	109

From Short CE: *Principles and practice of veterinary anesthesia,* Baltimore, 1987, Williams & Wilkins.

2. *Saline solutions.* Physiologic saline (0.85% saline) and half-strength saline contain only sodium and chloride ions in water. These solutions may be preferred over lactated Ringer's for some animals (for example, patients suffering from liver disease). Very concentrated (up to 7%) saline solutions, which are also called hypertonic saline, may be administered to patients in shock along with one of the other crystalloids previously mentioned. Hypertonic saline is never administered alone.

3. *Dextrose solutions.* Solutions of 2.5% or 5% dextrose in water are commonly used in animals suffering from hypoglycemia and in animals receiving insulin. Dextrose solutions are also useful in neonatal animals and in debilitated animals, both of which benefit from a ready source of calories during anesthesia.

The anesthetist must exercise caution when administering drugs and crystalloid fluids concurrently because undesirable interactions may occur. Diazepam, for example, precipitates in almost any fluid. Sodium bicarbonate and whole blood should not be mixed with fluids containing calcium.

Some patients require the administration of *colloid* solutions, which are not water based and have a specific gravity much higher than that of crystalloid solutions. Examples of colloid solutions include the following:

- *Plasma or blood.* Transfusions of plasma or blood are particularly useful in treating animals that are suffering from acute blood loss or severe anemia. Patients with extensive burns may also suffer severe plasma loss, and a plasma transfusion may be required. Plasma or blood is also useful in hypoproteinemic animals and patients with coagulation disorders.
- *Synthetic colloids.* Patients in shock are sometimes given synthetic colloids such as dextran, pentastarch, and hetastarch. Unlike crystalloid solutions, colloid solutions remain in circulation and help maintain circulating blood volume for a considerable time.

Other Preanesthetic Patient Care

On occasion the veterinarian may direct the technician or another staff member to provide specific preoperative care. Some patients require the administration of medication such as insulin injections or anticonvulsant medication. Antibiotics may be required for animals that have infections or that are scheduled for surgery involving a contaminated area (such as the gastrointestinal tract). The technician should obtain specific instructions from the veterinarian on the route, dose, and type of medication to be administered to each patient.

■ PREANESTHETIC AGENTS

Preanesthetic agents are drugs that are administered to an animal before general anesthesia. The most commonly used preanesthetic agents are atropine, acepromazine, xylazine, medetomidine, diazepam, and opioid agents. Either a single drug or a combination of drugs may be administered to an animal. Suggested dosages of the common preanesthetic agents for use in dogs and cats are given in Table 1-5.

Reasons for the Use of Preanesthetic Agents

The potential benefits associated with the use of preanesthetic agents are summarized in Table 1-6. The most important reasons for the administration of preanesthetic agents are the following:

1. To calm or sedate an excited or vicious animal. Sedation not only enhances patient comfort, but also simplifies the task of the anesthetist. However, not every patient requires sedation; in the case of debilitated, injured, or sick animals, even light sedation may cause excessive central nervous system (CNS) depression. Conversely, some vicious animals may be unaffected by even high doses

TABLE 1-5

Suggested Dosage Ranges of Common Preanesthetic Medications for Use in Healthy Dogs and Cats (For analgesic dosages, see Tables 8-3 and 8-4.)

Drug	Route	Canine Dosage (mg/kg)	Feline Dosage (mg/kg)
Acepromazine	SC, IM, IV	0.04-0.2 SC or IM 0.02-0.05 IV Maximum 3 mg Use with caution in boxers	Same
	oral	1-3 mg/kg	Same
Atropine	SC, IM, IV	0.02-0.04	Same
Butorphanol	SC, IM	0.1-0.5	Same
	IV	0.05	Same
Diazepam	IM	0.2-0.4 (not always effective)	Same
	IV	0.1-0.5 (max 10 mg)	Same
Glycopyrrolate	SC, IM	0.01-0.02	Same
Medetomidine	IM	20-40 µg/kg	10-40 µg/kg
(See also Table 1-8.)	IV	10-20 µg/kg	10-20 µg/kg
Meperidine	SC, IM	3-5	5
Midazolam	IM, IV	0.2, max 10 mg	Not recommended as sole agent
Morphine	SC, IM	0.25-1.0	0.1-0.3 (May produce excitement.)
Oxymorphone	IM	0.1-0.3	Same
	IV	0.05-0.10 Maximum 3 mg	0.02 Maximum 1 mg
Xylazine	IM	1-2	Same
	IV	0.2-0.5	Same

Data from Morgan RV: *AAHA formulary,* Denver, 1988, American Animal Hospital Association; Muir WW III, Hubbell JAE: *Handbook of veterinary anesthesia,* St Louis, 1989, Mosby; Warren RG: *Small animal anesthesia,* St Louis, 1983, Mosby; Ko JCH: Anesthetic potency: how to use medetomidine and atipamezole, *Vet Tech* 18(10):695-702, 1997.

of tranquilizing medications. For most patients, however, sedation allows an easier and smoother induction and recovery.

2. To reduce or eliminate possible noxious side effects resulting from the use of general anesthetics. General anesthetics, such as barbiturates, ketamine, and the inhalation anesthetics halothane, isoflurane, and methoxyflurane, may cause undesirable side effects in addition to their anesthetic action. For example, ketamine causes excessive salivation in some patients. Cardiac arrhythmias are sometimes seen in animals given the inhalation anesthetic halothane. Some opioid drugs (that is, narcotics) may induce bradycardia, vomiting, diarrhea, and flatulence. Preanesthetic agents, particularly the anticholinergics atropine and glycopyrrolate, are commonly given to prevent these unwanted effects.

3. To reduce the amount of general anesthetic required to induce anesthesia. The administration of preanesthetic tranquilizers and opioids causes significant sedation in most veterinary patients. Although this level of sedation is insufficient to allow surgery, the animal may require the administration of only a small quantity of general anesthetic to produce true anesthesia. Reduction of the amount of general anesthetic given to the patient minimizes the adverse side effects of the general anesthetic on the respiratory and cardiovascular systems. This approach to anesthesia, in which low doses of several preanesthetic and general anesthetic agents are used in combination to achieve a satisfactory anesthetic state, is termed *balanced anesthesia.*
4. To decrease pain and discomfort in the postoperative period. If the period of anesthesia is brief, drugs given during the preanesthetic period may exert some analgesic effect even during the recovery period.
5. Preanesthetic drugs have many uses, even in animals that are not undergoing anesthesia. For example, tranquilizers are used to calm patients for transport, physical examination, and minor procedures. They are helpful in preventing animals from chewing wounds and bandages. Phenothiazines are useful antiemetics for animals with gastrointestinal disease.

Preanesthetic agents are chosen from one or more of several classes of drugs, including tranquilizers, opioids (narcotics), and anticholinergics. The type of drug or combination of drugs is chosen by the veterinarian based on the nature of the procedure; the veterinarian's personal preference; and the patient's species, physical status, and temperament. The timing of the administration of the drug will also vary among patients. If possible, the veterinarian will usually elect to administer a preanesthetic well before the general anesthetic is given to allow ample time for the preanesthetic to gradually exert its effects. Drugs with a sedative effect, such as acepromazine and opioids, are most effective if the animal is left undisturbed until the full effect of the drug is evident. It is sometimes necessary, however, to give preanesthetic drugs at the same time as the general anesthetic, in the form of an intravenous or intramuscular injection. Caution should be used when giving any preanesthetic or general anesthetic drug by intravenous injection because the potential for adverse side effects is increased when this route is used. Response to oral administration is slow and unpredictable.

No preanesthetic agent is entirely free of side effects, and no single agent is safe for every animal. Table 1-7 gives a summary of the precautions and contraindications associated with the commonly used preanesthetic agents. The anesthetist should also be aware that all preanesthetics except glycopyrrolate cross the placental barrier, and adverse side effects may be observed in the newborn animal if the agents are administered shortly before birth. Because of the potential for side effects, the veterinarian may elect to omit one or more preanesthetics from the anesthetic protocol, particularly in neonatal or geriatric animals.

Anticholinergics (Parasympatholytics)

Two anticholinergic agents commonly used in veterinary medicine are atropine and glycopyrrolate (Robinul-V). Atropine is derived from the deadly nightshade plant and glycopyrrolate is a synthetic quaternary ammonium derivative of atropine. Both drugs may be given by the intravenous (IV), intramuscular (IM), or subcutaneous

TABLE 1-6

Benefits Associated with the Use of Selected Preanesthetic Agents

What the Preanesthetic Can Do	Which Preanesthetic?
Tranquilize or sedate the animal to facilitate catheterization, masking, or injection of an induction agent; reduce patient apprehension	1. Phenothiazines (acepromazine) 2. Thiazines (xylazine, medetomidine) 3. Opioids (meperidine, butorphanol, oxymorphone) 4. Benzodiazepines (diazepam, midazolam: debilitated animals only)
Decrease amount of general anesthetic required	All of the above
Muscle relaxation	1. Xylazine, medetomidine 2. Diazepam, midazolam
Induce vomiting in unfasted animal	1. Xylazine (cats) 2. Morphine (dogs)
Minimize bradycardia that occurs during intubation, handling of viscera, or as side effect of many anesthetics	1. Atropine 2. Glycopyrrolate
Minimize salivation	1. Atropine 2. Glycopyrrolate
Decrease gastrointestinal tract (GIT) motility, thereby preventing vomiting, diarrhea, and flatulence that may occur with some opioids	1. Atropine 2. Glycopyrrolate
Provide intraoperative or postoperative analgesia	1. Opioids 2. Nonsteroidal antiinflammatory agents (NSAIDs)
Prevent intraoperative or postoperative seizures	1. Diazepam

(SC) routes. As is common for anesthetic agents, the SC and IM dosages are considerably greater than the IV dosage. Atropine is available in several concentrations, including 0.5 mg/ml (1/120 grain/ml), 2.2 mg/ml, and 15 mg/ml. It is important to ensure that the atropine drawn into the syringe is the same concentration as that used to calculate the dose, or an incorrect amount may be administered. For example, an anesthetist who calculates a dose of 0.5 ml of atropine using a concentration of 0.5 mg/ml might cause atropine toxicity in a patient if the 0.5 ml is drawn from a bottle containing the drug at a concentration of 15 mg/ml.

Mode of action.   Anticholinergic drugs such as atropine exert their effect by blocking certain receptors for the neurotransmitter acetylcholine. Acetylcholine is produced by the parasympathetic part of the autonomic nervous system and is the transmitter at both the *nicotinic* and *muscarinic* receptors (Fig. 1-4). Atropine blocks the action of acetylcholine at the muscarinic receptors, which are the terminal ends of the parasympathetic nervous system. It therefore acts to reverse parasympathetic effects. Atropine has no effect on the nicotinic receptors.

The muscarinic receptors are found in the heart, gastrointestinal tract, bronchi, several secretory glands, and the iris of the eye, and it is in these locations that the

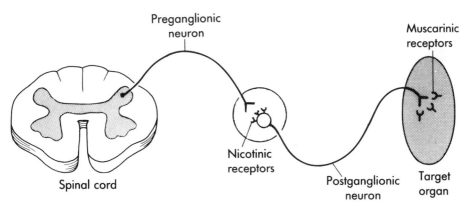

FIG. 1-4 Schematic view of the parasympathetic nervous system. Preganglionic neuron releases acetylcholine at the nicotinic receptors. Postganglionic neuron releases acetylcholine at the muscarinic receptors of the target organ. Atropine affects only the muscarinic receptors.

TABLE 1-7

Precautions for the Use of Selected Preanesthetic Agents

Anesthetic or Preanesthetic	Use with Caution in Which Situations?
Atropine	Tachycardia (heart rate over 140 in a dog, 180 in a cat)
	Constipation or obstruction
Acepromazine	Hypotension (shock)
	Seizure disorders, head trauma
	Hypothermia
Diazepam	Cesarean section
	Neonatal patients
Xylazine and medetomidine	Cardiovascular disease or respiratory disease
	Debilitated animals
	Neonates or geriatrics
	Pregnant animals
	Large dogs prone to bloat
Opioids	Respiratory disease
	Head trauma or spinal cord injury
	Chest injury
	Shock

effect of atropine is readily observed by the anesthetist (Fig. 1-5). When the parasympathetic system is activated (as often occurs during anesthesia), the muscarinic receptors are stimulated by acetylcholine. This is undesirable because it may result in bradycardia, pupil constriction, gastrointestinal stimulation, and salivation. By blocking the muscarinic receptors, atropine helps to prevent these parasympathetic effects.

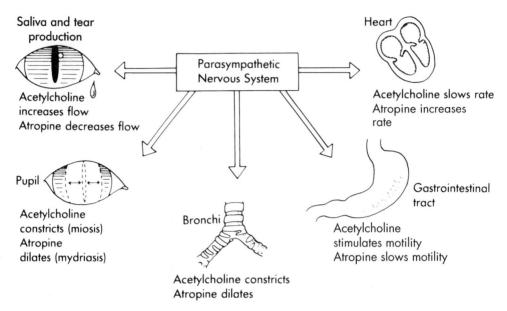

FIG. 1-5   Effect of atropine on the parasympathetic nervous system.

Method of use.   The onset of atropine action occurs approximately 20 minutes after SC injection, and therefore it should be administered at least 20 to 30 minutes before anesthetic induction. Atropine may be mixed in a syringe and administered intravenously with most other preanesthetic and anesthetic agents, including acepromazine and ketamine (but not diazepam). Because the onset of action is rapid after IV administration of atropine, it offers almost immediate protection when given in this way. The duration of effect of atropine is 60 to 90 minutes (less if strong parasympathetic tone is present). It is common to see bradycardia at the end of a long anesthesia, due in part to the loss of atropine activity.

Effects of atropine.   Atropine has many effects that make it a valuable drug in veterinary anesthesia, although its use is not without hazard.

1. Atropine blocks stimulation of the vagus nerve. Several anesthetic procedures and agents may stimulate the vagus nerve, which is an important part of the parasympathetic nervous system. Procedures that stimulate the vagus nerve include endotracheal intubation, handling of the viscera during surgery, and the administration of several commonly used anesthetic agents (including inhalation agents, xylazine, and some opioids). Stimulation of the vagus nerve is undesirable during anesthesia because it causes increased parasympathetic activity, resulting in bradycardia and reduced cardiac output. By blocking the stimulation of the vagus nerve, atropine prevents bradycardia and, in some cases, may cause the heart rate to increase. For this reason, atropine is said to "protect the heart" during anesthesia.

2. Atropine reduces salivation (antisialogogic activity). Several anesthetic agents, particularly ketamine, stimulate the parasympathetic nerves that promote sali-

vation. This may predispose the animal to aspiration of saliva and possible upper airway blockage. Atropine markedly reduces the production of saliva and, for this reason, is commonly given in conjunction with ketamine.

3. Atropine reduces gastrointestinal activity. Some anesthetic agents (particularly the opioids) increase the peristaltic movement of the gastrointestinal tract, leading to flatulence, vomiting, and diarrhea. Atropine counters these effects by inhibiting intestinal peristalsis. This action also accounts for the inclusion of atropine in several popular antidiarrheal preparations.

4. Atropine causes pupil dilation (mydriasis). This effect is not commonly seen when dogs are given the usual preanesthetic doses of atropine. In cats, however, mydriasis may occur even at the preanesthetic dosage rates. Mydriasis has been associated with temporary visual disturbances and may also predispose the animal to retinal damage if the eyes are exposed to bright light for a considerable time. The anesthetist should also be aware that animals given atropine may show reduced pupillary light reflex because of the mydriatic effect.

5. Atropine reduces tear secretions. In the awake animal, the cornea of the eye is lubricated by the secretion of tears. Atropine causes a marked reduction in tear production, and the corneas of animals receiving atropine should be protected from dessication by the instillation of ophthalmic ointment. This effect is particularly important when an anesthetic agent such as ketamine is used in addition to atropine. (Animals anesthetized with ketamine do not close their eyelids, resulting in an even greater tendency toward corneal drying.)

6. Atropine promotes bronchodilation. Atropine dilates bronchioles in the lungs, increasing the diameter of these airways. This may be beneficial in some patients; however, an increase in the diameter of the airway results in increased "dead space." (See Chapter 2.)

7. The use of atropine may be associated with the production of thick mucus secretions within the airways, particularly in cats. This may predispose the animal to airway blockage, and for this reason some veterinarians avoid the use of atropine in cats.

The effects of glycopyrrolate are similar to those of atropine, but the duration of effect can be up to twice as long. Glycopyrrolate may have less tendency to cause tachycardia and cardiac arrhythmias than atropine. Glycopyrrolate also suppresses salivation more effectively than atropine. For these reasons glycopyrrolate may be preferable to atropine for some procedures in both the cat and the dog, despite its greater expense.

Atropine toxicity.   Although it would seem that there are many advantages to using the anticholinergic drugs, they may be contraindicated in some animals. They should not be given to animals with rapid heart rates because even faster heart rates may result. Atropine must be used with caution in animals that have clinical signs of congestive heart failure because the heart is already working to its maximum capacity in these animals and tachycardia could be dangerous. Anticholinergics should be avoided in animals with constipation or ileus because these drugs will further reduce peristaltic action of the intestines.

An overdose of atropine may cause drowsiness in some animals and excitement in others. It may also cause dry mucous membranes and thirst, dilated pupils, and tachycardia. As previously mentioned, atropine toxicity may arise when an incorrect concentration of the drug is administered. Dogs are more susceptible to atropine toxicity than are cats. Atropine overdose can be treated with physostigmine at a dose of 0.02 mg/kg to a maximum of 0.5 mg/animal IV over several minutes. The dosage can be repeated every 5 to 10 minutes if required to a total maximum dose of 2 mg/animal.

Because of the potential for adverse side effects when atropine is administered, some veterinarians omit atropine from their anesthetic protocols. Other veterinarians, however, continue to advocate the routine use of atropine or glycopyrrolate preanesthesia, particularly when ketamine, opioids, xylazine, or medetomidine is to be administered. Atropine is commonly mixed with acepromazine and meperidine or butorphanol for preanesthetic sedation. (See page 38.) Atropine may also be used to treat bradycardia or profuse salivation that arises during or after anesthesia.

Tranquilizers and Sedatives

This broad group of drugs includes the phenothiazines, benzodiazepines, and thiazine derivatives. In general, agents from each of these classes act on the central nervous system, resulting in a more tranquil or calmer animal. These drugs may also cause ataxia and prolapse of the nictitating membrane (also called the third eyelid, Fig. 1-6). Most of these drugs have no analgesic effects. Thus a dog that appears quiet after sedation may suddenly become alert or aggressive when exposed to a painful stimulus.

Phenothiazines

The phenothiazine group of drugs includes such agents as acepromazine (also known as acetylpromazine) maleate, chlorpromazine hydrochloride, and triflupromazine hy-

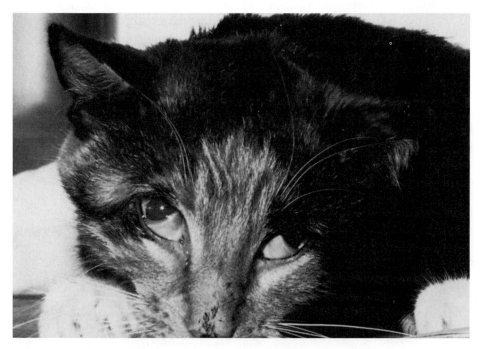

FIG. 1-6   Prolapse of the third eyelid. (From Warren RG: *Small animal anesthesia,* St Louis, 1983, Mosby.)

drochloride. Phenothiazines are probably the most commonly used agents for pre-anesthetic sedation. Because they do not cause respiratory depression and have minimal adverse effects on the heart, they are considered to have a wide margin of safety. They are effective in many species and may be given in combination with other agents, such as atropine, opioids, and ketamine. Phenothiazines may be administered orally, subcutaneously, intramuscularly, or (with caution) intravenously.

Effects of phenothiazines.   Phenothiazines have the following clinical effects:

1. *Sedation.* Phenothiazines affect the reticular activating center of the brain, causing sedation. This is the chief reason for the use of phenothiazines as preanesthetic agents.

2. *Antiemetic effect.* Phenothiazines, even at very low doses, help prevent vomiting during the anesthetic period. They are also used to prevent vomiting caused by gastrointestinal disease or motion sickness.

3. *Antiarrhythmic effect.* Some drugs, including epinephrine and halothane, have a potential to cause cardiac arrhythmias, which may result in decreased cardiac output. Phenothiazines antagonize this effect and are therefore considered to be antiarrhythmic.

4. *Antihistamine effect.* Histamine is a chemical released by the body as part of the allergic response. Phenothiazines prevent the release of histamine and therefore help reduce allergic reactions. For this reason, phenothiazines should not be used to sedate animals that are to undergo allergy testing.

5. *Peripheral vasodilation.* Phenothiazine agents dilate blood vessels, particularly when given by the IV route. Vasodilation may result in increased heat loss, leading to hypothermia. Even more seriously, vasodilation may lead to a fall in blood pressure (hypotension). Consequently, phenothiazines are not the preanesthetic agents of choice for animals in shock. Animals that experience significant hypotension as a result of phenothiazine administration should be given IV fluid replacement to raise blood pressure. The veterinarian may also prescribe drugs that increase blood pressure by constricting the arteries, including alpha sympathomimetics such as phenylephrine.

6. *Reduction of the threshold for seizures.* Phenothiazines predispose animals to seizure activity. For this reason a veterinarian may elect to omit acepromazine when anesthetizing an animal with a history of epilepsy or recent head trauma, or an animal undergoing a procedure such as myelography that may result in postoperative seizures.

7. *Effects on personality.* Occasionally, the administration of a phenothiazine or other tranquilizing agent (such as diazepam or xylazine) may induce excitement rather than sedation. This effect may persist into the postanesthetic period but usually resolves within 48 hours. Owners should be warned that personality changes sometimes occur after the administration of tranquilizing agents, and care should be used when handling patients returning home within 48 hours of anesthesia.

Phenothiazines have no analgesic (pain relieving) effect. Patients that are restless or excited because they are in pain are better managed with an opioid or nonsteroidal antiinflammatory drug.

As is evident from the discussion above, the use of phenothiazines is not without risk. Recently it has been suggested that the manufacturer's recommended dose for acepromazine is higher than that actually required for preanesthesia, and should be reduced by 50% or more to minimize the danger of side effects. High doses of phenothiazine drugs do not result in increased levels of sedation and may induce significant hypotension. The anesthetist should be particularly aware that phenothiazines have increased potency in geriatric animals, neonates, and animals with liver dysfunction, and the dose should be reduced by at least one half in these patients. It has also been noted by some that boxers may be more sensitive to phenothiazines and that the dosage may need to be reduced in this breed.

Benzodiazepines

The benzodiazepine group includes diazepam (Valium) as well as zolazepam (a component of Telazol), midazolam (Versed), and lorazepam (Ativan). Diazepam, although commonly used in veterinary anesthesia as a preanesthetic or combination induction agent, is not licensed in the United States or Canada for use in animals.

Effects of benzodiazepines. Benzodiazepines probably exert their effects through the release of endogenous GABA, an inhibitory neurotransmitter in the brain. Their usefulness to the anesthetist arises from the following properties:

1. *Antianxiety and calming effect.* Benzodiazepines, unlike phenothiazines, do not sedate or tranquilize animals. Animals given diazepam do not usually appear drowsy; instead, the animal appears less anxious, but still alert. Diazepam can be used as a sole premedication in very debilitated or geriatric animals; however, its use as the sole premedication agent in healthy young animals is often disappointing. Diazepam sedation in young dogs is unreliable and, with its normal inhibitions and anxieties removed by the drug, the animal may become more difficult to control. The anesthetist should also be aware that benzodiazepines, like phenothiazines, have no analgesic effect and will not be effective in calming animals that are experiencing pain.

2. *Skeletal muscle relaxation.* Benzodiazepines induce excellent skeletal muscle relaxation and often are used to counteract the muscle rigidity seen with dissociative agents such as ketamine.

3. *Anticonvulsant activity.* Diazepam is an excellent anticonvulsant drug and for this reason is commonly given in combination with agents that have a potential to cause seizures, including ketamine and local anesthetics. It is often the preanesthetic of choice for animals suffering from seizure disorders. Often it is also used as a preanesthetic for animals that are to undergo a diagnostic or surgical procedure of the spinal cord or brain (such as a cerebrospinal fluid tap or myelography) because it helps prevent postoperative seizures. Diazepam commonly is given intravenously as a treatment for many types of seizures, including those that occur in the postanesthetic period.

4. *Minimal adverse effects.* At therapeutic dosages, benzodiazepines have minimal adverse effects on the cardiovascular and respiratory systems and therefore have a high margin of safety. This property makes them particularly useful for anesthesia of high-risk and geriatric animals. If adverse effects are seen after the use of a benzodiazepine, flumazenil can be administered to reverse these agents (dose: 0.075-0.1 mg/kg).

Benzodiazepines should be used with caution in neonates and in animals with known liver dysfunction because these agents are poorly metabolized in these patients.

5. *Other properties.* It is interesting to note that benzodiazepine agents are used for a variety of purposes in veterinary medicine other than anesthesia. Diazepam and midazolam are effective appetite stimulants in cats, and oral diazepam is sometimes used to modify undesirable behavior such as inappropriate urination in cats. Both of these effects may arise from the action of benzodiazepine agents on neurotransmitters within the brain.

Method of use—diazepam.   The most effective and least painful way to administer diazepam is by the IV route, rather than the IM or SC* routes. When given as a sole agent intravenously, diazepam should be injected slowly because rapid administration may cause cardiac arrhythmias. Unfortunately diazepam is not water soluble, so it is not compatible with most other preanesthetic agents. It should not be mixed in a single syringe with atropine, acepromazine, barbiturates, or opioids because a precipitate may result. The only anesthetic agent that is physically compatible with diazepam is ketamine. Ketamine and diazepam can be mixed together in equal volumes in the same syringe, but prolonged storage is not recommended.

Diazepam is light sensitive, and for this reason is often provided in brown glass vials. If stored in a clear glass container, diazepam should be kept in a safe or other location away from light.

Because of its tendency to cause excitement and belligerence in healthy animals, diazepam is seldom used as a sole premedicating agent, except in very old or debilitated animals. More commonly, it is used in combination with drugs that induce anesthesia. Although it is not possible to induce anesthesia in a healthy animal through the use of diazepam alone, diazepam is an effective inducing agent when supplemented by other agents. In particular, the combination of ketamine and diazepam has gained wide acceptance as a safe and effective IV induction agent in small animals. Diazepam may also be administered concurrently with opioids or ultrashort-acting barbiturates (provided separate syringes are used) to achieve safe, smooth induction of high-risk patients.

Diazepam is classified as a controlled drug in Canada and the United States. Some potential for human abuse and theft exists, so this drug should be stored in a secure location, and appropriate records must be kept.

Method of use—midazolam.   Midazolam, a recently introduced benzodiazepine agent, appears to have some advantages over diazepam. It is water soluble and therefore can be mixed with other preanesthetic agents. It is less irritating to tissues than diazepam, and is also more reliably absorbed after IM injection. Effects are usually apparent within 3 minutes of IM injection.

Like diazepam, midazolam may induce minimal sedation when used on its own, and may in fact cause excitation in healthy cats and dogs. If midazolam is used as the sole preanesthetic agent, the patient often becomes more difficult to restrain. In feline patients, it is more useful to give midazolam in combination with ketamine (0.2 mg/kg midazolam and 10 mg/kg ketamine IM offers 30 to 40 minutes of sedation.)

Midazolam has minimal cardiovascular effects, but may cause transient respiratory depression. This drug has no analgesic effects.

---

*Diazepam can also be administered through a feeding tube passed into the rectum, at twice the IV dose. This provides rapid sedation for seizuring dogs and cats, in which IV access may be difficult.

Thiazine Derivatives

Xylazine (Rompun, Anased) is the most commonly used thiazine derivative. It has a wide range of applications in veterinary anesthesia. Medetomidine (Domitor), detomidine (Dormosedan), and romifidine are other thiazine derivatives used in veterinary anesthesia.

Pharmacologically, thiazine derivatives are classified as alpha-2 adrenoreceptor agonists. The site of action is receptors (alpha-2 adrenoreceptors) found on sympathetic nerves within the brain. Xylazine and other alpha-2 adrenoreceptor agonists stimulate these receptors, causing a decrease in the level of the neurotransmitter norepinephrine released within the brain. The result is sedation and analgesia. Muscle relaxation is created by inhibiting reflexes within the central nervous system. When combined with other tranquilizers or analgesic agents, the result tends to be additive in nature.

Both xylazine and medetomidine may have the potential to cause severe cardiovascular and respiratory complications. It is recommended that standard doses of these drugs be given only to young, healthy patients. Careful monitoring of patient status is essential after receiving these drugs. Fortunately, reversing agents are available for both xylazine and medetomidine, and can be used if adverse effects are seen.

Method of use—xylazine.   Xylazine is supplied as a 2.0% solution (20 mg/ml) for small animal use and as a 10% solution (100 mg/ml) for equine use. The 10% solution can be diluted with sterile water for use in small animals.

Xylazine can be used alone or in combination with ketamine, opioids, and many other agents. The required doses of other agents are reduced when they are given in combination with xylazine, particularly barbiturates (up to 80% reduction) and inhalation agents (up to 50% reduction). Whether given alone or in combination with other agents, xylazine can be administered IM or IV. Subcutaneous injections have much less effect and are generally avoided. Xylazine can be absorbed through skin abrasions and mucous membranes, and technicians handling xylazine should ensure that any of the drug spilled on human or animal skin is immediately washed off.

Effects of xylazine.   Xylazine is a potent sedative and muscle relaxant. Unlike phenothiazine or benzodiazepine agents, xylazine also has some analgesic effect. When combined with other tranquilizers, ketamine, opioid agents, or nitrous oxide, xylazine may provide sufficient analgesia and sedation to allow minor surgical procedures. Analgesia, however, is short-lived (approximately 20 minutes) and should be supplemented with other agents if a prolonged effect is required. The sedative effect of IM xylazine may last several hours in some patients.

Xylazine has considerable potential for adverse side effects and has been associated with a higher rate of anesthetic complications and death than other commonly used preanesthetic agents. Adverse side effects are reported most commonly after IV administration and include the following:

1. Xylazine may induce profound cardiovascular changes, particularly when given intravenously or when used without atropine. Bradycardia and second-degree heart block (faulty conduction of the electrical impulse between the right atrium and the ventricles) is commonly seen, and hypotension (low blood pressure) also may occur. Xylazine also sensitizes the heart to the arrhythmogenic effect of epinephrine. Because of these serious effects on the cardiovas-

cular system, the use of xylazine should be avoided in any animal that is debilitated or suffering from cardiac or respiratory disease. To reduce adverse cardiac effects, atropine can be given IM or SC as a premedication or reserved for those animals showing a significant (greater than 33%) drop in heart rate. However, it is not always effective in preventing or treating the cardiovascular side effects of xylazine and may in fact increase the workload of the heart.

2. Respiratory effects of xylazine vary from animal to animal and among species. After the administration of xylazine, some animals show respiratory depression, whereas others show no ill effects. Severe hypoventilation and cyanosis may occasionally arise from the use of xylazine, particularly in brachycephalic dogs. As a general rule, xylazine should not be administered to animals showing signs of respiratory disease.

3. Xylazine causes vomiting in up to 50% of dogs and 90% of cats. The emetic action of xylazine appears to be unpleasant for the animal but may be somewhat reduced if the animal is premedicated with atropine.

4. Xylazine has been reported to cause bloat in ruminants and in dogs. For this reason it should not be used as a preanesthetic in breeds of dogs prone to gastric dilation and torsion, such as German shepherds, Great Danes, Saint Bernards, and other large, deep-chested dogs.

5. Xylazine has been associated with temporary behavior and personality changes in both dogs and cats. This effect also has been reported for other preanesthetic agents, including acepromazine, opioids, and diazepam.

6. Xylazine is metabolized in the liver, and its metabolites are excreted in the urine. Adequate hepatic and renal function are therefore important requirements for any animal receiving this drug.

7. Xylazine may cause long-lasting sedation in some animals.

8. Xylazine reduces the secretion of insulin by the pancreas. Animals sedated with this drug may show transient hyperglycemia, which is not harmful to the animal but may confuse the interpretation of blood samples collected during this period. Hyperglycemia can also lead to transient osmotic diuresis, which may be harmful in dehydrated patients.

Medetomidine.   Given the adverse effects associated with xylazine use, attention has recently focused on another thiazine derivative, medetomidine (Domitor, available as a 1-mg/ml solution). Medetomidine has an affinity 10 times greater than xylazine for the alpha-2 receptors (those that mediate the sedative effects) and less affinity than xylazine for alpha-1 receptors (those that mediate many of the adverse side effects). As a result, medetomidine has greater potency and fewer adverse side effects than xylazine, including less tendency to cause vomiting. Otherwise, the clinical effects of medetomidine are similar to xylazine and include sedation, muscle relaxation, and analgesia.

In the United States, medetomidine is approved for IM or IV use only in the dog, but in Europe it is also approved for use in cats at a higher dose rate. Onset of action of medetomidine is within 1 minute after IV administration and within 5 minutes after IM administration. It reaches peak serum concentration 15 to 20 minutes after IM injection. Biotransformation takes place in the liver, with subsequent elimination by the kidney. Duration of sedation is 45 to 90 minutes, unless reversed with atipamezole. At equivalent doses, medetomidine will cause a longer duration of sedation and analgesia than xylazine.

TABLE 1-8	
Dosage for Medetomidine	
Dogs (sedation)	20-40 µg/kg IV or 30-40 µg/kg IM
Dogs (supplement IV ketamine/ diazepam)	5 µg/kg IV
Dogs (minor to moderate surgical procedures)	30 µg/kg +3 mg/kg ketamine IM or IV (Can mix in the same syringe)
Cats (induction)	60 µg/kg medetomidine + 5 µg/kg ketamine, IM or IV
Dogs (minor surgical procedures)	20-40 µg/kg + 0.2 mg/kg butorphanol IM (Can mix in the same syringe)
Dogs (immobilization and sedation)	20-30 µg/kg +0.25 mg/kg morphine IM* (Can mix in the same syringe)
Dogs (immobilization and sedation)	20-30 µg/kg +0.05 mg/kg oxymorphone IM* (Can mix in the same syringe)
Dogs (as a sedative/analgesic during gas anesthesia, for example if patient is moving in response to surgical manipulation)	1-2 µg/kg IV

Adapted from Ko JCH: Anesthetic potency: how to use medetomidine and atipamezole, *Vet Tech* 18(10):695-702, 1997.
*An anticholinergic is recommended.

The normal dosages are given in Table 1-8, with lower doses used for preanesthetic sedation and higher doses for immobilization. Dosages higher than those recommended do not result in greater sedation but will prolong the effect of the drug.

Medetomidine has also been used in microdose quantities (5 µg/kg) to supplement ketamine/diazepam induction of anesthesia. The addition of medetomidine improves the quality of induction and extends the duration of anesthesia compared with ketamine/diazepam alone. The combination of medetomidine and ketamine provides more effective analgesia and muscle relaxation than xylazine/ketamine or ketamine/diazepam. However, administration of oxygen is strongly recommended when this combination is given because some animals appear to develop severe hypoxemia.

Medetomidine can also be used in conjunction with inhalation agents and with injectable anesthetic drugs such as ketamine, propofol, and barbiturates.

As with xylazine, the use of medetomidine is associated with increased risk of cardiovascular and respiratory depression. In cats, the heart rate consistently decreases as much as 50% after injection of medetomidine (80 to 100 µg/kg). Transient hypertension, followed by hypotension, is common. Respiratory depression and cyanosis may occur as with xylazine. Cyanosis is apparently the result of decreased blood flow to peripheral tissues rather than low blood oxygen values. Spontaneous muscle twitching, vomiting, and hypothermia have also been reported after medetomidine administration. Urination is common 90 to 120 minutes after injection as a result of a diuretic effect of the drug.

As with xylazine, use of an anticholinergic with medetomidine may be advisable to reduce bradycardic effects.

Use of reversing agents.   Because of the adverse cardiovascular side effects and long duration of sedation that can occur after xylazine or medetomidine administration, use of a reversing agent is often advisable. Yohimbine (Yobine), given intravenously at a dose of 0.1 mg/kg IV, is an effective reversing agent for xylazine. Reversal of sedation and the cardiovascular effects of xylazine occurs within a few minutes of IV administration of yohimbine. Tolazoline, given IV at a dose rate of 1 to 2 mg/kg, is also an effective reversing agent. Yohimbine and tolazoline are associated with occasional unwanted side effects, including rapid arousal, excitement, rage, and tremors. Tolazoline may also cause vasodilation and hypotension.

Medetomidine has a specific antagonist, atipamezole (Antisedan), which is given at a dosage rate of 0.1 to 0.4 mg/kg. Atipamezole may be given IM or IV, although it is currently only approved for IM administration in the United States. The dosage for atipamezole is 5 times that of medetomidine; however, because the formulation of atipamezole is 5 times more concentrated than medetomidine (atipamezole 5 mg/ml, medetomidine 1 mg/ml), equal volumes of the two drugs should be administered. It is suggested that if the initial dose of IM atipamezole is not effective, administration of an amount equivalent to one half of the IM dose should be given by the IV route 5 minutes after the first injection. Atipamezole will reverse all of the clinical effects of medetomidine, both detrimental (bradycardia) and beneficial (analgesia). To maintain analgesia it may be appropriate to administer another analgesic agent, such as butorphanol, just before the reversal of medetomidine.

Opioids (Narcotics)

The term "narcotic" has long been applied to the class of drugs derived from morphine. This term has been replaced with "opiate" or "opioid" depending upon whether the drug is a natural chemical (opiate) or synthetically derived (opioid). The term "narcotic" is properly reserved for those agents that induce physical dependence and addiction and are therefore subject to stringent regulations regarding storage, use, and record keeping. Several opioids, such as buprenorphine, have little tendency to induce physical dependence and therefore are not considered to be narcotics. For the purposes of this text, the term "opioid" will be used for all members of this class, both narcotic and nonnarcotic.

Opioids are a versatile class of drugs that may be used as preanesthetics, induction agents, and analgesics. This chapter will discuss the general characteristics of this class of drugs, with emphasis on their use as preanesthetics and as neuroleptanalgesics. Information on the use of opioids as induction agents is found in Chapter 3, and detailed information on specific opioid agents and their use in postoperative analgesia is presented in Chapter 8.

Mode of action.   A great deal of research has been done to determine the site of opioid action within the nervous system. Opioid receptors are found on neurons throughout the body. The natural stimulants of these receptors are chemicals produced by the body, such as endorphins and enkephalins. The effects of opioids are chiefly the result of their action on receptors located in the brain and spinal cord. At

TABLE 1-9

Effect of Opioid Drugs on Receptors

Receptor	Effects	Agonists	Antagonists or Minimal Effect
Mu (μ)	Respiratory depression Euphoria Addiction Analgesia Sedation Miosis	Morphine Meperidine Fentanyl Oxymorphone Buprenorphine (partial)	Naloxone Butorphanol
Kappa (κ)	Analgesia Sedation Respiratory depression Miosis	Morphine Meperidine Fentanyl Oxymorphone Butorphanol	Naloxone
Sigma (σ)	Hallucinations Euphoria/dysphoria	Morphine Meperidine Fentanyl Oxymorphone Butorphanol	Naloxone
Delta (δ)	Analgesia Motor dysfunction	Morphine Fentanyl Meperidine	

Modified from Orsini J: Butorphanol tartrate: pharmacology and clinical indications, *Compendium* 10:849, Oct. 1988.

least four types of opioid receptors have been identified: mu (μ), kappa (κ), sigma (σ), and delta (δ). Opioid agents differ in their action at each of these sites and therefore in their overall effects on the body (Table 1-9).

An opioid agent may act as an agonist (stimulating agent) or antagonist (blocking agent) at each type of receptor. Some agents (including morphine, oxymorphone, and fentanyl) are pure *agonists*, in that they stimulate all receptors. Other agents (for example butorphanol) are considered *mixed agonists/antagonists* in that they block one type of receptor and stimulate another type. Still other opioids (for example, naloxone) block all types of receptors and are therefore considered to be pure *antagonists*. These antagonists have little clinical effect on their own, but are sometimes used to reverse the effects of the pure agonists and the mixed agonists/antagonists.

Beneficial effects.   Opioid agents have two effects on the nervous system that account for their use in veterinary anesthesia:

1. *Central nervous system (CNS) effects.* Depending on the dose, the particular opioid agent, and the species in which the agent is used, an opioid agent may cause CNS depression or excitement. In dogs the predominant effect is sedation. Most animals exhibit a combination of CNS depression and analgesia within 60 seconds of intravenous administration of opioids. Although swallowing may persist, endotracheal intubation is often possible. If high doses are given (particularly to a sick animal), a hypnotic state may be pro-

duced in which the patient appears profoundly sedated yet can be aroused by sufficient stimulation. Hypnosis is typically more profound than the sedation seen with acepromazine, xylazine, or diazepam. Recovery is often slow (up to 6 hours in some animals) unless a reversing agent is given.

Unlike dogs, cats may react to some opioids by exhibiting bizarre behavior patterns, including anxiety or mania, particularly if the drug is given intravenously. For this reason, some opioids (for example, morphine) must be used at very low doses in cats. Dogs that are not painful may also show excitement (for example, whining and barking) after opioid administration, particularly if a tranquilizing agent is not used concurrently.

2. *Analgesia.* Opioids have long been considered to be the most effective agents known to medicine for the treatment of pain. The potency varies between members of the class: pure agonists such as morphine and oxymorphone are more effective for treatment of severe pain than the mixed agonist/antagonists such as butorphanol.

With the routine use of general anesthetics that have limited analgesic properties (for example, isoflurane, halothane, propofol, and barbiturates) and the current emphasis on prevention of postoperative pain, the analgesic effect of opioids remains one of the chief reasons for their use in veterinary medicine. (See Chapter 8 for more information on the use of opioids for pain control.)

Method of use.   Opioid agents are used in many ways in veterinary anesthesia:

1. They are a common component of preanesthetic mixtures. Typically, these are a mixture of an anticholinergic (such as atropine or glycopyrrolate), a tranquilizer (such as acepromazine), and an opioid (particularly meperidine or butorphanol; see formulas in Box 1-1). These preanesthetic "cocktails" are mixed together in advance and given to the patient by SC or IM injection before anesthetic induction. An opioid is included in these mixtures for its analgesic effects and to potentiate the sedative properties of acepromazine.

2. Opioids are used to prevent and treat postoperative pain. (See Chapter 8.)

3. Opioid agents are sometimes used at higher dosages and in combination with a tranquilizer to achieve the state of profound sedation and analgesia termed *neuroleptanalgesia.* Animals that are given these agents lie quietly in lateral recumbency but can be aroused by sufficient noise or surgical stimulation. Neuroleptanalgesia using an opioid/tranquilizer combination is commonly used for procedures that require significant CNS depression and analgesia but not general anesthesia. Examples include dentistry, minor surgery such as porcupine quill removal, and diagnostic procedures such as endoscopy or radiography. Neuroleptanalgesic combinations can also be used to induce anesthesia. (See Chapter 3.)

Neuroleptanalgesic combinations may be used in both the cat and dog and can be prepared within the clinic using tranquilizing agents (such as acepromazine, xylazine, or diazepam) and opioids (such as morphine, meperidine, oxymorphone, or butorphanol). In some cases, the drugs are mixed in the same syringe; or, they may be injected separately by the IM or IV route after pretreatment with atropine. Safe use of neuroleptic agents by the IV route requires slow injection over 1 to 2 minutes because hypotension or CNS stimulation may occur if a large bolus is given. For all neuroleptanalgesic

Box 1-1 Formulas for Preanesthetic Mixtures

PREMIX
Contains per ml:

1 mg acepromazine
0.2 mg atropine
20 mg meperidine

To make up a 20-ml solution, mix together the following:

Acepromazine	2 ml of 10 mg/ml solution = 20 mg
Atropine	8 ml of 0.5 mg/ml solution = 4 mg
Meperidine	4 ml of 100 mg/ml of solution = 400 mg

Make the mixture up to 20 ml by adding 6 ml of sterile saline.
For dosage rates for cats and dogs, see the chart below.

BAA (Butorphanol-Ace-Atropine)
Contains per ml:

1 mg acepromazine
0.2 mg atropine
2 mg butorphanol

To make up a 20-ml solution, mix together the following:

Acepromazine	2 ml of 10 mg/ml solution = 20 mg
Atropine	8 ml of 0.5 mg/ml solution = 4 mg
Butorphanol	4 ml of 10 mg/ml solution = 40 mg

Make the mixture up to 20 ml by adding 6 ml of sterile saline.
NOTE: Sedation is usually greater than for Premix. Alternatively, the acepromazine can be reduced to half this dose (1 ml of 10 mg/ml solution = 10 mg, in 20 ml of total solution) for sedation comparable to Premix. For minimal sedation or for use in geriatric animals, reduce acepromazine to one fourth of this dose (0.5 ml of 10 mg/ml solution = 5 mg).

DOSAGE RATES FOR CATS (FOR BAA OR PREMIX)

WT (kg)	1	2	3	4	5	6	7	8	9	10
Dose (ml)	0.2	0.35	0.45	0.55	0.65	0.75	0.85	0.95	1	1.1

combinations, the opioid component can be reversed using naloxone or another narcotic antagonist. However, the tranquilizer component cannot be reversed, unless a specific antagonist such as yohimbine is available. The ability to partially reverse neuroleptanalgesia allows its use in geriatric and other higher-risk patients, provided ventilatory support is available in case of severe respiratory depression.

Adverse effects.   Because of associated side effects, opioids must be administered with caution.

1. *Effect on respiratory function.* The most serious side effect is the tendency of these drugs to depress respiration, particularly when used with a tranquilizing agent. When given at high dose rates, opioids cause a decrease in both respiratory rate and tidal volume, resulting in decreased blood oxygen lev-

Box 1-1 Formulas for Preanesthetic Mixtures—cont'd

DOSAGE RATES FOR DOGS (FOR BAA OR PREMIX)

WT (kg)	1	2	3	4	5	6	7	8	9	10
Dose (ml)	0.1	0.15	0.2	0.25	0.3	0.35	0.4	0.45	0.5	0.55
WT (kg)	11	12	13	14	15	16	17	18	19	20
Dose (ml)	0.6	0.65	0.65	0.7	0.75	0.8	0.8	0.85	0.9	0.95
WT (kg)	21	22	23	24	25	26	27	28	29	30
Dose (ml)	0.95	1	1	1.1	1.1	1.2	1.2	1.2	1.2	1.3
WT (kg)	31	32	33	34	35	36	37	38	39	40
Dose (ml)	1.3	1.3	1.4	1.4	1.4	1.5	1.5	1.5	1.6	1.6
WT (kg)	41	42	43	44	45	46	47	48	49	50
Dose (ml)	1.6	1.7	1.7	1.7	1.7	1.7	1.8	1.8	1.9	1.9
WT (kg)	51	52	53	54	55	56	57	58	59	60
Dose (ml)	1.9	1.9	2	2	2	2	2.1	2.1	2.1	2.2
WT (kg)	61	62	63	64	65	66	67	68	69	70
Dose (ml)	2.2	2.2	2.2	2.3	2.3	2.3	2.3	2.4	2.4	2.4
WT (kg)	71	72	73	74	75	76	77	78	79	80
Dose (ml)	2.4	2.5	2.5	2.5	2.5	2.6	2.6	2.6	2.7	2.7

Data courtesy of Doris Dyson, Ontario Veterinary College, Guelph, Ontario; and Donald Sawyer Education Services, Okemos, Mich.
BAA, Butorphanol-Ace-Atropine.

els (PaO_2) and increased carbon dioxide levels ($PaCO_2$). Respiratory efforts may become inadequate to reduce blood carbon dioxide levels, resulting in significant respiratory acidosis. The respiratory depression seen is dose dependent for most opioid agents, meaning the effect is more pronounced at high doses. Some opioids (for example, butorphanol) show a "ceiling effect" in that high doses show no greater depression of respiration than do low doses.

The tendency of opioids to depress respiration is potentially so severe that high doses of an opioid agent should not be given unless the anesthetist is able to support respiration by manually bagging the animal or by use of a ventilator. If respiratory arrest occurs, it is usually possible to maintain the animal with manual support of respiration until the effect of the opioid has been antagonized with naloxone or has worn off.

Interestingly, despite the tendency of opioids to depress respiration, some animals pant after opioid administration. This results from a direct effect of opioids on the temperature-regulating center of the brain, which mistakenly interprets normal body temperature as being elevated.

2. *Effect on gastrointestinal function.* The effect of opioids on the gastrointestinal tract is twofold. The initial effect of many agents is an increase in peristaltic movement, resulting in diarrhea, vomiting, and flatulence. Pretreatment with atropine or acepromazine usually moderates this effect. After the initial stimulation of peristalsis, a prolonged period of gastrointestinal stasis may occur, resulting in constipation.

3. *Physical dependence* (addiction). Prolonged use of some opioid agents can lead to physical dependence. Human patients given morphine develop tolerance for its effects in approximately 2 to 3 weeks. Physical dependence is seen after 3 weeks of intermittent use. Not all opioids are addictive: those with minimal or antagonistic activity at mu receptors (for example, butorphanol) have less potential for causing physical dependence.

Other reported effects of opioid agents include:

- Bradycardia (less pronounced in animals pretreated with atropine)
- Hypotension after rapid intravenous administration (as a result of vasodilation)
- Cough suppression
- Miosis in dogs and mydriasis in cats
- Increased responsiveness to noise
- Excessive salivation

Reversibility.   One advantage of the opioid class as a whole is the reversibility of these agents. Several narcotic antagonists (reversing agents) are available, including naloxone hydrochloride (Narcan), levallorphan tartrate, nalorphine hydrochloride, and nalbuphine (Nubaine). Technically, levallorphan and nalorphine are classified as mixed agonist/antagonists, whereas naloxone is a pure antagonist. Butorphanol (a mixed agonist/antagonist) has also been used to reverse pure opioid agonists such as morphine. Of these drugs, naloxone is the preferred reversing agent because it is the most effective and causes the least respiratory depression. Narcotic antagonists are effective in reversing opioid agents only, and cannot be used to reverse the effects of phenothiazines, thiazine derivatives, and other nonopioid agents.

Narcotic antagonists exert their effect by binding to opioid receptors and thus acting as blocking agents. By displacing other opioid agents from receptors, they reverse the agonist effect of those agents. Reversal of sedation, respiratory depression, hypotension, bradycardia, and gastrointestinal effects occurs within minutes of IV injection of the antagonist. Unfortunately, reversal of analgesia also occurs. Reversal of analgesia can be avoided by titrating the dose of reversing agent such that respiratory depression is only partially relieved, allowing an acceptable level of analgesia to be maintained; or by using a reversing agent such as butorphanol that has, in itself, some analgesic effect.

Reversal of opioid effects through the use of an antagonist is too expensive for routine anesthesia. However, the technique is extremely useful in emergency overdose situations. Narcotic antagonists are also used for rapid reversal of anesthesia in the compromised or geriatric patient. They are also helpful in reviving neonates delivered by a cesarean section when the operation is performed under opioid agents. One drop of naloxone, placed under the tongue of each puppy or kitten, is usually sufficient to reverse the respiratory depression caused by fentanyl, morphine, or other opioids given to the mother.

When used as a reversing agent, naloxone is given at a dose rate of 0.04 mg/kg IV, SC, or IM, every 2 hours as needed. The calculated dose should be diluted in 10 ml of saline and slowly given IV until the desired level of reversal is achieved. The remainder of the calculated dose can be given SC. The effects of narcotic antagonists are usually observed within 30 seconds of IV injection.

Reversing agents may not remove all sedative effects in some animals, and additional doses are usually ineffective in such cases. In fact, repeated doses of some reversing agents may cause CNS and respiratory depression through overload and stimulation of opioid receptors. Occasionally, animals treated with reversing agents may show symptoms of sympathetic system activity, including tachycardia and cardiac arrhythmias.

Regulatory considerations.   Most opioid agents are subject to government regulation regarding purchase, handling, and dispensing. The need for detailed record-keeping and the potential for abuse or theft of opioid agents is a significant disadvantage of this class of drugs. In the United States, the Controlled Substances Act assigns each opioid to one of five drug schedules according to each drug's potential for abuse. In a similar way, Canadian legislation has classified each opiate as a narcotic, controlled, or prescription drug. Agents classified as narcotics in Canada, or as Schedule II substances in the United States, cannot be dispensed or drawn into a syringe except under the direct supervision of a licensed veterinarian. Regulated substances should be kept in a cabinet, safe, or other locked storage place and should not be left on counter tops or in other public areas. After withdrawing a dose from a bottle of controlled substance, the bottle should be immediately returned to locked storage. Usage must be accurately recorded in a drug logbook, and inventory must be periodically checked to ensure that no drug is unaccounted for.

✔ **KEY POINTS**

1. The technician's duties during the preanesthetic period may include obtaining an adequate patient history, performing a physical examination, and performing diagnostic tests, as requested by the veterinarian.
2. Preanesthetic care of the patient may include fasting and intravenous catheterization. Preparation of equipment and administration of drugs are also the responsibility of the anesthetist.
3. No single anesthetic protocol is ideal for all patients. Rather, the anesthetic techniques and agents used are tailored to the needs of the individual patient.

Factors such as previous or concurrent illness; patient age, temperament and species; nature of the procedure; and preference of the veterinarian are all considered in determining the choice of anesthetic protocol.

4. Diagnostic tests such as the complete blood count (CBC) and urinalysis may provide valuable information regarding the patient's ability to tolerate anesthesia. Procedures such as radiography, electrocardiography, and blood gas determination also may be useful in selected patients but are seldom done on a routine basis.

5. The risk of anesthesia to the patient should be assessed before initiating the procedure. The patient should be assigned to a class based on physical condition, as outlined by the American Society of Anesthesiologists.

6. The patient should be in stable condition, when possible, before being anesthetized; preexisting problems such as dehydration or shock should be corrected.

7. Although intravenous (IV) catheterization offers enhanced patient safety and convenience for the anesthetist, this procedure is associated with the risk of accidental overhydration. A fluid infusion rate of 10 ml/kg/hr is considered safe for most patients.

8. Preanesthetic agents increase the safety and convenience of anesthesia by reducing the dose of general anesthetic needed, by preventing bradycardia and other parasympathetic effects, and by reducing patient stress and discomfort. All preanesthetic agents, however, have side effects that may be harmful in some patients.

9. Anticholinergics (such as atropine and glycopyrrolate) help prevent bradycardia, bronchoconstriction, excessive salivation, and gastrointestinal activity. They are particularly recommended for use in animals that are to receive xylazine, opioids, or ketamine. Anticholinergic agents may be harmful when used in animals with preexisting tachycardia, constipation, or ileus.

10. Tranquilizing agents include phenothiazines, benzodiazepines, and thiazine derivatives. Phenothiazines have a wide margin of safety but may cause hypotension in some patients. Benzodiazepines have a calming effect on geriatric and debilitated animals and are excellent for prevention and treatment of seizures. Thiazine derivatives are extremely potent and produce excellent muscle relaxation but may cause serious cardiovascular and respiratory complications in some patients.

11. Opioids may be used as preanesthetic agents, as induction agents, as postoperative analgesics, and (in combination with tranquilizers) as neuroleptanalgesics. Their greatest advantage is the profound analgesia they produce in most patients. They have the potential to cause adverse side effects on the cardiovascular, respiratory, and gastrointestinal systems, and prolonged administration may be associated with addiction. Their use is subject to government regulation regarding purchase, handling, and dispensing.

12. The action of some preanesthetic agents may be reversed through the use of specific agents such as yohimbine, atipamezole, and naloxone.

REVIEW QUESTIONS

1. Given the busy nature of a veterinary practice, it is probably best to assume that the same anesthetic protocol should be used on all patients.
   True   False
2. The following question would be a good example of how to ask a question: "Your dog does not exercise much, does he, Mrs. Jones?"
   Agree   Disagree
3. Different species may have different physiologies in regard to the metabolism of drugs.
   True   False
4. An obese dog will require more anesthetic than a normal weight dog of the same breed.
   True   False
5. Blood tests such as ALT have minimal value for an anesthetist.
   True   False
6. It is always best to withhold food and water from any patient scheduled to receive a general anesthetic for at least 12 hours before the scheduled procedure.
   True   False
7. Which of the following is not a crystalloid solution?
   a. Lactated Ringer's
   b. Normal saline
   c. Dextran
   d. 5% dextrose
8. Which of the following is not a valid reason for administering a preanesthetic medication?
   a. It reduces the amount of general anesthetic required for induction.
   b. It may calm an excited animal.
   c. It may reduce possible noxious side effects from the general anesthetic.
   d. It increases patient safety by allowing the animal to stay under the general anesthetic for a longer time.
9. Most preanesthetics will not cross the placental barrier.
   True   False
10. It is recommended that atropine not be given to an animal that has tachycardia.
    True   False
11. Anticholinergic drugs such as atropine block the release of acetylcholine at the:
    a. Muscarinic receptors of the parasympathetic system
    b. Nicotinic receptors of the parasympathetic system
    c. Muscarinic receptors of the sympathetic system
    d. Nicotinic receptors of the sympathetic system
12. Phenothiazine tranquilizers such as acepromazine sedate the animal and give some analgesia.
    True   False
13. In general, the opioids can have a significant effect on the cardiovascular and respiratory systems, causing bradycardia and respiratory depression.
    True   False

14. A patient that is anemic or moderately dehydrated would be classified as a _____ anesthetic risk.
    a. Class I
    b. Class II
    c. Class III
    d. Class IV
    e. Class V

For the following questions, more than one answer may be correct.

15. The suggested minimum data base for any patient may include:
    a. History
    b. Physical examination
    c. Diagnostic tests
    d. Name of the required procedure
16. Disadvantages or adverse side effects of opioids include:
    a. No analgesia
    b. Respiratory depression
    c. A tendency to cause bloat
    d. Bradycardia
17. Effects that atropine may have on the body include:
    a. Decreased salivation
    b. Increased vagal tone
    c. Decreased gastrointestinal motility
    d. Mydriasis
18. Clinical signs that are associated with atropine toxicity include:
    a. Excitability
    b. Miosis
    c. Tachycardia
    d. Dry mucous membranes
19. Effects that one may see after premedication with the phenothiazine tranquilizers include:
    a. Sedation
    b. Antiarrhythmic effect
    c. Peripheral vasodilation
    d. Reduced salivation
    e. Reduced seizure threshold
20. Characteristic effects of the benzodiazepines include:
    a. Pronounced sedation in young animals
    b. Muscle relaxation
    c. Significant decrease in respiratory function
    d. Minimal effect on cardiovascular system
21. Physical effects that may be seen after administration of xylazine include:
    a. Bradycardia
    b. Mydriasis
    c. Bloat
    d. Hypoventilation
    e. Vomiting

22. Effects of opioid administration include the following:
    a. Analgesia
    b. Increased sensitivity to noise
    c. Panting
    d. Decreased tear production
23. Opioids may be reversed with:
    a. Atipamezole
    b. Naloxone
    c. Atropine
    d. Yohimbine
24. Which of the following drugs will most likely precipitate out when mixed with other drugs or solutions?
    a. Atropine
    b. Acepromazine
    c. Diazepam
    d. Butorphanol
25. A neuroleptanalgesic is a combination of:
    a. An opioid and an anticholinergic
    b. An anticholinergic and a tranquilizer
    c. An opioid and a tranquilizer
    d. An anticholinergic and a benzodiazepine

Answers for Chapter 1

1. False   **2.** Disagree   **3.** True   **4.** False   **5.** False   **6.** False
7. c   **8.** d   **9.** False   **10.** True   **11.** a   **12.** False   **13.** True
14. c   **15.** a, b, c, d   **16.** b, d   **17.** a, c, d   **18.** a, c, d   **19.** a, b, c, e
20. b, d   **21.** a, c, d, e   **22.** a, b, c   **23.** b   **24.** c   **25.** c

Selected Readings

HASKINS SC: Opinions in small animal anesthesia, *Vet Clin North Am Small Anim Pract* 22(2): 326-469, 1992.

KO JCH: Xylazine, detomidine, medetomidine and their antagonists, *Vet Tech* 18(3):209-217, 1997.

KO JCH: Anesthetic potency: how to use medetomidine and atipamezole, *Vet Tech* 18(10):695-702, 1997.

MAMA K: New drugs in feline anesthesia, *Compendium* 20(2):125-137, 1998.

MUIR WW III, HUBBELL JAE, et al.: *Handbook of veterinary anesthesia*, St Louis, 1995, Mosby.

PADDLEFORD RR: *Manual of small animal anesthesia*, New York, 1988, Churchill Livingstone.

SHORT CE: *Principles and practice of veterinary anesthesia*, Baltimore, 1987, Williams & Wilkins.

WARREN RG: *Small animal anesthesia*, St Louis, 1983, Mosby.

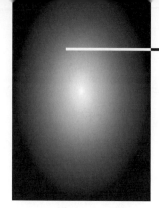

CHAPTER **2**

General Anesthesia

PERFORMANCE OBJECTIVES

After completion of this chapter, the reader will be able to:

- Define or explain the following terms: general anesthesia, balanced anesthesia, titration, induction, endotracheal intubation, hyperventilation, tachypnea, apneustic breathing, hypostatic congestion, atelectasis, cyanosis, bagging, dead space, hypertension, hypotension, vital sign, and reflex.
- Identify and describe the components of general anesthesia, including the various stages and planes.
- Understand the techniques, advantages, and disadvantages of IV, IM, and inhalation anesthesia.
- Describe the technique of endotracheal intubation and understand the advantages and disadvantages of this procedure.
- State the rationale for monitoring an anesthetized patient and know the various parameters that should be monitored.
- Describe appropriate ways to position an animal during anesthesia.
- State the various tasks or duties that need to be performed during the recovery period.
- Understand the concept of patient safety as it relates to general anesthetics.

T
hrough the use of the preanesthetic drugs described in Chapter 1, the anesthetist is able to tranquilize (and in the case of neuroleptanalgesics, profoundly sedate) the small animal patient. This level of CNS depression is adequate for minor procedures; however, a state of *general anesthesia* is usually required for major surgeries. This chapter describes the components of general anesthesia, including induction, maintenance, and recovery. The classical stages and planes of general anesthesia and the anesthetic procedures and monitoring associated with each stage are also described.

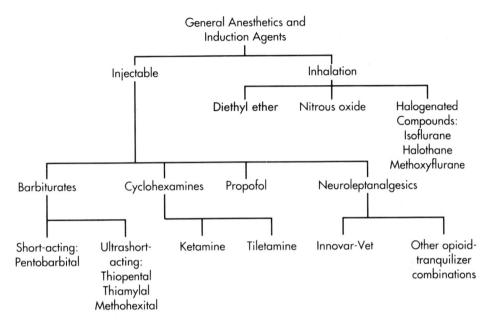

FIG. 2-1   Past and present agents used in general anesthesia.

■ DEFINITION OF GENERAL ANESTHESIA

General anesthesia is a state of controlled and reversible unconsciousness characterized by lack of pain sensation (*analgesia*), lack of memory (*amnesia*), and relatively depressed reflex responses. Ideally, this state is achieved without significantly affecting the patient's vital systems, particularly respiration and circulation.

In any given patient, general anesthesia may be accomplished through the use of injectable anesthetics, inhalation anesthetics, or both (Fig. 2-1). *Injectable anesthetics* include barbiturates (for example, thiopental sodium, thiamylal sodium, methohexital, and pentobarbital sodium); cyclohexamines (for example, ketamine, tiletamine); and propofol. Neuroleptanalgesic agents may also be used to induce anesthesia. *Inhalation anesthetics* used in veterinary medicine include diethyl ether, halothane, methoxyflurane, isoflurane, enflurane, sevoflurane, desflurane, and nitrous oxide. Patients may be anesthetized with one drug or with several agents used in combination in a technique called *balanced anesthesia*. The characteristics of general anesthesia are covered in this chapter, and the properties, advantages, and disadvantages of specific agents are discussed in detail in Chapter 3.

■ COMPONENTS OF GENERAL ANESTHESIA

General anesthesia is brought about through the use of techniques and agents chosen by the veterinarian and together called the *anesthetic protocol*. The administration of a general anesthetic to any animal varies according to such parameters as temperament and physical status of the patient, nature of the procedure to be done, cost and availability of various drugs, and preference of the veterinarian.

Regardless of the anesthetic protocol chosen, any anesthetic procedure may be divided into the following components: preanesthesia, induction, maintenance, and recovery.

Preanesthesia

The preanesthetic period is the time immediately preceding anesthesia in which patient data are collected, the patient is fasted, and preanesthetic drugs are administered. This period is discussed in Chapter 1.

Induction

The process by which an animal leaves the normal conscious state and enters an unconscious state is known as *induction*. Usually, the induction process is initiated only after the animal has received premedication drugs, as ordered by the veterinarian, and enough time has lapsed for these drugs to take effect. This is a minimum of 10 minutes if the drugs are given by the intramuscular (IM) route and 20 minutes if the subcutaneous (SC) route is used. Occasionally, premedications and induction agents may be administered simultaneously (for example, when acepromazine, atropine, and ketamine are mixed in a syringe and given intravenously to a cat).

The induction agent may be administered to the patient either by injection or inhalation. When injection is used, it is often followed by intubation with an endotracheal tube to allow the administration of an inhalation (gas) anesthetic by means of an anesthetic machine. Alternatively, the animal may be directly induced by means of a gas anesthetic delivered by a mask or anesthetic chamber, and no injectable anesthetic is necessary.

Initially, the animal may show signs of incoordination or excitement, followed by progressive relaxation and unconsciousness. The onset of general anesthesia is also characterized by the loss of some protective reflexes, including the abilities to swallow and cough.

Maintenance

Following the induction period, the animal enters the *maintenance period,* during which a stable level of anesthetic depth is achieved. Surgery and other procedures are commonly performed during this period. As with induction, a predictable sequence of events occurs during the maintenance period, including the onset of analgesia, skeletal muscle relaxation and cessation of movement, further loss of protective reflexes including the palpebral (eye blink) reflex, and the occurrence of mild respiratory and cardiovascular depression. If anesthetic depth increases, the patient may show more severe respiratory and cardiovascular depression, and in the unusual event of an anesthetic overdose, respiratory and cardiac arrest can occur.

Recovery

The maintenance period ends and recovery begins when the concentration of anesthetic in the brain begins to decrease. The method by which the anesthetic is eliminated from the brain and circulatory system varies according to the anesthetic agent:

- Injectable drugs are commonly removed from the blood by the liver and undergo metabolism by liver enzymes. The metabolites are excreted by the urinary system. Some drugs do not undergo metabolism and are excreted unchanged by the kidneys (for example, ketamine in the cat).
- In the case of short-acting thiobarbiturates, the level of anesthetic in the brain falls as the drug is rapidly redistributed to other tissues, especially muscle and eventually fat. This redistribution results in lower levels of the drug in the brain and thus the recovery of the patient. In this case, the patient awakens from the anesthetic even though the drug is still present in the body.
- Inhalation agents are eliminated mainly through the respiratory tract as anesthetic molecules leave the brain, entering first the blood and then the alveoli of the lung.
- Recovery from either injectable or inhalation anesthesia may be hastened by the action of analeptic agents such as doxapram. Some injectable agents (for example, opioids, medetomidine, and xylazine) have specific reversing agents, as discussed in Chapter 1.

However it is achieved, recovery from anesthesia is in many respects the reverse of the induction process. Reflex activity, muscle tone, and sensitivity to pain are regained as consciousness returns.

■ SAFETY OF GENERAL ANESTHESIA

General anesthesia is not without risk. The administration of any anesthetic may affect the patient's vital centers, which are the areas of the brain that control cardiovascular and respiratory function and thermoregulation. Death may occur if the activity of these centers is not maintained throughout anesthesia. It is therefore vitally important that the animal be closely monitored during induction, maintenance, and recovery from any general anesthetic. Particular attention should be focused on heart rate, pulse quality, ventilation, and mucous membrane color.

The anesthetist may use several strategies to increase the safety of anesthesia and minimize the adverse effects of general anesthetic agents:

- Preanesthetic drugs such as atropine or acepromazine may be given to prevent bradycardia and cardiac arrhythmias during general anesthesia.
- Preanesthetic sedatives such as xylazine, acepromazine, and opioids help reduce the dose of general anesthetic required to induce and maintain anesthesia, thus minimizing the adverse side effects of the general anesthetic agent. For example, a patient preanesthetized with acepromazine will require significantly less barbiturate to induce unconsciousness than an animal that has not received preanesthetic medication. In some patients, multiple general anesthetic and preanesthetic agents (such as a combination of nitrous oxide, an opioid, and a muscle relaxant) may be used in a balanced anesthesia technique to further minimize the required dose of each agent used.
- All injectable drug dosages should be double-checked before administration to the animal, and the anesthetist should ensure that the concentration of an agent drawn into a syringe is the same as that used for the drug calculations. It is a good idea to label all syringes containing injectable anesthetic agents with the name of the patient, the name of the drugs, and the drug concentration.

- When inducing an animal or maintaining an animal already under anesthesia, only the minimum dose of drug needed to achieve the desired level of anesthesia should be administered. Many injectable agents are given "to effect," which means that only the amount of injectable anesthetic necessary to produce unconsciousness is given, rather than administering the entire dose calculated on a milligram per kilogram basis. This technique is necessary because the amount of drug needed to induce or maintain anesthesia cannot be accurately predicted for a given patient. Most dogs, for example, will achieve a moderately deep state of anesthesia after receiving 15 mg of thiopental sodium per kg body weight. A few dogs will reach a comparable anesthetic depth after receiving only 10 mg/kg thiopental sodium, and others will require 20 mg/kg to reach the same depth. Because the anesthetist can seldom predict the exact dose that a given patient will require, it is safer to give the drug as a series of bolus injections, observing the animal for signs of anesthesia and discontinuing the administration of anesthetic when the desired depth is reached. This process is known as *titration*.

Factors that may affect the animal's response to a general anesthetic include age, breed, physical condition, preanesthetic drugs given, and the ability of the patient's liver and kidney to metabolize and excrete the drugs. For example, the amount of thiobarbiturate required to induce a quiet, older dog may be one half or less of the dose required for an active 2-year-old dog, despite the fact that the dogs weigh the same. Similarly, a cat with a urinary obstruction may be deeply anesthetized after receiving less than 10 mg of IV ketamine, whereas a healthy cat may require 30 mg of IV ketamine to reach the same depth of anesthesia.

Just as the amount of drug required to *induce* anesthesia varies between patients, so also varies the amount of inhalation or injectable agent required to *maintain* anesthesia. At a given concentration of halothane gas, for example, one patient may show brisk reflexes and appear to be only lightly anesthetized, whereas another may show the absence of all reflexes and a relatively slow heart rate, indicating deep anesthesia. The knowledgeable anesthetist monitors the patient closely and alters the amount of anesthetic given to suit the patient's requirements, rather than relying solely on a calculated dose recommended by a textbook.

- Close observation of a patient during the recovery period is also critical. Various untoward events, such as vomiting, laryngospasm, and convulsions, may occur during the recovery period. Hypothermia is also of concern to the anesthetist because recovery from anesthesia may be delayed if the animal's temperature has been allowed to fall below the normal range. Problems that may be encountered during the recovery period are described in Chapter 6.

■ CLASSICAL STAGES AND PLANES OF ANESTHESIA

During the course of general anesthesia, the animal passes through a series of anesthetic stages and planes roughly correlated with changes in anesthetic depth. With the induction of anesthesia, the patient enters stage I. As anesthetic depth increases, the animal passes through stage II and stage III (the anesthetic depth most appropriate for surgical procedures) and, in some cases, may enter stage IV. These stages and planes are summarized in Table 2-1. Although they were first developed and based on work done with the anesthetic agent diethyl ether, the stages may be adapted to describe the effect of other agents, including both injectable and inhalation anesthetics. The signs listed in the table will vary somewhat, depending on the agent used and the individual patient's response.

Stage I

Immediately after the administration of an inhalation or injectable agent, the animal enters the initial stage of anesthesia, stage I. Animals in this stage are conscious but disoriented and show reduced sensitivity to pain. Respiration and heart rate are normal, and all reflexes are present.

Stage II

Stage II begins with the loss of consciousness. All reflexes are still present and, in fact, may appear exaggerated. The animal is able to chew and swallow, and yawning is common. The pupils are dilated but will constrict in response to intense light.

As the higher centers of the brain release voluntary control of body functions, the animal may exhibit excitement in the form of rapid movement of the limbs, vocalization, and struggling. Breathing may be irregular, and the animal may appear to be holding its breath. Although animals in stage II may appear to be "fighting" the anesthesia, the actions are not under conscious control. Rather, they are thought to occur because the anesthetic selectively depresses neurons in the brain that normally inhibit and control the function of motor neurons.

Throughout stage II, care should be taken to prevent the struggling patient from injuring itself, the restrainer, or the anesthetist. To limit the duration of this "excitement" stage, it is desirable that the patient's depth be increased as quickly as possible. This is done by continuing the administration of anesthetic until stage III is reached. Stage II ends when the animal shows signs of muscle relaxation, slower respiration rate, and decreased reflex activity.

Observation of stage II is dependent on the rate of induction and the use of premedication drugs. Premedicated animals that are rapidly induced with an injectable anesthetic usually pass directly from stage I to stage III.

Stage III

The third stage is subdivided into four planes, representing increasing anesthetic depth from plane 1 through plane 4. In *plane 1* the respiratory pattern becomes regular, and involuntary limb movements cease. The eyeballs start to rotate ventrally, the pupils may become partially constricted, and the pupillary response to bright light is diminished. The gagging and swallowing reflexes are depressed such that an endotracheal tube may be successfully passed, allowing the patient to be connected to a gas anesthetic machine. Other reflexes (such as the palpebral reflex) are present; however, responses are less brisk than in stage II. Although appearing to be unconscious, the patient will not tolerate surgical procedures at this light plane of anesthesia and will move or otherwise react to a painful stimulus.

Animals in *plane 2* of stage III are generally considered to be at medium depth of anesthesia, suitable for most surgical procedures. Surgical stimulation may

TABLE 2-1

Depth indicators of anesthetic stages and planes

Stage of Anesthesia	Behavior	Respiration	Cardiovascular Function	Response to Surgery	Depth
I	Disoriented	Normal, may be panting; respiration rate 20-30 breaths/min	Heart rate unchanged	Struggle	Not anesthetized
II *"Excitement stage"*	Excitement: struggling, vocalization, paddling, chewing, yawning	Irregular, may hold breath or hyperventilate	Heart rate may increase	Struggle	Not anesthetized
III—PLANE 1 *Light anesthesia*	Anesthetized	Regular; rate 12-20 breaths/min	Pulse strong; Heart rate >90 bpm	May respond with movement	Light
III—PLANE 2 *Medium (surgical) anesthesia*		Regular (may be shallow); rate 12-16 breaths/min	Heart rate >90 bpm	Heart and respiration rates may increase	Moderate
III—PLANE 3 *Deep anesthesia*		Shallow; rate <12 breaths/min	Heart rate 60-90 bpm; CRT increased; pulse less strong	None	Deep
III—PLANE 4		Jerky	Heart rate <60 bpm; prolonged CRT; pale mucous membranes	None	Overdose
IV	Moribund	Apnea	Cardiovascular collapse	None	Dying

evoke a mild response such as increased heart rate or respiration rate, but the patient usually remains unconscious and immobile. The pupillary light response is sluggish, the eyeballs may be central or rotated, and the pupils are slightly dilated. The respirations are regular but shallow, with a respiratory rate between 12 and 16 breaths per minute in the dog and slightly higher in the cat. Heart rate and blood

Eyeball Position	Pupil Size	Pupil Response to Light	Muscle Tone	Reflex Response
Central	Normal	Yes	Good	All present
Central, may be nystagmus	May be dilated	Yes	Good	All present, may be exaggerated
Central or rotated, may be nystagmus	Normal	Yes	Good	Swallowing poor or absent, others present but diminished
Often rotated ventrally	Slightly dilated	Sluggish	Relaxed	Patellar, ear flick, palpebral, and corneal may be present; others absent
Usually central, may rotate ventrally	Moderately dilated	Very sluggish or absent	Greatly reduced	All reflexes diminished or absent
Central	Widely dilated	Unresponsive	Flaccid	No reflex activity
Central	Widely dilated	Unresponsive	Flaccid	No reflex activity

pressure are mildly decreased. The skeletal muscle tone becomes more relaxed, and many of the normal protective reflexes (for example, pedal and palpebral) are diminished or lost.

In *plane 3* of stage III, the patient appears to be deeply anesthetized. Significant depression of circulation and respiration is often present, and for this reason plane

3 is considered to be excessively deep for most surgical procedures. The respiratory rate is less than 12 breaths per minute, and respirations are shallow. Ventilation assistance in the form of "bagging" with the reservoir bag or assistance from a mechanical ventilator may be desirable in some patients. Heart rate is also notably reduced in patients at this plane, even in the presence of surgical stimulation. Pulse strength may be reduced because of a fall in blood pressure. The capillary refill time may be increased to 1.5 to 2 seconds. The pupillary light reflex is poor throughout this plane and may be absent. The eyeballs become central, and the pupils are moderately dilated. Reflex activity is often totally absent. Skeletal muscle relaxation is marked, to the degree that no resistance occurs when the mouth is opened (that is, jaw tone is slack).

Plane 4 of stage III can be recognized by a "rocking boat" ventilatory pattern. This type of ventilation is characterized by spasmodic, jerky inspirations, caused by a lack of coordination of the intercostal and abdominal muscles and the diaphragm. Plane 4 is also characterized by fully dilated pupils and the absence of a pupillary light reflex. The eyes may be dry because of the absence of lacrimal secretions. Muscle tone is flaccid. More importantly, there is obvious depression of the cardiovascular system as marked by a dramatic drop in heart rate and blood pressure, accompanied by pale mucous membranes and a prolonged capillary refill time. The patient in this plane is too deeply anesthetized for safety and is in danger of imminent respiratory and cardiac arrest.

Stage IV

If anesthetic depth is increased past stage III, plane 4, the animal enters stage IV of anesthesia. At this stage there is a cessation of respiration, quickly followed by total circulatory collapse and death. Immediate resuscitation is necessary to save the patient's life.

Overview of Anesthetic Stages and Planes

Although these stages and planes appear easy to differentiate on paper, they are not well defined in every animal. A given patient may show some signs that indicate stage III, plane 2 anesthesia and other signs that indicate stage III, plane 3. The anesthetist must assess as many parameters as possible to come to a conclusion regarding the patient's depth of anesthesia. (See page 95 for examples of depth assessment.)

The appearance of the anesthetic stages and planes also varies between anesthetic agents. Methoxyflurane, for example, produces greater respiratory depression than halothane. An animal in stage III, plane 3 of methoxyflurane anesthesia may have a respiratory rate of 8 breaths per minute, whereas the same animal at the same plane of anesthesia might have a respiratory rate of 12 breaths per minute when anesthetized with halothane.

What, then, is the ideal depth of anesthesia? This question has no easy answer. The anesthetist must ensure that the patient does not perceive a surgical stimulus. At the same time, the anesthetist must avoid excessive anesthetic depth, which may result in depression of the cardiovascular and respiratory systems. The skills involved in achieving successful induction, maintenance, and recovery of anesthetized animals are discussed in the remainder of this chapter.

■ INDUCTION TECHNIQUES AND AGENTS
Induction Using Injectable Agents

Anesthesia may be induced by either intravenous or intramuscular injection of general anesthetic agents.

Induction by intravenous injection. One of the most common induction methods involves the intravenous (IV) injection of an anesthetic drug. Thiopental sodium, ketamine, propofol, etomidate, and oxymorphone/acepromazine are examples of inducing agents that are given intravenously. Typically, a standard dose of the agent is calculated and drawn into a syringe, then administered as needed to induce unconsciousness. This allows endotracheal intubation of the animal without resistance. (For a detailed outline of some induction techniques, see Procedure 2-1.) Once intubated, the animal may be maintained at a moderate or a deep level of anesthesia through the administration of an inhalation anesthetic. The use of inhalation anesthetic is not always necessary, however, because it is possible to perform minor surgical and short diagnostic procedures (such as quill removal and radiography) under injectable anesthesia alone.

The duration of anesthesia varies with the injectable agent used, but is usually less than 20 minutes. If necessary, anesthesia may be prolonged by repeated administration of the intravenous agent. However, with the exception of propofol, repeated dosing is generally discouraged because it may lead to the accumulation of large amounts of anesthetic within the body and result in a prolonged recovery. If more than 20 minutes of anesthesia is required, it is usually preferable to maintain anesthesia using gas inhalation anesthetics.

Induction by intramuscular injection. Some induction agents, including ketamine and tiletamine-zolazepam (Telazol), may be administered by intramuscular (IM) injection. This method is useful for animals in which IV injections are difficult, such as ferrets and very young puppies and kittens. Inhalant induction through the use of a mask or anesthetic chamber may also be used in these animals.

Intramuscular agents are also useful in anesthesia of animals that cannot be handled (for example, vicious domestic animals, wild animals, and captive animals in zoos). Because it is difficult to approach and handle these animals, the agent is usually administered by means of a blowpipe or tranquilizing gun, or through the use of restraint equipment such as a squeeze cage or rabies pole. Agents that can be administered by this method include ketamine/xylazine mixtures, tiletamine/zolazepam, neuroleptanalgesics, and opiates (particularly etorphine and carfentanyl).

Induction by IM injection differs from IV induction in several important respects:

1. For most agents, the anesthesia dose required for induction by IM injection is 2 to 3 times the IV induction dose.
2. It is difficult to titrate drugs given by the IM route, so usually the entire calculated dose is given.
3. Drugs administered by the IM route require several minutes to reach the brain at a concentration high enough to induce anesthesia. IM induction of anesthesia is therefore characterized by a relatively slow onset of anesthesia. In contrast, drugs administered intravenously take effect much more quickly.

PROCEDURE 2-1
Intravenous Induction of Anesthesia

The method of administering an intravenous drug for the purpose of IV induction varies depending upon the agent used and the veterinarian's preference. In most cases, the patient is premedicated with a tranquilizer (and in some cases, an anticholinergic). Premedication reduces the dose of anesthetic required and allows smoother induction.

1. Thiopental: To reduce the chance of sloughing from perivascular injection of a thiobarbiturate, an indwelling catheter can be used (Fig. 2-2). Inject one half of the calculated dose over a 10- to 15-second period (bolus injection). This technique allows rapid induction of stage III anesthesia with minimal stage II excitement. If intubation is not possible after 30 seconds following injection, a second dose (one fourth of the calculated dose) may be given. This method of administration is continued until the desired depth is reached. Use caution in patients with systemic disorders (such as acidosis or hypoproteinemia) because they may require a much smaller dose than healthy patients.

2. Ketamine/tranquilizer mixtures: In contrast to the bolus induction technique used with barbiturates, ketamine mixtures (that is, ketamine/diazepam, ketamine/acepromazine, and ketamine/xylazine) can be injected slowly (over 30 to 60 seconds). Slow injection minimizes the toxic effects of these anesthetic agents upon the cardiovascular and respiratory systems. Bolus injection techniques can also be used: for example, one third to one half of the calculated dose of ketamine/diazepam can be given IV over a 15- to 30-second period, with further increments every 45 seconds until the desired depth is reached.

3. Propofol can be given by slow IV injection (one third of the calcuclated dose every 30 seconds) to induce anesthesia. More rapid induction may be useful in uncooperative patients, but is more likely to induce apnea.

FIG. 2-2   Use of an intravenous catheter for injection of a barbiturate. **A,** Intravenous catheter showing metal stylet used for placement of catheter in vein. **B,** Surgical preparation of cephalic vein. **C,** Insertion of catheter into vein. **D,** Catheter is advanced over stylet. **E** and **F,** Taping of catheter in place. **G,** Injection of drug into catheter cap.

PROCEDURE 2-1
Intravenous Induction of Anesthesia—*cont'd*

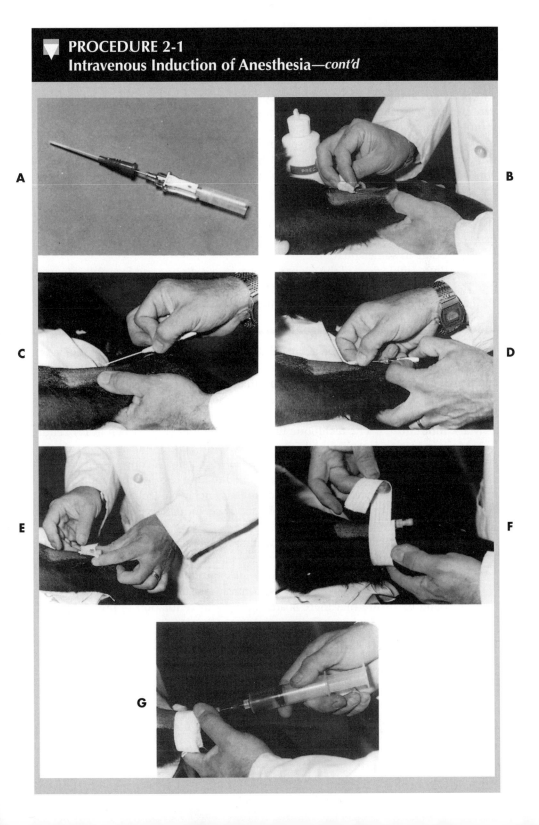

4. IM administration is characterized by a lengthy recovery period because the animal requires considerable time to metabolize the relatively large dose of drug given by this route.

The characteristics of intramuscular and intravenous anesthesia are illustrated by the use of ketamine, an anesthetic commonly used in cats. When given intravenously at a dose of 5 mg/kg, induction of anesthesia occurs in less than 1 minute. Alternatively, the drug can be given intramuscularly at a dose of 15 mg/kg, inducing anesthesia in 3 to 5 minutes. Recovery from IV ketamine administration is usually rapid, and healthy animals often appear fully recovered within 1 to 2 hours. In contrast, complete recovery from IM ketamine administration may require 8 to 12 hours.

Induction by oral administration.   Anesthesia may result when some agents (for example, ketamine) are given orally. This route of administration constitutes extra-label use of these agents. Oral administration is not used routinely, but it may be appropriate in some situations.

Typically, a single dose of the agent is drawn into a syringe and forcefully squirted into the animal's mouth. Care should be taken to avoid aspiration of the material by the patient. Alternatively, the agent can be mixed with a small amount of food.

Induction Using Inhalation Agents

Induction of anesthesia may be achieved through the use of rapid-acting inhalation anesthetics, such as halothane or isoflurane. Nitrous oxide is occasionally used to supplement the anesthetic effect of other inhalation agents. The gas anesthetic contained in an anesthetic machine is administered to an awake patient by means of a face mask or anesthetic chamber.

Mask induction.   The technique for mask induction is described in Procedure 2-2. Mask induction is well suited for use with rapid-acting inhalation anesthetics, such as isoflurane; it is more difficult to achieve with a slow-acting anesthetic, such as methoxyflurane. Mask induction is considered to have less risk than induction using injectable agents because the anesthetist can quickly control the animal's depth by adjusting the vaporizer setting. If problems arise, induction can be discontinued immediately.

There are several cautions associated with the use of this technique for induction:
- One drawback of mask induction is the potential for significant operating room pollution. Waste anesthetic gas readily leaks around the mask and is released into the room air. It is helpful to use a mask that fits snugly over the patient's face, and to ensure that there is adequate room ventilation to prevent inhalation of waste gas by hospital personnel. (see Chapter 5.)
- Another potential drawback is the risk of stressing the patient if the animal resists the use of a mask. Struggling may cause the release of epinephrine, which predisposes the patient to potentially fatal cardiac arrhythmias. To avoid this, it is advisable to use mask induction only on the calm or sedated patient.
- Mask induction may not be appropriate for patients with poor respiratory function because of the slow induction time. It is also unsuitable for patients at risk of vomiting during the induction procedure.

▼ PROCEDURE 2-2
Mask Induction

1. Use either a malleable black rubber mask or a clear plastic mask with a rubber diaphragm for mask induction. The mask should fit tightly on the animal's face to reduce leakage of waste gas and to minimize dead space.
2. Connect the mask to the Y piece of an anesthetic machine and hold in place over the animal's muzzle (Fig. 2-3).

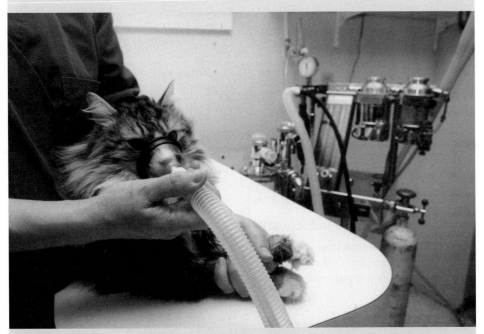

FIG. 2-3   Mask induction of a cat.

3. Give 100% oxygen for 2 to 3 minutes to allow the patient to adjust to the mask and to increase the amount of oxygen in the blood.
4. Set the anesthetic vaporizer to deliver 0.5% isoflurane or halothane. The oxygen flow rate should be set at 30 times the patient's tidal volume as a minimum or 3 to 4 liters per minute (because higher flow rates help speed induction).
5. Gradually increase the concentration of anesthetic by small increments (for example, increasing the vaporizer setting by 0.5% every 30 seconds) until an anesthetic concentration of 3% to 4% is reached.
6. This method is often well accepted by cats and small dogs, although some struggling may be seen after 2 to 3 minutes, possibly corresponding to stage II excitement. Induction of stage III, plane I anesthesia usually requires 5 to 10 minutes, depending on the agent used.

- The anesthetist must ensure that the mask does not occlude the patient's nostrils, as might happen with a cat or brachycephalic patient if the mask is too tight.

It is possible to maintain anesthesia by using a mask throughout the surgical procedure. However, many anesthetists prefer to intubate the patient with an endotracheal tube after induction.

Anesthetic chamber induction. Induction of anesthesia also can be achieved through the use of an anesthetic chamber (Procedure 2-3 and Fig. 2-4). Anesthetic chambers allow the induction of even the most uncooperative animal, but they are also associated with several problems:

- The technique is obviously suited only for use in small patients.
- One major disadvantage to this technique is the difficulty in monitoring the patient's heart rate, respirations, and other vital signs.
- As with mask induction, there is some risk of vomiting, especially in the nonfasted patient.
- There is considerable risk of exposure of hospital personnel to waste anesthetic gas, particularly when removing the patient from the chamber. To avoid waste gas exposure, the chamber must be equipped with a scavenger, and the anesthetic gas should be evacuated before the chamber is opened.
- Both mask and chamber inductions should be avoided in animals for which rapid induction and immediate endotracheal intubation are desired. This category includes all brachycephalic dogs, animals that have not been fasted, and animals with respiratory problems, including those with pleural effusion, diaphragmatic hernia, and pulmonary edema.

Monitoring During the Induction Period

Regardless of the induction method chosen, monitoring of the patient is of paramount importance throughout the induction period. The heart rate, pulse strength, respiratory rate and depth, mucous membrane color, and capillary refill time should

---

▼ PROCEDURE 2-3
Induction of Anesthesia Using an Anesthetic Chamber

1. To induce anesthesia using an anesthetic chamber, place the conscious animal inside the chamber, which contains ordinary room air. The chamber should be large enough for the patient to lie down with its neck extended.
2. Deliver oxygen gas combined with an inhalation anesthetic to the chamber by means of an air inlet. Typically, a high concentration of anesthetic (4% to 5%) and a high flow rate of oxygen (3 to 5 liters per minute) are used.
3. Observe the behavior of the patient and remove the patient from the chamber when the patient loses its ability to stand (loss of righting reflex). This can be tested by rocking the chamber gently.
4. If the patient is too lightly anesthetized to be intubated immediately after being removed from the chamber, use a mask to induce a deeper level of anesthesia.

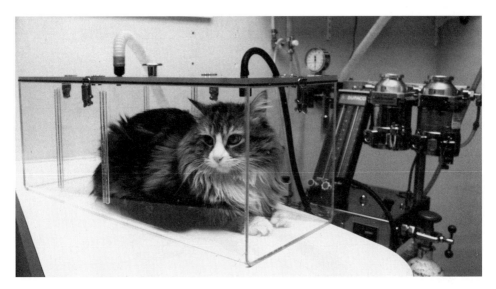

FIG. 2-4   Induction chamber.

be checked frequently by the anesthetist to ensure patient safety. The animal's reflexes and jaw tone should also be monitored because they indicate the depth of anesthesia. Endotracheal intubation may be attempted after the patient shows no signs of resistance, gagging, or swallowing when the tongue is grasped and the mouth is opened.

■ ENDOTRACHEAL INTUBATION

Once anesthesia is induced in the patient, the anesthetist may choose to place a breathing tube (endotracheal tube) in the patient's airway. This tube conducts air directly from the oral cavity to the trachea, bypassing the nasal passages and pharynx (Fig. 2-5).

Advantages of Endotracheal Intubation

Anesthesia with endotracheal intubation offers several advantages over anesthesia in the nonintubated animal:
- If a gas anesthetic machine is to be used, intubation of the patient allows more efficient delivery of the anesthetic gas to the animal than does a mask. Because gas flow rates can be lowered if an endotracheal tube is in place, intubation results in reduced exposure of hospital personnel to waste anesthetic gas.
- Intubation improves the overall efficiency of respiration by reducing the amount of dead space within the respiratory passages. Dead space describes those portions of the breathing passages that contain air but in which no gas exchange can occur (that is, the mouth, nasal passages, pharynx, bronchi, and trachea). By minimizing dead space, the endotracheal tube ensures that a larger proportion of the gas delivered to the patient reaches the exchange surface in the alveoli.
- Intubation allows the anesthetist to deliver oxygen directly to the patient when respiration must be assisted. Forced delivery of oxygen (with or without an

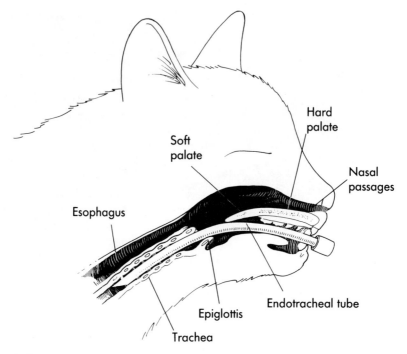

FIG. 2-5   Intubation of a cat, showing anatomy.

inhalation anesthetic) to a patient can be achieved by squeezing the reservoir bag of the anesthetic machine or through the use of a ventilator. The assisted delivery of oxygen to the patient by these means is called *intermittent positive pressure ventilation* (IPPV) and is discussed in Chapter 7. This type of ventilation support may be essential to a patient that is having trouble breathing adequately during anesthesia. Positive pressure ventilation through an endotracheal tube is also necessary in animals that have been given neuromuscular blocking agents.

■ The presence of an endotracheal tube with an inflated cuff reduces the risk of aspiration of vomitus, blood, saliva, or other material that may be present in the oral cavity or breathing passages. This material may collect during any procedure; however, the risk of aspiration is particularly high during oral surgery or dentistry and in patients that have not been fasted. Because of the usefulness of an endotracheal tube in maintaining a patent airway, it is customary to leave it in place throughout anesthesia and into the recovery period, removing it only when the animal regains the swallowing reflex.

Problems Associated with Endotracheal Intubation

There are several problems and hazards associated with endotracheal intubation:

■ As discussed in Chapter 1, intubation may stimulate the activity of the vagus nerve and cause an increase in parasympathetic system tone, particularly in dogs. This, in turn, may cause bradycardia, hypotension (low blood pressure), and cardiac arrhythmias. Occasionally, cardiac arrest may occur, particularly in an animal with preexisting cardiovascular disease. Atropine given in the pre-anesthetic period is helpful in preventing parasympathetic stimulation.

- Some species and breeds are difficult to intubate. Brachycephalic dogs, for example, have a large amount of redundant tissue within the oral cavity. This tissue falls over the back of the pharynx when the animal's mouth is opened, obscuring the entrance to the trachea (the glottis). Despite this difficulty, it is important to intubate these animals, because otherwise it may be impossible to maintain an open airway during anesthesia. The use of a laryngoscope may be helpful to visualize the oropharynx in these patients. (See Chapter 4.)

- Overzealous efforts to intubate an animal may damage the larynx, pharynx, or soft palate. Particular care should be used when intubating cats, which have a narrow glottis that is easily traumatized. If the tissues of the larynx are irritated during intubation, reflex closure of the laryngeal cartilages may occur. This condition, called *laryngospasm*, may result in blockage of the airway, which must be relieved or asphyxiation will result. To prevent laryngospasm, the anesthetist should avoid trauma to the laryngeal area during intubation. In cats it is also common procedure to spray the larynx with lidocaine to help desensitize the laryngeal tissues and reduce the risk of laryngospasm. Some anesthetists prefer to use lidocaine gel as a lubricant on the endotracheal tube. Although this will not work quick enough to desensitize the vocal cords during intubation, it may allow the vocal cords to remain desensitized postanesthesia and thus reduce the chance of excess coughing and laryngospasm after extubation. Treatment of laryngospasm is discussed in Chapter 6.

- Certain food animal species and exotic and laboratory animal species are difficult to intubate because the mouth cannot be opened wide enough to allow the anesthetist to see the pharynx or glottis. "Blind" intubation is necessary in these species.

- If the endotracheal tube is inserted too far into the breathing passages, it may enter one bronchus, resulting in the ventilation of only one lung (Fig. 2-6). The tip of the tube should lie midway between the larynx and the thoracic inlet. Palpation of the thoracic inlet while gently moving the tube can assure the anesthetist of correct insertion depth of the tube. Alternatively, the length of the

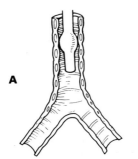
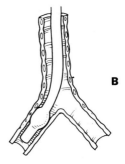

A   B

FIG. 2-6   Placement of endotracheal tube in trachea. **A,** Correct placement. **B,** Endotracheal tube advanced into bronchus (incorrect placement).

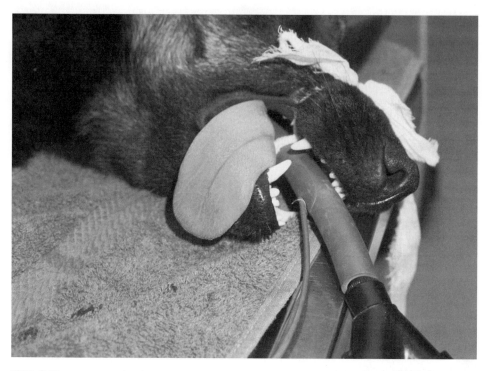

FIG. 2-7   Excessive dead space (endotracheal tube too long or not advanced sufficiently).

tube can be "premeasured" by determining the distance between the nose and the thoracic inlet of the patient before anesthesia.

- Many commercially available tubes are designed for human use and are too long for veterinary patients, particularly cats. If an excessively long tube is used, a large portion may extend forward past the animal's incisors, increasing the amount of dead space (Fig. 2-7). The endotracheal tube should be adjusted or trimmed so that the end of the tube is as close as possible to the animal's incisors. When shortening a tube, care must be taken to avoid cutting into the cuff inflation apparatus.

- Pressure necrosis may result if the cuff of the endotracheal tube is excessively inflated. (See Procedure 2-4, endotracheal intubation, for infusing the correct amount of air into the cuff.) Cats are particularly sensitive to pressure necrosis from endotracheal tubes, and it is sometimes recommended that noncuffed tubes or tubes with low-pressure cuffs be used with this species. Some anesthetists suggest that if tubes with high-pressure cuffs are used, the cuff should be inflated for no longer than 30 minutes before being deflated and moved to a new location in the trachea.

- Endotracheal tubes may become obstructed by saliva, mucus, blood, or foreign material such as gauze. Mucus, blood, or other such material may also occlude the distal end of the tube after use, making this a hazard for the next patient if the tube is not cleaned properly. Obstruction may also occur if the tube is

Text continues on p. 70

PROCEDURE 2-4
Endotracheal Intubation

1. Gather all necessary materials together before inducing the patient. Select several endotracheal tubes of varying sizes and check them for holes, loose connectors, and excessive wear. Test the cuff of each tube to make sure it remains inflated when air is introduced. Record the amount of air required to inflate the cuff.

2. Determine the length of the tube required by measuring the distance from the incisor teeth to the thoracic inlet. Estimate the diameter of the tube required by palpating the trachea. (See Chapter 4.)

3. Lubricate the tube with a sterile lubricant such as water soluble jelly. In cats, use a lubricant containing a local anesthetic, such as xylocaine, to decrease the incidence of laryngospasm. It is also customary to spray a topical anesthetic on the vocal cords of feline patients before intubation. Delay the intubation 1 to 2 minutes to allow the spray to take effect. Commercial laryngeal sprays are available, or 1% lidocaine may be drawn into a tuberculin syringe and aerosolized through a 26-gauge needle. (Cetacaine was previously used for this purpose, but its use has been largely discontinued because of its tendency to induce methemoglobinemia.) Whatever agent is used, administer only a small amount of topical anesthetic (0.1 ml).

4. When the animal reaches an appropriate plane of anesthesia, open the mouth to allow intubation. An animal showing signs of resistance (such as gagging and swallowing) is too lightly anesthetized to be intubated. The animal is usually restrained in sternal recumbency, although intubation in lateral or dorsal recumbency is preferred by some anesthetists. Extend the neck and raise the head so that the head and neck are in a straight line (Fig. 2-8). The animal's trunk should be propped upright and not allowed to sag laterally. Hold the upper jaw stationary, with the lips pulled dorsally, and push the lower jaw down by pulling the animal's tongue forward and down. It is often advisable to use a mouth gag to reduce the chance of being inadvertently bitten by the patient. The tongue may be held out by either the assistant or the person intubating the animal. Open the mouth wide enough to allow the anesthetist to clearly see the epiglottis, which normally lies over the entrance to the trachea. (See Fig. 2-8.) The restrainer should not push on the animal's ventral neck and head region, as this may obscure the laryngeal anatomy, making intubation difficult.

5. A laryngoscope is often used to assist intubation. This instrument consists of a handle, a smooth blade (which may be curved or straight), and a light source (either a small bulb lamp or a fiberoptic source). Laryngoscopes facilitate intubation by illuminating the pharyngeal area and by moving the epiglottis aside, exposing the glottis and vocal cords. The laryngoscope blade is first used to disengage the soft palate from the epiglottis. It is then gently placed at the back of the tongue, adjacent to the base of the epiglottis (in the

Continued

PROCEDURE 2-4
Endotracheal Intubation—cont'd

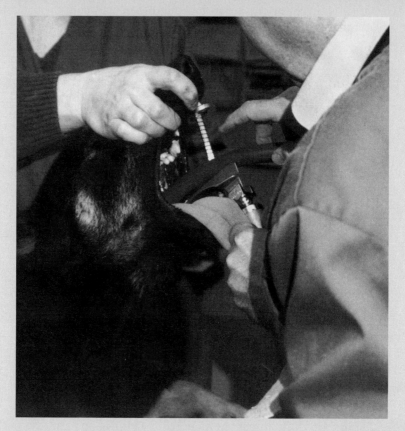

FIG. 2-8   Position of animal for intubation.

case of a curved laryngoscope blade, Fig. 2-9) or on the tip of the epiglottis itself (straight laryngoscope blade). This pulls the epiglottis forward and down, allowing the anesthetist to view the entrance to the trachea.

As an alternative to a laryngoscope, some anesthetists use the index finger of one hand to depress the epiglottis and guide the endotracheal tube into the trachea. This method of intubation carries some risk of being bitten by the patient if anesthetic depth is not sufficient. It is also possible to blindly intubate the animal by passing the tube into the mouth (which is held open with a mouth gag) while extending the tongue with the other hand. In this method, the tube is passed along the roof of the mouth, over the epiglottis, and into the entrance to the trachea. Significant trauma to pharyngeal and laryngeal tissues is possible with this technique, and esophageal intubation is common.

6. Insert the endotracheal tube past the vocal folds and into the trachea. This may be difficult in cats because the vocal cords are often positioned such that

PROCEDURE 2-4
Endotracheal Intubation—cont'd

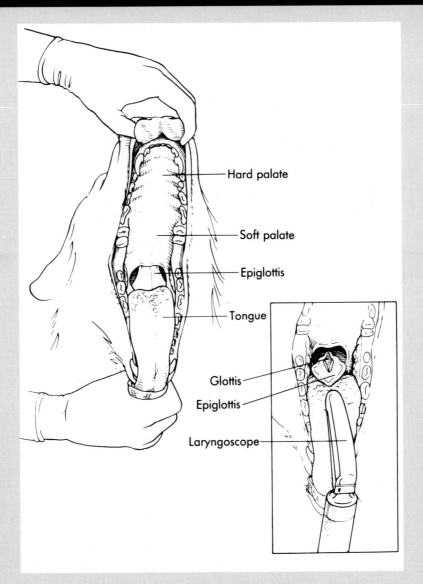

Hard palate

Soft palate

Epiglottis

Tongue

Glottis

Epiglottis

Laryngoscope

FIG. 2-9 Anatomy of the pharynx. When epiglottis is depressed, glottis is exposed. Endotracheal tube is advanced through glottis.

Continued

they close off the glottis. Intubation in cats is best accomplished by timing the advancement of the tube to coincide with exhalation (when the vocal cords separate and the glottis is open). The endotracheal tube should not be

PROCEDURE 2-4
Endotracheal Intubation—cont'd

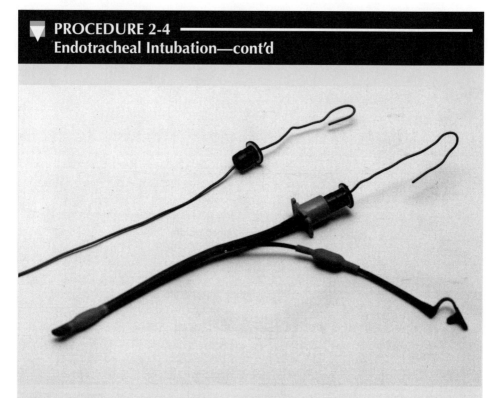

FIG. 2-10   Stylet and endotracheal tube (with stylet in place).

forced through the vocal cords, but gently rotated, if resistance is encountered. The tube should be advanced such that the curve of the tube matches that of the patient's neck.

When a small tube is advanced, problems may arise due to bending of the tube during insertion. A thin steel or wooden rod may be inserted into the tube to act as a stylet and prevent bending (Fig. 2-10). The stylet should not protrude beyond the end of the tube because it may traumatize the laryngeal tissues.

7. Ensure that the tube enters the trachea and not the esophagus. The entrance to the esophagus lies just dorsal to the entrance to the trachea and, although difficult to see, it easily accommodates an endotracheal tube. Accidental intubation of the esophagus results in delivery of anesthetic and oxygen to the stomach rather than to the lungs, and the patient is unlikely to remain anesthetized if this occurs. Esophageal intubation can usually be avoided if the anesthetist visualizes the entrance to the trachea throughout the intubation procedure and ensures that the tube clearly enters that location.

PROCEDURE 2-4
Endotracheal Intubation—cont'd

8. Once the endotracheal tube is in place, confirm its presence within the trachea (rather than the esophagus). This can be done in one of several ways:
   - The mouth can be opened and the entrance to the trachea observed. The tube can be seen to emerge from the glottis if it is in the correct location.
   - In long-nosed breeds, it is possible to palpate the tube with the index finger at the point at which it enters the larynx.
   - A cough may be heard as the tube is inserted. The cough reflex is a normal response to endotracheal intubation, particularly at a light plane of anesthesia. It usually indicates that the tube is entering the correct passageway to the trachea.
   - During expiration, the animal's breath can be felt as it exits the endotracheal tube. If the tube is in the trachea, a tuft of hair placed at the end of the endotracheal tube will also move with the animal's exhalations. Either way, the anesthetist is assured that the tube has been placed in the breathing passages and not in the esophagus.
   - Once the tube is connected to an anesthetic machine, the reservoir bag and unidirectional valves should move during inspiration and expiration if the tube is correctly placed.
   - The anesthetist may palpate the animal's cervical region, ensuring that only one firm tubular structure is present, which is the trachea containing the endotracheal tube. (The esophagus normally cannot be palpated.) Palpation of two firm tubular structures usually indicates that the endotracheal tube is in the esophagus, and the trachea and the tube are being palpated separately. It is often possible to palpate the beveled end of the tube within the trachea, confirming its location.
   - Vocalization is impossible if an endotracheal tube is correctly placed. Growling or whining usually indicates that the tube is in the esophagus and must be removed and reinserted in the correct location.
9. Secure the endotracheal tube in place using a piece of gauze tied around the tube and behind the animal's head or on top of its nose (Fig. 2-11).
10. Inflate the cuff of the endotracheal tube. Then check for leakage of anesthetic gas around the cuff. This is done by gently squeezing the reservoir bag. If only a tiny hiss is heard, the cuff is adequately inflated. If there is a loud hiss, indicating that air is leaking around the tube, more air should be infused into the cuff or a larger size endotracheal tube used. If no hiss is heard, consider deflating the cuff slightly, as it may be exerting excessive pressure on the tracheal mucosa.

Continued

PROCEDURE 2-4
Endotracheal Intubation—cont'd

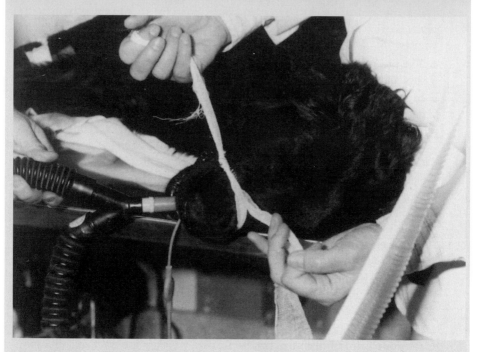

FIG. 2-11   Use of plain gauze to tie endotracheal tube in place.

kinked or twisted or if the end is occluded against the wall of the trachea. If this arises, obstruction of the endotracheal tube may cause a functional upper airway obstruction in the patient, which is a serious anesthetic emergency.

- Intubated animals require careful monitoring during recovery to ensure that the tube is removed when the animal begins to swallow. If the patient regains consciousness with the tube in place, the tube may be damaged by the patient chewing on it. In fact, patients have been known to chew tubes in half and aspirate the distal portion into the airway. Obviously, the presence of such a tracheal foreign body would be difficult to explain to the owner.

- Although endotracheal tubes used in human anesthesia are routinely discarded after a single use, it is common in veterinary practice for tubes to be used on several patients. Tubes must therefore be thoroughly disinfected between patients to prevent the spread of infectious diseases such as tracheobronchitis ("kennel cough"). The disinfection procedure, however, may also pose a problem to the patient. If endotracheal tubes are soaked in a cold disinfectant solution for too long a period, or in a solution that is concentrated, the rubber will become impregnated with the disinfectant. When next used, the disinfectant still in the endotracheal tube will irritate tracheal mucosa.

This can result in the patient coughing after anesthesia, or even cause the tracheal mucosa to slough.

- Despite all precautions, an animal may cough for a day or two after anesthesia because of minor irritation from the tube's presence in the trachea and larynx. Animal owners should be warned that it is common for animals to cough for 1 to 2 days after anesthesia if an endotracheal tube is used.

Because of the hazards associated with the use of endotracheal tubes, and for reasons of convenience, not all animals undergo endotracheal intubation during anesthesia. If an endotracheal tube is not used, the inhalation agent is delivered by mask throughout the procedure. Animals lightly anesthetized with intramuscular or intravenous agents for the performance of short procedures also may not require the use of an endotracheal tube if the animal maintains the ability to swallow throughout the anesthesia. Despite these exceptions, intubation is recommended for safety reasons if inhalation anesthetics are used or if a lengthy procedure is performed with the patient under injectable anesthesia.

Endotracheal tubes are further discussed in Chapter 4. Details of the intubation procedure are given in Procedure 2-4.

■ MAINTENANCE OF ANESTHESIA

Following successful induction of anesthesia, the animal enters a period in which anesthetic depth is adequate for surgical procedures. During this *maintenance period*, the anesthetist has two important tasks. First, the animal must be monitored closely to ensure that the vital signs (particularly heart rate and respiration) remain within acceptable limits. Second, the anesthetist must maintain the animal at an appropriate anesthetic depth (that is, one that is neither too light nor too deep). The importance of these two tasks can hardly be overemphasized. Failure to maintain an adequate depth of anesthesia may result in the animal's perception of pain and premature arousal from anesthesia. On the other hand, maintaining an animal at an excessive depth of anesthesia may lead to a slow recovery or an anesthetic overdose. Attention to vital signs is even more crucial because failure to monitor and maintain vital signs within acceptable limits may result in death or permanent brain damage.

The key to effective and safe anesthesia during the maintenance period is adequate monitoring. The word *monitor* comes from the Latin *monere*, meaning "to warn." The anesthetist who closely monitors the animal under anesthesia will usually receive ample warning of problems as they arise. Although continuous monitoring of the anesthetized patient by a veterinary technician is not practical in many veterinary clinics, an attempt should be made to observe and evaluate the healthy anesthetized patient at least once every 3 to 5 minutes. This allows rapid but thorough assessment of depth, cardiovascular and respiratory status, and other parameters (Box 2-1). High-risk patients should be checked at more frequent intervals or, if possible, monitored continuously.

Although the anesthetist must observe both vital signs and reflexes, it is important to differentiate between the two. The term *vital sign* refers to those parameters that indicate the response of the animal's homeostatic mechanisms to anesthesia, including heart rate, respiration rate, and capillary refill time. The patient's vital signs indicate how well the patient is maintaining basic circulatory and respiratory function during anesthesia. The term *reflex* refers to an involuntary response to a

---

Box 2-1 Parameters to Be Monitored During Anesthesia

PARAMETERS TO BE ASSESSED AT LEAST EVERY 5 MINUTES THROUGHOUT ANESTHESIA
Respiration rate, depth, and character (assess both reservoir bag movement and chest movements)
Mucous membrane color and capillary refill time (CRT)
Heart rate
Pulse strength and rate
Jaw tone, eye position, and palpebral reflex activity
Oxygen flow rate and oxygen tank pressure
Intravenous catheter placement and fluid administration rate
Patient's temperature (may be adequate to palpate paws and ears)

---

stimulus (such as a pinprick or tap). Reflex responses give the anesthetist valuable information on the depth of anesthesia but do not convey information on the patient's homeostatic mechanisms.

Monitoring Vital Signs

Vital signs may be monitored by the anesthetist's senses (that is, touch, hearing, and sight) or through the use of electronic devices such as an ECG machine or pulse oximeter. This section describes the parameters that can be monitored by the anesthetist without special instrumentation.

Vital signs that should be monitored during anesthesia include heart rate and rhythm, pulse pressure, capillary refill time, mucous membrane color, blood loss, respiratory rate and depth, and thermoregulation. Other vital signs that may be of interest but that require special monitors (discussed in the next section) include blood oxygenation, expired CO_2, ECG, and blood pressure.

Heart rate and rhythm. The minimum acceptable heart rate for anesthetized patients is 60 beats per minute (bpm) in the dog and 100 bpm in the cat. Lower heart rates may indicate excessive anesthetic depth or some other problem and should be brought to the veterinarian's attention immediately. Heart rates of 60 to 120 bpm are common during anesthesia (compared to 60 to 180 bpm in the normal awake dog and 110 to 220 bpm in the normal awake cat). The decreased heart rate normally seen in an anesthetized animal is the result of the depressant effect of most anesthetics on heart rate and myocardial function. A few drugs (for example, atropine, ketamine, and tiletamine) have the opposite effect and can raise heart rates.

Cardiac rhythm also may be affected by anesthetic agents, particularly halothane and xylazine. Disturbances in cardiac rhythm should be brought to the attention of the veterinarian for assessment.

Cardiac monitoring may be achieved in several ways, including direct palpation of the chest wall or pulse, auscultation of the chest using a stethoscope, use of an electrocardiogram (ECG), and use of an esophageal stethoscope. Several types of heart monitors are available that detect the patient's pulse or ECG and transmit information to the anesthetist by an audible beep, a flash of light, or a digital readout. Some monitors can be adjusted to sound an alarm when the heart rate moves above or below limits set by the anesthetist.

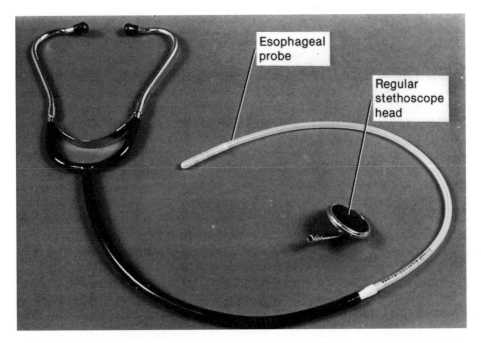

FIG. 2-12 Esophageal stethoscope. (From Warren RG: *Small animal anesthesia*, St Louis, 1983, Mosby.)

Use of an esophageal stethoscope allows auscultation of the heart even if the patient's chest area is covered with surgical drapes and conventional auscultation is difficult. The esophageal stethoscope consists of a thin, flexible tube attached to a regular stethoscope. The tube is lubricated with a small amount of water or lubricating jelly and is inserted through the oral cavity into the patient's esophagus. The tube is advanced until an audible heartbeat is detected through the earpieces (Fig. 2-12) or through an attached audio monitor. Insertion of the esophageal stethoscope is usually delayed until after the endotracheal tube is in place to minimize the danger of the stethoscope accidentally entering the trachea.

The presence of a beating heart does not necessarily imply that circulation is adequate. Heartbeat should be assessed in conjunction with pulse strength or measured blood pressure values.

Capillary refill time. The capillary refill time (CRT) is the rate of return of color to a mucous membrane after the application of gentle digital pressure. (See Fig. 2-13.) The CRT reflects the perfusion of the tissues with blood. Pressure on the mucous membranes compresses the small capillaries and blocks blood flow to that area. When the pressure is released, the capillaries rapidly refill with blood and the color returns, provided the heart is able to generate sufficient blood pressure. However, a short CRT is not an infallible indication that the circulation is adequate; in fact, a normal CRT may be observed shortly after euthanasia in some animals.

A prolonged CRT (more than 2 seconds) may indicate hypotension resulting from excessive anesthetic depth or circulatory shock. CRT is usually prolonged in patients in which the systolic blood pressure is less than 80 mm Hg. If systolic blood

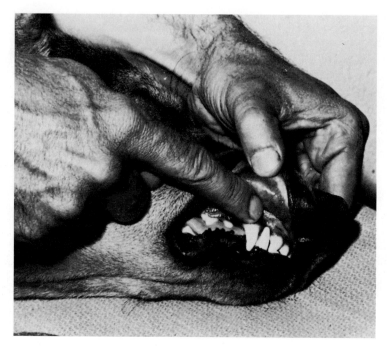

FIG. 2-13   Assessing gingiva for capillary refill time and mucous membrane color. (From Warren RG: *Small animal anesthesia,* St Louis, 1983, Mosby.)

pressure drops below 50 mm Hg, the capillaries may not refill at all. Animals suffering from this degree of hypotension will usually feel cold and have pale mucous membranes. Other factors that may also cause prolonged capillary refill time or poor perfusion include hypothermia, vasodilation, and cardiac failure.

Mucous membrane color.   The most convenient location for observing mucous membrane color is the gingiva (Fig. 2-13). In the case of dogs with pigmented gingiva, other sites may be used, including the tongue, buccal mucous membrane, conjunctiva of the lower eyelid, or the mucous membrane lining the prepuce or vulva. Pale mucous membranes may indicate blood loss or anemia or may result from poor perfusion (as may occur with prolonged anesthesia). Purple or blue mucous membranes indicate cyanosis, a shortage of oxygen in the tissues. Cyanosis during anesthesia is usually the result of respiratory failure or upper airway obstruction and must be addressed immediately.

Pulse strength.   Although the technician can only obtain an accurate reading of blood pressure through the use of special instruments, it is possible to roughly estimate blood pressure by palpating a major artery and determining the strength of the pulse. The pulse can be detected at any one of several locations, including the lingual (Fig. 2-14), femoral, carotid, and dorsal pedal arteries. The pulse should be strong and synchronized with the heartbeat. Difficulty in detecting a palpable pulse may indicate low blood pressure. Unfortunately, natural variation in pulse strength among normal animals somewhat limits the usefulness of this method of blood pressure monitoring.

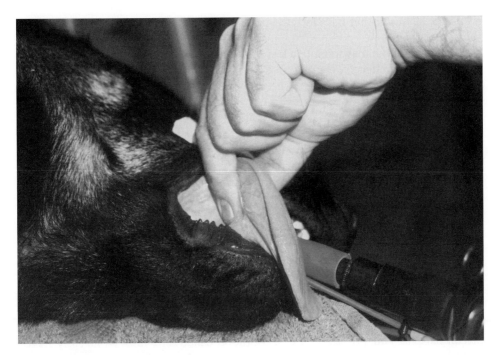

FIG. 2-14 Palpation of the lingual artery.

A rough estimate of blood pressure is also given by capillary refill time, although it is a somewhat insensitive test. CRT is noticeably prolonged when the patient's blood pressure drops.

Blood pressure is important to the anesthetist because it reflects the adequacy of blood circulation throughout the body. Decreased blood pressure is called *hypotension*, and an increase in blood pressure is termed *hypertension*. Hypotension during anesthesia may indicate any of the following:

- Excessive anesthetic depth. Blood pressure is influenced by both general anesthetics and preanesthetic drugs. Increasing the depth of inhalation anesthesia usually results in a fall in blood pressure.
- Excessive vasodilation. Certain preanesthetic drugs (that is, acepromazine and xylazine) may also reduce blood pressure by causing the blood vessels to dilate. Animals that are dehydrated or hypotensive (most commonly as the result of circulatory shock) before anesthesia are at particular risk of suffering a further drop in blood pressure when given these agents.
- Cardiac insufficiency.
- Excessive blood loss, leading to hypovolemia.

Accurate monitoring of blood pressure requires the use of instruments and is discussed on page 79.

Blood loss.   Blood loss, if excessive, predisposes the patient to shock and anesthetic complications. Blood loss in major surgery may be estimated by counting used sponges. One fully soaked 3 × 3 inch sponge holds 5 to 6 ml of blood. The true amount of blood lost may be up to twice this figure because it is difficult to measure the blood that has clotted, been retained by surgical drapes, or pooled at the surgery site.

A healthy animal may tolerate a loss of up to 15% of its blood volume without serious circulatory effects. This is approximately 13 ml/kg in dogs and cats.

Respiration rate and depth.   The animal's respiration rate may be monitored by observing movements of the reservoir bag or of the animal's chest. Normal respiration rate in a conscious animal is 10 to 30 breaths per minute in the dog and 25 to 40 breaths per minute in the cat. At a moderate depth of anesthesia, the normal rate is 8 to 20 breaths per minute, although rates up to 50 may be seen. During the maintenance period, respiratory rates less than 8 breaths per minute may indicate excessive anesthetic depth and should be reported to the veterinarian.

The anesthetist must monitor not only the respiratory rate, but also the depth and character of the breathing. With increasing depth of anesthesia, there is normally a decrease not only in the rate, but also in the volume of air taken with each breath (tidal volume). This decrease in respiratory rate and volume is sometimes called *hypoventilation*. Tidal volume decreases by at least 25% in most anesthetized animals, largely because most preanesthetic and general anesthetic drugs decrease the ability of the intercostal muscles to expand the thorax on inspiration. As the animal's breaths become more shallow (that is, as tidal volume decreases), some alveoli in the lung may not receive amounts of air adequate to sustain inflation. As a result, these alveoli partially collapse, leading to a condition called *atelectasis*. In its early stages, atelectasis can be reversed by gentle inflation of the lungs by the anesthetist. In this procedure, called *bagging*, the reservoir bag of the anesthetic machine is carefully squeezed, forcing air into the patient's breathing passages. When bagging a patient, the anesthetist should closely observe the animal's chest to ensure that it rises only slightly. This prevents overinflation of the lungs. Some anesthetists routinely bag every patient under inhalation anesthesia once every 5 minutes. Alternatively, atelectasis may be prevented by mechanical ventilation of the patient through the use of a ventilator. (See Chapter 7.)

In contrast to the hypoventilation observed in many anesthetized patients, the anesthetist may occasionally note rapid and deep respirations in some anesthetized patients. An increase in respiratory rate is called *tachypnea*, whereas an increase in depth is termed *hyperventilation*. Tachypnea must be differentiated from panting, in which the breathing is rapid but shallow and air intake is through the open mouth. Panting is a common side effect of some opioid drugs, particularly oxymorphone.

True hyperventilation and tachypnea have many possible causes. They are a normal response to increased carbon dioxide (CO_2) in the blood or metabolic acidosis. When an anesthetic machine is used, hyperventilation may indicate that the CO_2 is not being adequately removed from the breathing circuit by the CO_2 absorber. Rapid respirations may also result from an underlying disease, such as pulmonary edema. Hyperventilation is also commonly seen as a response to a mild surgical stimulus. For example, it is often seen when the surgeon pulls on the suspensory ligament of the ovary during an ovariohysterectomy. An elevated respiratory rate may also indicate a progression from moderate to light anesthesia and is one of the first signs of arousal from anesthesia.

Not only the respiratory rate and depth but also the type of respiration may be significant. The anesthetized animal's breathing should be smooth and regular, with both thoracic and diaphragmatic components. Difficult or labored breathing may indicate the presence of an airway obstruction. As previously mentioned, "rocking boat" respiration is another abnormal breathing pattern noted in very deep anesthesia.

The time relationship between inspiration and expiration may vary also. Normal inspiration lasts 1 to 1.5 seconds and expiration lasts 2 to 3 seconds. Animals anesthetized with ketamine may exhibit an *apneustic* respiratory pattern, in which inspiration is followed by a prolonged pause before expiration.

Auscultation of the chest may yield useful information, not only about cardiac function but also about respiratory function. Normal respiratory sounds are almost inaudible in the dog and cat: harsh noises, whistles, or squeaks may indicate narrow or obstructed airways or the presence of fluid in the airways or alveoli.

As evident from this discussion, the rate, depth, and type of respirations must be closely monitored by the anesthetist. A change in any of these parameters may be the first warning of a change in anesthetic depth or of the onset of an anesthetic problem.

Thermoregulation. Throughout anesthesia, the animal's temperature should be maintained as close as possible to the normal range for that species. Although body temperature does not change minute by minute, there is usually an overall drop of temperature with time during anesthesia. Temperature loss is greatest in the first 20 minutes, and the anesthetist should be concerned with preventing temperature loss from the moment of induction. Prolonged general anesthesia may reduce the patient's temperature by 3° C or more. Several factors contribute to this effect:

- Animals are routinely shaved before surgery, and the skin may be washed with antiseptic and alcohol solutions that cool by evaporation.
- The anesthetized animal cannot generate heat by shivering or muscle activity.
- The metabolic rate of an anesthetized animal is less than that of a conscious animal, resulting in less heat generation.
- During the course of surgery, a body cavity may be opened and the viscera exposed to air at room temperature.
- Several preanesthetic and general anesthetic agents cause vasodilation, resulting in an increased rate of heat loss.
- Pediatric and geriatric animals are less able to thermoregulate themselves and are therefore predisposed to hypothermia.

One unfortunate result of hypothermia is prolonged recovery from anesthesia. Hypothermia slows the rate at which liver enzymes metabolize anesthetic drugs, allowing the drugs to remain active in the body for a longer time. In addition, shivering (which is seen in recovering animals) may increase the patient's oxygen demands during the recovery period.

During anesthesia, rectal temperature should be monitored every 30 minutes. If the rectum is covered by surgery drapes or is otherwise inaccessible to the anesthetist, a rough estimate of body temperature can be obtained by touching the patient's paws or ears. Temperature also may be measured using special thermometers designed for use in the ear canal or esophagus.

Prevention of hypothermia may involve such measures as administering warm IV fluids (rather than fluids at room temperature or refrigerated fluids) and the use of a circulating warm water heating pad (Fig. 2-15), hot water bottles wrapped in towels, bubble packing, and foil wraps. It is also important to ensure a comfortable air temperature in the surgery room itself. Patients should not be placed on a stainless

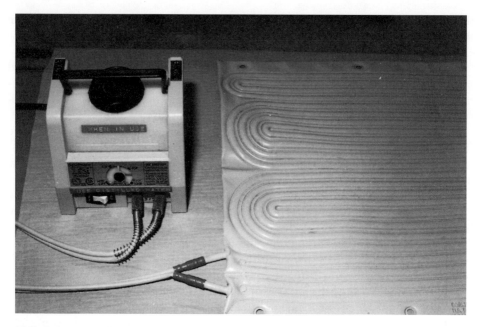

FIG. 2-15   Circulating warm water heating pad.

steel table or trough unless an insulating layer of newspaper, towels, or a heating pad is provided. Electric heating pads should be avoided, as burns are sometimes associated with their use.

Hyperthermia (increased body temperature) is occasionally seen in anesthetized small animals, particularly in susceptible dogs anesthetized with ketamine, halothane, or succinylcholine. Although rare, this syndrome, called malignant hyperthermia, may be fatal if not promptly relieved through the application of cold wet towels and the use of drugs such as dantrolene.

Use of Instruments to Monitor Vital Signs

Although a competent technician can safely monitor most patients without the use of specialized instruments, the use of monitoring devices may be of significant benefit to the anesthetist. Instruments offer continuous monitoring, whereas the technician in a busy veterinary practice is seldom able to sit with the patient throughout the anesthetic period. Instruments also allow precise quantitative measurement of parameters such as blood pressure and the percent of oxygen saturation in the patient's hemoglobin.

On the other hand, electronic monitoring, although convenient, should not be relied on to give a complete picture of patient status. Instruments are subject to power failure, interference from artifacts, and a loss of contact with the patient. Instrumentation cannot replace the presence of a skilled and conscientious anesthetist.

This section describes the instruments that can be used to monitor the following vital signs: blood pressure (Doppler flow probe or oscillometer), central venous pressure, blood gases (PaO_2 and $PaCO_2$), SaO_2 (pulse oximetry), expired CO_2 (capnography), and electrocardiography.

Blood pressure. As described in the previous section (see page 74), the anesthetist can make a rough estimate of blood pressure through manual palpation of a peripheral pulse. Blood pressure monitors allow more accurate determination of blood pressure.

It should be recognized that the term "blood pressure" refers only to *arterial* blood pressure. The pressure of blood in the veins is measured by other techniques. (See the section on central venous pressure.)

Several terms are used to describe various types of arterial blood pressure. *Systolic pressure* is produced by the contraction of the ventricles and propels blood through the aorta and major arteries. It is the highest pressure that is exerted throughout the cardiac cycle, and can be manually felt as the pulse of an artery. *Diastolic pressure* is the pressure that remains when the heart is in its resting phase, between contractions. It is the lowest pressure that is exerted throughout the cardiac cycle. All instruments that monitor blood pressure are able to measure systolic blood pressure, and some are able to measure diastolic pressure as well.

Normal systolic pressure in the dog and cat is approximately 120 mm Hg, and normal diastolic pressure is 80 mm Hg (together indicated as 120/80). The mean (average) arterial blood pressure is 94 mm Hg. Minimal acceptable blood pressure is 80/40 (mean, 60 mm Hg).

There are two methods of blood pressure monitoring by means of instruments: *direct monitoring* and *indirect monitoring*. In direct blood pressure monitoring, the reading is obtained by means of a catheter inserted into an artery. In the case of indirect blood pressure monitoring, a probe is placed on the outside surface of the animal (usually on a leg or the tail).

Direct blood pressure monitoring is infrequently performed in veterinary practice, although it is common in research and referral institutions. An indwelling catheter is placed in the femoral or dorsal pedal artery by means of a surgical cutdown or percutaneous insertion technique. The catheter is connected to a manometer or pressure transducer to display the measured pressure.

In practice, it is most common to determine blood pressure by indirect methods, using an external device placed around the patient's leg to detect the strength of a pulse in a peripheral artery. A sphygmomanometer, blood pressure cuff, and Doppler flow probe are commonly used for this purpose. Alternatively, an oscillometer may be used.

Most indirect blood pressure monitors, whether used on humans or animals, are based on the same principle: if a cuff is placed snugly around a limb and is inflated, an artery lying beneath the cuff will be compressed. When the cuff applies a pressure that is higher than the systolic blood pressure, blood flow through the artery stops. When the cuff pressure is slowly released, blood flow will resume when the cuff pressure equals the systolic blood pressure.

Various types of equipment are used to detect the returning blood flow and indicate the pressure at which it occurs (the systolic blood pressure):

1. The noise made by the returning blood flow may be auscultated with a stethoscope. (This is the basis of sphygmomanometry in humans but is difficult to do accurately in a dog or cat.)
2. A Doppler flow probe may detect an ultrasound echo from red blood cells passing through the vessel (Fig. 2-16).

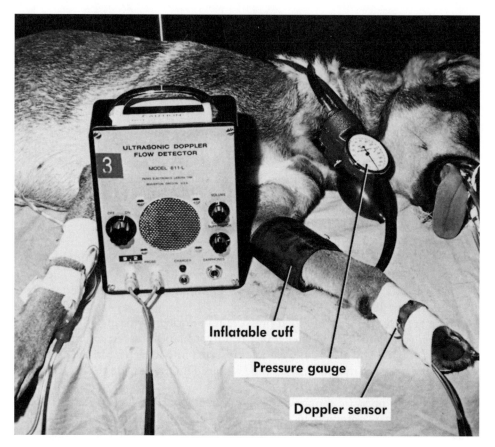

FIG. 2-16 Doppler blood pressure monitor. (From Warren RG: *Small animal anesthesia,* St Louis, 1983, Mosby.)

3. An oscillometer can detect the distention of the limb due to the volume of blood entering the limb with each heartbeat.

Regardless of the instrumentation used, systolic blood pressure is normally indicated by a pressure dial (manometer) or by a digital display.

The Doppler flow probe is the most affordable blood pressure monitoring device that can be used on veterinary patients. (See Procedure 2-5 for details of the technique for measuring blood pressure using a Doppler device.) Like the human sphygmomanometer, a cuff is placed around the extremity (that is, a foreleg, hind leg, or tail). A probe is placed just distal to the cuff at a location where the pulse can be felt. In the awake animal, the probe is most commonly placed just proximal to the large pad on the forelimb or hind limb to evaluate the metacarpal or metatarsal artery. It is also possible to place the probe over the ventral aspect of the tail to evaluate the coccygeal artery. Once the location has been selected, the probe is secured loosely to the area with adhesive tape. Wherever the probe is placed, it is important that excessive pressure not be applied when it is secured to the limb. This can collapse the artery, and thus no sound will be heard.

PROCEDURE 2-5
Measuring Indirect Blood Pressure Using a Doppler Probe

1. Clip any hair from the area where the probe will be placed.
2. Apply ultrasound gel to the concave portion of the probe.
3. Place cuff over the limb proximal to where probe will be placed.
4. Place probe over area to be evaluated (coccygeal, metacarpal, or metatarsal artery).
5. Inflate cuff until no sound is heard.
6. The pressure gauge should be placed at the level of the right atrium, otherwise incorrect pressure readings will be taken. For every 2 cm that the gauge is above or below the right atrium, 1 mm Hg should be added or subtracted, respectively.
7. Slowly release pressure from cuff until the first "swishing" sound is heard. This occurs at the systolic pressure.
8. Continue to release pressure. If a change in sound is noted (for example, less pulsation, more constant, or change in frequency), this is the diastolic pressure. (This is not always apparent with this technique.)
9. Five readings are taken. The highest and lowest are discarded and the remaining readings are averaged to find the value of the systolic pressure.

The probe emits a series of high-frequency sound waves. When the sound waves encounter a pulsating artery, the frequency is changed. This is detected by the instrument, which converts the sound wave into a "swishing" sound audible to the attendant.

As the cuff is inflated around the limb, the pressure will occlude the flow of blood through the artery distal to the cuff. This will mean no sound is detected by the sensor. As the pressure is released, blood will begin to flow through the arteries. This blood flow will be picked up by the sensor probe and converted into an audible sound. The pressure read on the manometer when the blood flow is first detected is the systolic pressure. Some people believe that the diastolic pressure can be measured when the sound frequency changes; however, it is often difficult to detect this change.

When using a Doppler to measure blood pressure in cats, a correction factor of 14 mm Hg should be added to the reading to determine the true systolic pressure. The sphygmomanometer reading correlates more accurately with mean blood pressure than with systolic blood pressure in cats. Like most instruments, the Doppler is subject to technical errors such as the following:

- The use of a cuff that is too large or too small will give false readings. The width of the cuff should be no more than 40% of the circumference of the leg around which the cuff is being wrapped.
- The sensor probe must be placed with the concave portion of the probe lying on the patient's skin.

- Ultrasound gel should be used on the probe to augment sound wave transmission. Lubricating jelly should not be used because the chloride ions in the jelly can remove the protective barrier of the probe. The probe should be cleaned with damp gauze after use so that the gel doesn't dry on the probe.

Blood pressure can also be measured using an oscillometer. This technique relies on pressure oscillations within the cuff bladder. These occur because the pulsation of the artery or arteriole causes changes in the volume of the limb around which the cuff is wrapped. The cuff is inflated and then slowly deflated by a computer. The computer measures the change in intracuff pressure as it reflects the size of the limb changes with each pulse. The computer calculates the systolic, mean, and diastolic pressures from these cuff pressure changes. Although this technique works well in large- and medium-sized dogs, it is often inaccurate in small patients and hypotensive patients.

Central venous pressure.   Just as blood pressure in an artery can be measured, it is possible to measure the pressure of blood flow in a large central vein such as the anterior vena cava. This value, the *central venous pressure* (CVP), allows the veterinarian to assess how well blood is returning to the heart and also the ability of the heart to receive and pump blood. This value is extremely helpful in monitoring animals for right-side heart failure because it measures the backup of blood in the vena cava that results from this condition. It is also useful in preventing overhydration in animals receiving IV fluids, because CVP values rise as blood volume increases.

CVP can be directly measured by inserting a long catheter percutaneously or by cutdown into the jugular vein. The catheter is advanced into the anterior vena cava and toward the heart so that the tip of the catheter lies close to the right atrium. The catheter is connected to a water manometer to obtain a measurement.

The manometer should be positioned such that "0" on the manometer is level with the right atrium (halfway between shoulder and sternum in sternal patients, and level with the sternum in laterally recumbent patients). If the catheter is correctly positioned, the meniscus of the fluid in the manometer should rise and fall with each breath. Normal CVP in dogs and cats is less than 8 cm H_2O pressure. Pressures over 12 to 15 cm H_2O (taken during exhalation) are considered elevated. It is usually more valuable to monitor trends over time rather than base an assessment on a single reading.

Blood gases.   Among the most important tasks of the anesthetist is to ensure that the patient is sufficiently oxygenated, that carbon dioxide levels are within acceptable limits, and that respiratory acidosis is minimized. Each of these parameters depends upon respiratory function, which can be roughly evaluated by observation of the rate, depth, and character of the patient's respirations. However, this method of monitoring may give an inaccurate impression of the patient's respiratory function: ventilation may appear normal, yet the animal may be suffering from significant respiratory depression.

Fortunately, accurate assessment of respiratory function is possible through the use of several techniques, including the use of blood gas analysis (PaO_2, $PaCO_2$ measurement), capnography, and pulse oximetry. These instruments indicate whether the patient is obtaining oxygen and delivering it to the tissues and how efficiently the lungs are eliminating carbon dioxide.

Before examining the ways in which oxygen, carbon dioxide, and blood pH are measured, it may be useful to review how oxygen and carbon dioxide are carried in the bloodstream.

Oxygen is carried through the blood in two forms: as a free molecule dissolved in plasma (measured by the oxygen partial pressure in the arteries, abbreviated PaO_2) and chemically combined with hemoglobin in red blood cells (measured as the percentage of hemoglobin saturated with oxygen, SaO_2). Each 100 ml of oxygenated blood contains about 20 ml of oxygen: 0.3 ml dissolved in plasma, and 19.7 ml joined to hemoglobin.

Both PaO_2 and SaO_2 can be measured, although by different instruments. Blood gas analyzers measure PaO_2; pulse oximeters measure SaO_2. Both indicate the degree of oxygenation of a patient (how well the lungs deliver oxygen to the blood). Most anesthetized animals show a greatly elevated PaO_2 (up to 500 mm Hg compared to the normal 90 to 115 mm Hg) because they are breathing almost 100% oxygen from the anesthetic machine, whereas the nonanesthetized animal breathes approximately 21% oxygen in room air. Similarly, SaO_2 readings on anesthetized animals are usually high (97% to 99%).

Low PaO_2 and SaO_2 values are sometimes observed during anesthesia. PaO_2 values below 60 mm Hg indicate significant hypoxia and the need for oxygen supplementation and possibly ventilation assistance to maintain minimal oxygen delivery to the tissues. Similarly, an SaO_2 reading below 90% suggests hypoxia and should be immediately investigated.

Carbon dioxide is transported through the blood in three ways. About 30% of the carbon dioxide joins with hemoglobin in the red blood cells. Approximately 10% is dissolved in plasma and can be measured as $PaCO_2$ (the CO_2 partial pressure in the arteries). The remainder reacts with water to form carbonic acid, which is quickly converted into bicarbonate and hydrogen ions according to the reaction:

$$CO_2 + H_2O \rightarrow H_2CO_3 \rightarrow HCO_3^- + H^+$$

The anesthetist can evaluate how well the patient is eliminating carbon dioxide by measuring $PaCO_2$ through blood gas determination. $PaCO_2$ is often elevated during anesthesia (45 to 60 mm Hg compared with less than 45 mm Hg in the awake patient) because the respiratory depression produced by most anesthetics causes the body to retain CO_2. In other words, the patient does not breathe often enough or deeply enough to eliminate the normal amount of carbon dioxide. $PaCO_2$ values over 60 mm Hg indicate a serious problem and the need to assist ventilation by bagging the patient or through the use of a ventilator. (See Chapter 7.)

Because of high carbon dioxide levels, anesthetized patients may also become significantly acidotic (that is, excess hydrogen ions are produced from carbon dioxide according to the equation above). Blood pH in anesthetized animals usually reflects this mild respiratory acidosis and is commonly 7.20 to 7.30, compared with the normal animal's blood pH of 7.35 to 7.45.

Blood pH measurement can be performed at the same time blood gas determinations are made to help the anesthetist determine the acid-base status of the body and the adequacy of the patient's respiration.

Determination of PaO_2 and $PaCO_2$.   Blood gas levels, although useful, are not commonly measured in practice. Sample collection must be done with care: blood

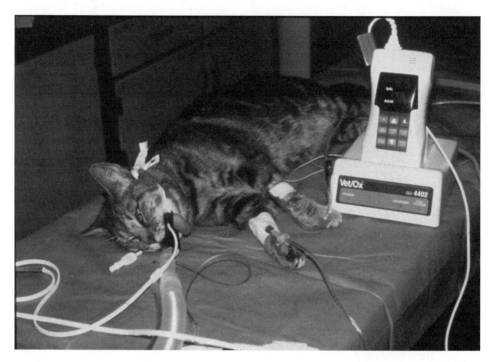

FIG. 2-17   Pulse oximeter monitoring cat through a lingual probe. (Photo courtesy of Dr. Jeff Ko.)

intended for blood gas analysis should be obtained from an artery if possible (as opposed to routine blood samples, which are taken from a vein). In certain situations, a venous sample may be used. For example, the lingual vein has extensive anastomoses with arteries in the tongue, and the blood gas values obtained from lingual vein samples are close to arterial values.

Once obtained, the blood sample must be stored on ice and values should be measured within 2 hours. Many veterinary biochemistry laboratories and some veterinary hospitals are equipped to perform these tests, and in areas where a veterinary laboratory is not readily available, a human hospital laboratory may be willing to accept samples from nonhuman patients.

Determination of SaO_2.   As with PaO_2, the patient's SaO_2 (that is, the amount of oxygen bound to hemoglobin, expressed as a percentage of the total capacity) indicates its level of oxygenation. SaO_2 can be measured with a pulse oximeter. This piece of equipment is reasonably inexpensive, noninvasive, and easy to use. Pulse oximeters are equipped with a probe or clip that is placed across a thin strip of the patient's tissue (Fig. 2-17). In anesthetized animals the tongue is commonly used, but the probe may also be applied to the earlobe, rectal mucosa, toe web, gingiva, underside of the base of the tail, ear pinna, lip, or any other area that is thin, hairless, and nonpigmented. Many commercially available pulse oximeters measure not only the SaO_2 but also the heart rate. Some units also display the ECG and expired CO_2 level.

Normal SaO_2 values should be above 95%; this is equivalent to a PaO_2 of 85 to 100 mm Hg. A value of 90% saturation is equivalent to a PaO_2 of 60 mm Hg and indicates borderline hypoxia. (For Sao_2 values between 75% and 90%, the Pao_2 in mm Hg is approximately equal to the Sao_2 value minus 30.) If the pulse oximeter reading is between 75% and 90%, hypoxia is likely present.

Pulse oximeters and blood gas analyzers allow early recognition of situations in which the patient is poorly oxygenated. A pulse oximeter reading of 90% to 95% indicates that the patient's hemoglobin is not fully saturated with oxygen and a respiratory or cardiovascular problem may be present. The patient will not become hypoxic until the reading falls to 90% or less, and it is hoped that the anesthetist will be able to correct the problem before this occurs. Without the use of pulse oximetry or blood gases, early hypoxia is difficult to assess because cyanosis only becomes apparent if values fall below 85% saturation.

If pulse oximeter or blood gas readings are abnormally low during anesthesia, the anesthetist should consider the following questions:

- Is the instrument working correctly? Readings may be affected by factors such as probe placement, external light sources, and motion. In some cases, the area being monitored is underperfused and readings may improve if the probe is moved to a different location.
- Is adequate oxygen being delivered to the patient? Inadequate oxygen delivery may result from esophageal intubation, an oxygen flow rate that is too low, endotracheal tube blockage, or an empty oxygen tank.
- Is oxygen being transferred from the alveoli to the blood? This process may be impeded by inadequate ventilation or preexisting lung disease.
- Is circulation adequate? Bradycardia, severe arrhythmias, or hypotension may decrease oxygenation.

Regardless of the cause, patients with subnormal Pao_2 or Sao_2 readings may require supplemental oxygen delivery or ventilation through bagging or the use of a ventilator.

Capnography.   Capnography is the technique of measuring the amount of carbon dioxide in the air as it is breathed in and out by the patient (Fig. 2-18). A monitor is placed between the endotracheal tube and the anesthetic circuit (mainstream capnography) or in a small tube off to one side of the junction of the endotracheal tube and the anesthetic circuit (side stream capnography). The instrument measures the carbon dioxide level of the air that passes this monitor on both inspiration and expiration and displays this information in graph form (Fig. 2-19). During inspiration, the amount of carbon dioxide should be zero unless there is some rebreathing taking place or the carbon dioxide absorber is not working properly (*A* to *B* on the graph). During expiration, the carbon dioxide content of the air rises (*B* to *C*) and should reach approximately 40 mm Hg at the end of expiration when the last volume of alveolar gas is exhaled (*C* to *D*). This value is called the *end tidal carbon dioxide* ($ETco_2$) and is important because it closely approximates $Paco_2$. The CO_2 level rapidly falls as expiration ends and inspiration begins (*D* to *E*).

The normal exhaled CO_2 level is 30 to 40 mm Hg. Hypercapnia (that is, higher than normal CO_2) is present if the $ETco_2$ is greater than 40 mm Hg. Hypocapnia (that is, lower than normal CO_2) is present if the $ETco_2$ is less than 30 mm Hg.

Low values for $ETco_2$ may occur with rapid respiratory rates, with hypoventilation or apnea, or if excessive dead air space dilutes the exhaled alveolar gas. Low

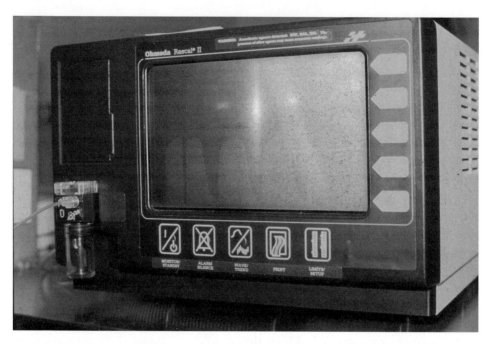

FIG. 2-18   Capnograph. (Photo courtesy of Dr. Jeff Ko.)

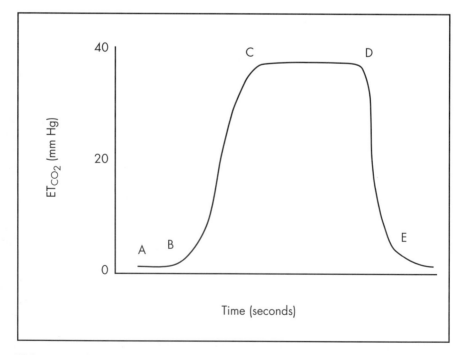

FIG. 2-19   Capnograph tracing. (From Wright B, Hellyer P: Respiratory monitoring during anesthesia: pulse oximetry and capnography, *Compendium* 18[10]:1083-1097, 1996.)

values may also be seen if the endotracheal tube is in the esophagus or bronchus or if the capnometer has been disconnected from the endotracheal tube.

Elevated carbon dioxide values may occur at any point in the graph. Elevated values during the inspiratory phase (See Fig. 2-19, *A-B*.) may occur because excessive carbon dioxide is being breathed in by the patient (for example, if the carbon dioxide absorber is depleted). Elevated CO_2 during the expiratory plateau is most commonly due to hypoventilation. (See Fig. 2-19, *C-D*.)

It can be seen that there may be a variety of reasons for hypercapnia or hypocapnia. Some of these need to be quickly corrected, whereas others may be self-limiting. It is important for the anesthesia technician to work with the veterinarian to properly identify problems and correct them when necessary.

Electrocardiography. Electrocardiography allows the anesthetist to monitor heart rate and rhythm on a continuous or intermittent basis. Veterinary technicians should be familiar with the procedure to set up an ECG machine and leads, as outlined in standard veterinary nursing references.

The anesthetist should be able to recognize the ECG patterns that signify an impending emergency. These include:

- *Tachycardia.* Heart rates greater than 180 bpm in a cat or a small dog, and 160 bpm in a large dog should be reported to the veterinarian. Tachycardia may result from the use of drugs (for example, ketamine and atropine) or may be a response to surgical stimulation. It may also be present because of a preexisting condition such as hyperthyroidism.

- *Bradycardia.* Heart rates of less than 60 bpm in a large dog, 70 bpm in a small dog, and 100 bpm in a cat should be reported to the veterinarian. Like tachycardia, bradycardia may be the result of drug administration (for example, xylazine, medetomidine, and opioids) or may indicate a problem with anesthesia (for example, excessive anesthetic depth, hypoxia, or hypothermia).

- *Heart block.* The presence of a heart block indicates that the electrical impulse that causes the heart to beat is not being transmitted throughout the heart. In second-degree heart block (Fig. 2-20), some P waves (atrial contractions) are not followed by QRS complexes (ventricular contractions). In third-degree heart block (Fig. 2-21), the atrial and ventricular contractions occur independently, and the P waves and QRS complexes are therefore unassociated. Both second- and third-degree heart block decrease the efficiency of cardiac contractions.

- *Premature ventricular contractions (PVCs).* A PVC is an impulse that arises from a focus in the ventricle and represents an ineffective and uncoordinated contraction. These often appear as bizarre, wide QRS complexes on the ECG tracing. Occasional PVCs are commonly seen in anesthetized animals, especially those induced with barbiturates. The appearance of frequent PVCs in an ECG tracing usually indicates that the heart is significantly compromised, and this should be brought to the attention of the veterinarian. Hypoxia is often a cause of PVCs in anesthetized animals, and in some cases may be successfully treated by increasing the delivery of oxygen to the patient. Lidocaine is sometimes given intravenously as a treatment for premature ventricular contractions.

- *Fibrillation.* Fibrillation is the contraction of small muscle bundles within the ventricles or atria. Ventricular fibrillation indicates that cardiac arrest has

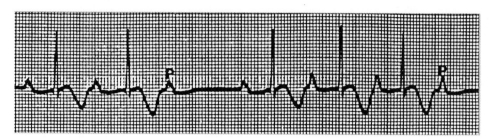

FIG. 2-20   ECG tracing showing second-degree heart block. (From Glaze K: Basic electro-cardiography, part III, *Vet Tech* 18[1]:25-33, 1997.)

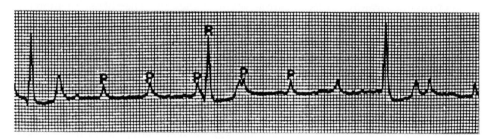

FIG. 2-21   ECG tracing showing third-degree heart block. (From Glaze K: Basic electrocardiography, part III, *Vet Tech* 18[1]:25-33, 1997.)

occurred. Ventricular fibrillation appears on an ECG tracing as an irregular undulating line, with complete absence of recognizable QRS complexes.

Reflexes and Other Indicators of Anesthetic Depth

The anesthetist should have at all times an accurate assessment of the patient's depth of anesthesia. Anesthetic depth is a complex balance between the action of the anesthetics and the patient's overall condition. Body temperature, ventilation, blood pH, and blood pressure all have a potent influence on the way in which an anesthetic affects the animal. It is therefore important to monitor the whole animal, assessing the apparent depth in light of the animal's vital signs.

Anesthetic depth is indicated in several ways. Reflex activity, muscle relaxation, heart and respiratory rates, pupil size, and eye rotation are all useful guides in determining how deeply or lightly the patient is anesthetized (Table 2-2). For some anesthetics (particularly cyclohexamine agents such as ketamine) it may be difficult for the anesthetist to determine the level of anesthetic depth; however, the following guidelines are useful for anesthesia induced by most general anesthetic agents.

Reflex activity.   All normal, conscious animals demonstrate predictable reflex responses to certain types of stimuli. One example is the cough reflex, in which the animal responds to the presence of foreign material in the trachea by forceful coughing. Reflex responses help protect the animal from injury (in the case of the cough reflex, by clearing upper airway obstructions and preventing aspiration of injurious materials). These protective reflexes are progressively depressed at increasing depths of anesthesia, such that an animal in stage III, plane 3 (or deeper anesthesia) may have few reflex responses or none. The reflexes most commonly monitored in veterinary anesthesia include the palpebral, swallowing, pedal, ear flick, corneal, and laryngeal reflexes.

TABLE 2-2			
Indicators of anesthetic depth			

		ANESTHETIC DEPTH	
SIGN	**Light**	**Medium**	**Deep**
Spontaneous movement	Maybe	No	No
Swallowing	Maybe	No	No
Vaporizer setting	Low	Medium (1.1-1.5 MAC)	High
Muscle tone	Normal	Moderate	None
Palpebral reflex	Active	Moderate	None
Eyeball position	Central	Ventromedial	Central
Pupillary light reflex	Present	May be present	Absent
Shivering	Maybe	No	No
Heart rate	Often elevated	Variable	Often decreased
Respiratory rate	Often elevated	8-30 breaths/min	Often decreased

Modified from Haskins SC: General guidelines for judging anesthetic depth, *Vet Clin North Am Small Anim Pract* 22(2):432-434, 1992.
MAC, Minimum alveolar concentration.

Palpebral reflex.   The palpebral reflex (blink reflex) can be tested by lightly tapping the medial or lateral canthus of the eye and observing whether the animal blinks in response (Fig. 2-22). Some anesthetists prefer to test this reflex by lightly stroking the hairs of the upper eyelid. In the conscious animal, this reflex helps protect the eye from injury. Most animals retain the palpebral reflex throughout stages I and II and partially through stage III, although individual and species variations exist. The stage at which the palpebral reflex is lost also varies among different anesthetic agents: at a surgical plane of anesthesia, it is usually present in barbiturate anesthesia, occasionally present in methoxyflurane anesthesia, but seldom present in halothane anesthesia. As with most reflexes, loss of the palpebral reflex indicates an increase in anesthetic depth, whereas return of the reflex usually indicates imminent arousal from anesthesia.

Swallowing reflex.   The swallowing reflex occurs spontaneously in awake animals; it is usually stimulated by the presence of saliva or food in the pharynx. Lightly anesthetized animals swallow frequently, and this reflex can be readily monitored by observing movement in the patient's ventral neck region. The swallowing reflex is lost at a medium depth of anesthesia and is usually regained just before the patient recovers consciousness. The return of the swallowing reflex during recovery usually indicates that it is safe to remove the endotracheal tube. Animals that vomit after this point usually will swallow rather than aspirate the vomited material, and the endotracheal tube is therefore no longer needed to protect the airway. (In fact, if the endotracheal tube is not removed at this point, the patient may soon begin to chew on it!)

Pedal reflex.   The pedal reflex is elicited by squeezing or pinching a digit or pad and observing whether the unconscious animal flexes the leg, withdrawing the paw

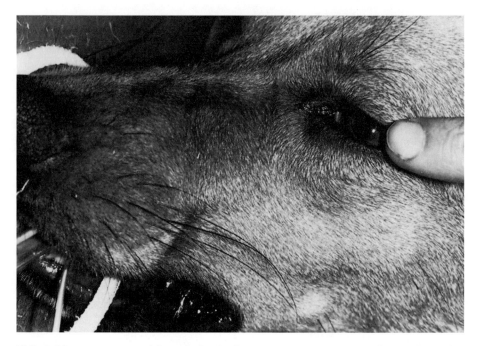

FIG. 2-22   Assessment of the palpebral reflex. (From Warren RG: *Small animal anesthesia,* St Louis, 1983, Mosby.)

from the examiner (Fig. 2-23). The pedal reflex is a good indicator of anesthetic depth in animals that have been given the general anesthetic pentobarbital. This indicator is not as useful in inhalation anesthesia, because the reflex is normally lost during induction.

Ear flick reflex.   The ear flick reflex (pinna reflex) is particularly useful in cats. It can be tested by gently touching the hairs on the inner surface of the pinna and observing the resultant twitch of the ear. This reflex may be retained well into stage III, particularly in cats anesthetized with ketamine. This reflex may be difficult to elicit in some animals and may be easily lost if tested too frequently within a short period.

Corneal reflex.   The corneal reflex can be tested by touching the cornea with a sterile object (a drop of water or artificial tear solution is commonly used) and noting whether the animal blinks and withdraws the eye into the orbital fossa. This reflex is not commonly tested in dogs and cats unless it is necessary to determine if the patient is too deeply anesthetized. This reflex is usually present until stage III, plane 4 anesthesia.

Laryngeal reflex.   The laryngeal reflex is stimulated when the larynx is touched by an object. The reflex response is an immediate closure of the epiglottis and vocal cords. This reflex normally protects the animal from aspiration of material into the trachea. The laryngeal reflex may be observed during intubation if the animal is not sufficiently anesthetized to allow the tube to be passed. It is easily elicited in cats, in which a sustained laryngeal reflex response is the cause of laryngospasm.

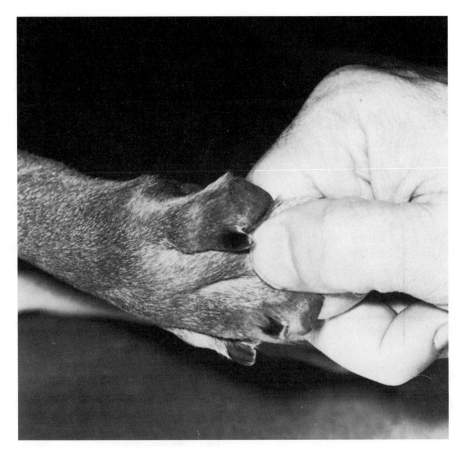

FIG. 2-23   Pedal reflex. (From Warren RG: *Small animal anesthesia,* St Louis, 1983, Mosby.)

Muscle tone.   Muscle tone is also a useful guide to anesthetic depth. With increasing depth, skeletal muscles become more relaxed and offer little resistance to movement. Among the muscles that can be readily assessed are the muscles of mastication, which control jaw tone. Jaw tone is assessed by attempting to open the jaws wide and estimating the amount of passive resistance (Fig. 2-24). Muscle tone also can be assessed by attempting to flex and extend the foreleg at the elbow and carpus. Anal tone also indicates skeletal muscle relaxation and may be assessed by noting the size of the rectal orifice. Some degree of muscle relaxation is desirable for most procedures; however, extreme muscle relaxation resulting in a flaccid jaw tone usually is unnecessary and may indicate excessive anesthetic depth.

The degree of muscle relaxation observed in the patient is dependent not only on anesthetic depth but also on the particular drugs given to the animal, some of which promote relaxation (for example, diazepam and xylazine) and some of which increase muscle tone (for example, ketamine and tiletamine). Specific muscle-paralyzing agents, such as succinylcholine, may be used in combination with general anesthetics to achieve pronounced muscle relaxation for certain procedures. (See

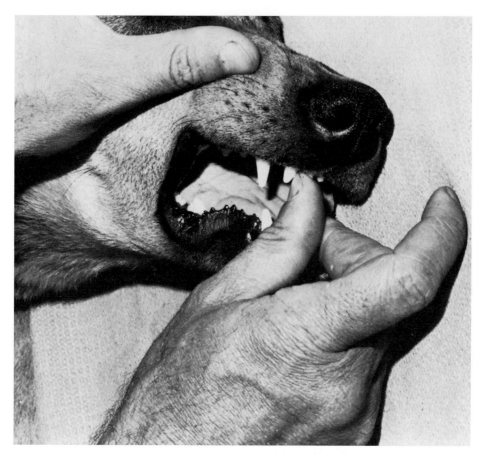

FIG. 2-24   Assessing jaw tone. (From Warren RG: *Small animal anesthesia,* St Louis, 1983, Mosby.)

Chapter 7.) This may be advantageous to the surgeon but gives the anesthetist one less parameter with which to monitor anesthetic depth.

Eye position and pupil size.   Eye position, pupil size, and the pupillary response to light also may indicate anesthetic depth, although there is considerable variation among individual animals. The eyeball itself is usually central in stage I anesthesia. It becomes eccentric in stage II, making the animal appear to be looking toward its chin (Fig. 2-25). As the animal approaches a surgical plane of anesthesia, the eyeball often becomes more central, and the central position is maintained through increasing depth of anesthesia. Some anesthetics (for example, ketamine) do not cause eye rotation, even at moderate anesthetic depth.

The size of the pupil also may reflect anesthetic depth: the anesthetized patient normally has dilated pupils (mydriasis) during stage II anesthesia; constricted pupils (miosis) when lightly anesthetized; and progressively greater pupil dilation as anesthetic depth increases. The ability of the pupil to constrict in response to light (pupillary light reflex) also diminishes with increasing depth of anesthesia and is usually absent at surgical anesthetic depth. Dilated, central pupils that are not responsive to

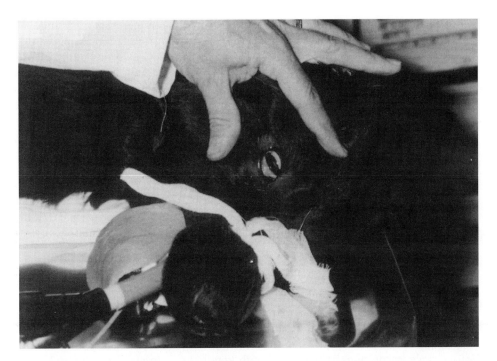

FIG. 2-25   Ventral rotation of the eyeball and prolapse of the third eyelid during anesthesia.

light may indicate a dangerously deep level of anesthesia. The anesthetist should be aware, however, that atropine can cause pupil dilation, particularly in cats. This interaction may confuse the interpretation of pupil size and the pupillary light reflex.

Salivary and lacrimal secretions.   The presence or absence of salivary and lacrimal secretions also may give clues regarding anesthetic depth, particularly in an animal that has not received anticholinergics. Production of tears and saliva diminishes with increasing anesthetic depth and is totally absent in deep surgical anesthesia. Because of the relative absence of tears and the subsequent danger of corneal drying, the use of ophthalmic drops or ointment is advised for all animals undergoing general anesthesia. Atropine ointment should not be used.

Heart and respiratory rates.   Heart and respiratory rates may be a valuable guide to anesthetic depth. Both parameters show a tendency to decrease as the animal enters deeper levels of anesthesia and a tendency to increase with lighter anesthesia. Caution should be used in interpreting both heart rate and respiratory rate because they are subject to many influences in addition to anesthetic depth. For example, an animal's heart rate increases in response to a fall in blood pressure. Heart rate is also elevated by the perception of a painful stimulus. Some preanesthetic and anesthetic drugs (for example, ketamine and atropine) increase heart rate, whereas most other agents decrease heart rate. Heart rate also may be affected by endotracheal intubation, which may cause bradycardia. Like heart rates, respiratory rates may reflect anesthetic depth but are influenced by other parameters, including the PaO_2, $PaCO_2$, and the anesthetic agent used.

Response to surgical stimulation. One other parameter that may indicate anesthetic depth is the response of the animal to surgical stimulation. As previously mentioned, certain procedures, such as manipulation of viscera or pulling on the suspensory ligament of the ovary, may result in a response that indicates a perception of pain, although the perception is not usually conscious. Animals perceiving surgical stimulation may show an increase in heart rate and blood pressure. The anesthetist should not necessarily interpret these signs as an indication that the animal's anesthetic depth is inadequate unless the increase in heart rate is considerable. Minor changes in heart rate during surgery are considered normal and, in fact, the absence of such a response may indicate an unnecessarily deep level of anesthesia. Increased respiratory rate or signs of voluntary movement by the patient, however, do indicate insufficient anesthetic depth and the perception of pain. Lacrimation, salivation, and sweating (most easily observed on the foot pads) also indicate that the patient may be perceiving a painful stimulus and that depth is inadequate.

Judging Anesthetic Depth

During the course of anesthesia, the anesthetist should monitor as many parameters as possible and weigh all available evidence before judging the anesthetic depth of the patient. No one piece of information is unfailingly reliable, and it is foolish to determine the anesthetic plane by monitoring only one reflex or vital sign. In addition, each animal is unique and has an individual response to increasing anesthetic depth. For example, some dogs anesthetized with ketamine maintain the palpebral reflex throughout stage III, whereas others lose this reflex as early as stage III, plane 2. If the palpebral reflex is used as the sole criterion for judging anesthetic depth, the animal that retains that reflex into deep anesthesia may be incorrectly judged to be only lightly anesthetized. Increasing the concentration of anesthetic delivered to such a patient might easily result in dangerously deep anesthesia. Observation of the other indicators of anesthetic depth would likely give the anesthetist a more balanced view of the situation and a more accurate assessment of true anesthetic depth. Examples of the use of judgment in interpreting anesthetic depth are given in Box 2-2.

Similarly, observation of the amount of anesthetic being delivered to the patient (for example, by the vaporizer of an anesthetic machine) does not in itself indicate the patient's anesthetic depth. Although high vaporizer settings result in increased delivery of anesthetic to the patient and, subsequently, an increase in patient depth, there is tremendous variation in patient response. One animal may be maintained at stable surgical anesthesia when given a concentration of 1% halothane gas, whereas another animal may require 2% halothane and still another may be satisfactorily maintained at 0.5% halothane. The concentration of anesthetic gas received by the animal also is not necessarily the concentration indicated by the vaporizer setting; it may vary with the oxygen flow rate and quality of ventilation received by the patient. (See Chapter 4.) Nevertheless, a consideration of the vaporizer setting and the length of time that the animal has been anesthetized may help the anesthetist decide if an animal is anesthetized too lightly or too deeply. The basic rule is that if there is doubt about the level of anesthesia in a particular patient, one should decrease the vaporizer setting and monitor the animal until such time as the anesthetic depth can be accurately determined.

Box 2-2 Examples of Depth Assessment

1. A mature cat has been anesthetized with thiopental given intravenously. The anesthetist notes that the cat appears unconscious and relaxed. The pulse is strong, and the heart rate is 144 bpm. The respirations are regular, and the rate is 20 breaths per minute. The pupils are centrally positioned. The palpebral reflex is brisk, but there is no pedal or ear flick reflex. The anesthetist wishes to intubate the animal. At this depth of anesthesia, is it possible? What other tests could the anesthetist perform to determine anesthetic depth?

   Answer: The cat appears to be in stage III, plane 1 anesthesia and may be deep enough to intubate. The anesthetist should assess the jaw tone and observe whether there is any resistance when the tongue is gently pulled before assuming that intubation is possible.

2. A 13-year-old dog has been anesthetized by mask induction with isoflurane. After intubation, it is maintained on 2% isoflurane. The anesthetist wishes to ensure that the dog is sufficiently anesthetized to allow removal of a large skin tumor. The dog's respirations are shallow, with a rate of 8 breaths per minute. The heart rate is 90 bpm. There is no response to surgery, and all reflexes are absent. The pupils are central; the jaw tone is slack. Is the animal adequately anesthetized for this procedure?

   Answer: The animal is indeed adequately anesthetized and, in fact, may be at an excessive anesthetic depth. Respiration rate is slow and tidal volume is low. The absence of all reflexes, the central pupils, and the slack jaw tone all indicate that the animal may be in stage III, plane 3 anesthesia. At this point, the anesthetist should consider reducing the isoflurane setting to 1.5% and monitoring the animal for signs of decreased depth. After doing this, the anesthetist should carefully monitor the animal for signs of pain perception (for example, increased respiratory rate, movement, lacrimation, and sweat on the foot pads) to ensure that the vaporizer setting is high enough for adequate analgesia. Ideally, the heart rate and respiratory rate will increase slightly but not enough to indicate imminent arousal. (In any case, arousal is unlikely if the animal is receiving 1.5% isoflurane.)

3. An 8-year-old dog has been anesthetized with atropine and ketamine/diazepam, given intravenously, and is now under halothane anesthesia. The dog's heart rate is 100 bpm and the respirations are 8 breaths per minute. The jaw tone appears moderate, but the pupils are central and show no response to light. No reflexes are present. Is the anesthetic depth appropriate?

   Answer: The anesthetist cannot be sure whether the anesthetic depth is appropriate or too deep because some parameters indicate stage III, plane 2 (heart rate, jaw tone) but others indicate stage III, plane 3 (respiratory rate, reflexes, pupil position and response to light). The patient has been given atropine and ketamine, which may have elevated the heart rate. At this point, the anesthetist should assume the patient is excessively deep and should reduce the concentration of halothane. At the same time, the anesthetist should monitor the patient for signs of arousal.

Recording Information During Anesthesia

Complete and accurate medical records are a legal requirement in veterinary practice. Most jurisdictions require that some form of anesthetic record be maintained (Fig. 2-26). In many cases, this record can be in the form of a logbook in which information is listed such as the date, client, and patient identification; preoperative physical status; nature of the procedure performed with the patient under anesthesia;

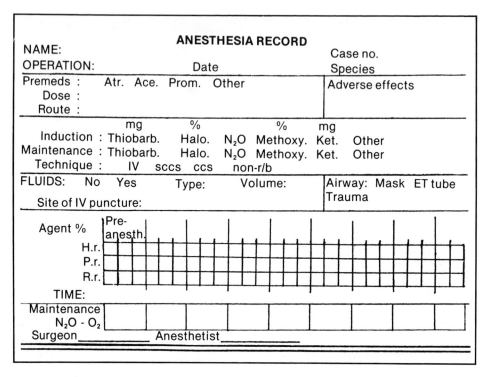

FIG. 2-26 Anesthetic record (short form). (From Warren RG: *Small animal anesthesia*, St Louis, 1983, Mosby.)

and the anesthetic protocol. A brief description of the animal's response to anesthesia should also be given. Records of this type allow the veterinarian to review the total number of anesthetic procedures that have been carried out in a given period, as well as review the number of deaths related to anesthesia or the number of animals that developed anesthetic complications. This information may be helpful in assessing the anesthetic protocols and procedures used by a practice.

Information regarding the anesthetic procedure also must be recorded in the patient's record. This allows the veterinarian to quickly review the animal's anesthetic history and may be helpful in determining the best anesthetic protocol to use for future procedures. For example, if the record indicates that the animal has undergone anesthesia with a barbiturate agent and experienced a lengthy recovery, the veterinarian may elect to anesthetize the dog with an alternative agent in the future. On the other hand, if a geriatric dog with congestive heart failure has been recently anesthetized without incident using a particular agent, the veterinarian would be justified in using the same agent for the next anesthesia.

In some situations, an anesthesia form such as that given in Fig. 2-27 is used to record a detailed description of an anesthetic procedure. Forms such as these contain information on the patient's preoperative status (for example, temperature, pulse, and respiration and the results of diagnostic tests), the anesthetic protocol used (including fluids administered and the amounts and concentrations of drugs

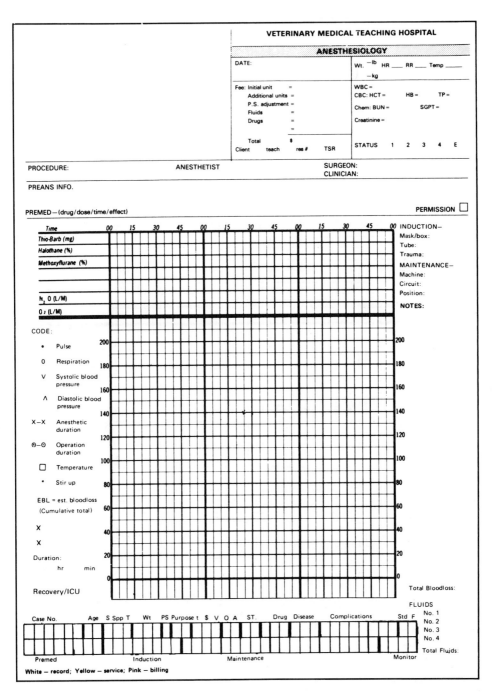

FIG. 2-27   A, Comprehensive anesthetic record. (From Warren RG: *Small animal anesthesia,* St Louis, 1983, Mosby.)

Continued

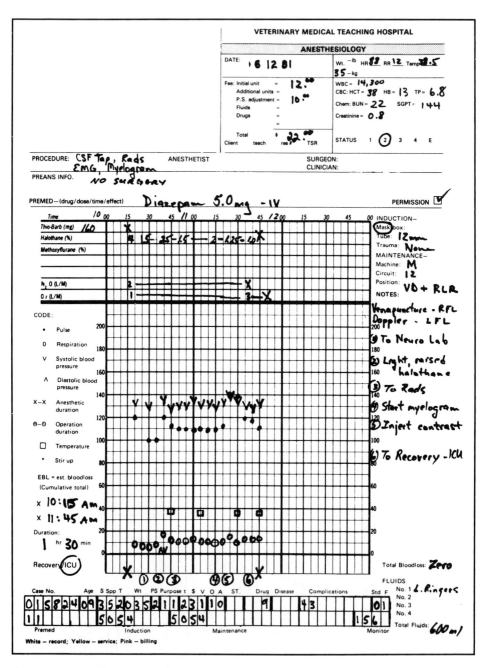

FIG. 2-27, cont'd.   B, Sample case.

given), and the patient's vital signs throughout anesthesia (for example, pulse, respiration, blood pressure, temperature, and lab results). The time at which anesthesia commenced and was terminated, the beginning and end of surgery, and the time required for recovery should also be indicated. Typically, the information is recorded chronologically to allow an overview of the patient's responses at every point throughout the procedure. Detailed records of this type are not commonly used in veterinary practice; however, they are useful in a teaching or research institution.

■ PATIENT POSITIONING AND COMFORT DURING ANESTHESIA

In addition to monitoring the patient's vital signs and reflexes as described, the anesthetist should ensure that the patient is not compromised by rough handling or careless positioning during the procedure. Examples of appropriate patient care during anesthesia include the following:

- During induction, the animal should be supported as it loses consciousness. Particular care should be taken to avoid striking the animal's head on the table during induction and when the animal is transferred to surgery.
- If an intubated patient is to be turned over, the endotracheal tube should be temporarily disconnected from the anesthetic machine. Rolling or twisting the animal while still connected to the machine may cause the endotracheal tube to twist and collapse, resulting in an airway obstruction (Fig. 2-28).

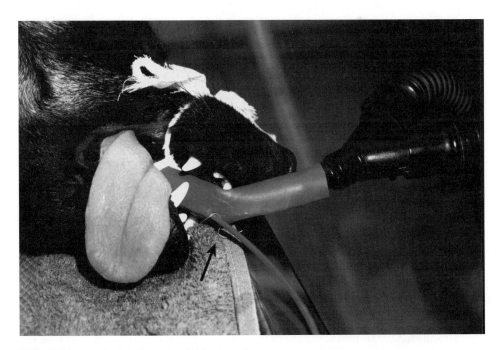

FIG. 2-28   Kinked endotracheal tube in a dog.

- Before the surgery preparation begins, the anesthetist must ensure that the patient's endotracheal tube is correctly placed (that is, not in the esophagus) and that it is large enough to prevent significant leakage of waste gas around the tube. Once the surgical preparation starts, it is difficult to position the animal to allow reintubation without compromising aseptic technique.
- The hoses of the anesthetic machine should be supported so that there is no drag on the endotracheal tube. This could result in tracheal trauma by the tube or inadvertent removal of the tube. Care should be used to avoid positions that kink or bend the endotracheal tube, and the position of the hoses and endotracheal tube should be checked during patient transfer and after repositioning. The reservoir bag should be placed so that it is clearly visible at all times.
- When positioning the animal on the surgery table, the anesthetist should ensure that the animal assumes as normal a posture as possible. In particular, overextension or hyperflexion of the neck and limbs should be avoided because they may result in permanent neurologic injury. Hyperflexion of the neck also may lead to endotracheal tube obstruction.
- Care should be taken when attaching restraining devices such as ropes or gauze ties to the patient. These devices must not be excessively tight, or blood circulation to the limbs may be compromised.
- Heavy drapes or instruments must not compress the chest of small patients because this may interfere with respiration.
- The practice of tilting the surgery table allows the surgeon easier access to some abdominal organs, particularly the uterus and ovaries. However, the anesthetist should be aware that tilting the table more than 15 degrees may cause the abdominal organs to significantly compress the diaphragm, which may compromise heart and lung function.

■ RECOVERY FROM GENERAL ANESTHESIA

The recovery period may be defined as the period between discontinuation of anesthetic administration (whether injectable or inhalation) and the time the animal is able to maintain sternal recumbency without support. The length of the recovery period depends on many factors, including the following:

1. The length of the anesthesia. As a general rule, the longer the period of anesthetic administration, the longer the expected recovery period.
2. The condition of the patient. Lengthy recoveries are seen in animals suffering from almost any debilitating disease (particularly liver and kidney disease).
3. The type of anesthetic given and the route of administration. Animals given inhalation agents typically show shorter recovery periods than do animals given injectable agents. Lengthy recoveries are particularly common if the injectable agent is given IM rather than IV.
4. The patient's temperature. Hypothermic patients are slow to metabolize and excrete anesthetic drugs.
5. The breed of the patient. Certain canine breeds (for example, greyhounds, salukis, Afghan hounds, whippets, and Russian wolfhounds) are slow to recover from certain anesthetic agents, especially barbiturates.

Stages of Recovery

An animal recovering from general anesthesia gradually progresses back through the same anesthetic stages that were experienced during induction. As the animal moves from deep to moderate to light anesthesia, vital signs and reflexes change in predictable ways. Heart rate, respiratory rate, and respiratory volume increase. The pupil, which had rotated ventrally, moves back to its normal central position (although it may rotate ventrally again and return to a central position before arousal). Reflex responses, including the palpebral, pedal, and ear flick, become stronger. The animal may shiver. The animal may swallow, chew, or attempt to lick.

Shortly after swallowing, the animal will normally show signs of consciousness, including voluntary movement of the head or limbs, opening the eyelids, and vocalization.

Anesthetist's Role in the Recovery Period

The recovery period is by no means a time of relaxation for the anesthetist. Anesthetic complications and death may occur during this period, even in animals that appear to have no problems during induction or maintenance. Ideally, recovery should occur in an area in which the animal can be watched on a continual basis. An emergency kit, monitoring equipment (for example, stethoscope, pulse oximeter, and thermometer), and oxygen should be readily available.

The duties of the anesthetist during the recovery period include monitoring and reassuring the patient, extubation and administering oxygen as necessary, preventing patient self-injury, and general nursing care.

Monitoring. Vital signs should be evaluated every 5 minutes during the recovery period. Particular attention should be given to mucous membrane color, capillary refill, and breathing. Periodic, thorough evaluation is necessary; observation from across the room is not adequate. For example, a recovering animal may have significant bradycardia and respiratory depression, yet show no signs that are evident to the casual observer.

Animals exhibiting abnormal vital signs or a delayed return to consciousness should be examined by the veterinarian. Conditions such as shock, hemorrhage, hypoglycemia, and hypothermia may be present and must be treated as soon as possible. It is also important that the recovering patient be closely monitored for problems such as vomiting, seizures, laryngospasm, and dyspnea. These are discussed in detail in Chapter 6.

When monitoring recovery from anesthesia, particularly in brachycephalic patients, the anesthetist must take care to ensure that the airway remains open and the tissues receive adequate oxygen. Brachycephalic and other relatively high-risk patients should be observed continuously until fully conscious.

It is advisable that IV catheters or butterflies, if present, should be removed only when the patient appears fully recovered. These catheters allow easy administration of fluids or drugs in the event the patient's condition requires them.

Administration of oxygen. If possible, oxygen should be provided for several minutes after the discontinuation of the anesthetic agent. If an anesthetic machine has been used for the procedure, it is customary to continue oxygen administration at a high flow rate (for example, 200 ml/kg/minute) for 5 minutes or until the animal swallows, at which time the patient must be disconnected from the machine and the endotracheal tube must be removed. If necessary, oxygen can be administered after extubation through a face mask or nasal cannula. Oxygen helps flush anesthetic out of the animal's system, allowing faster recovery. If the patient remains connected to the anesthetic machine, expired waste gas will be evacuated by the scavenger, rather than breathed out into the room. Periodic bagging with pure oxygen is advisable for as long as the recovering patient is connected to the machine because this helps re-inflate collapsed alveoli and increases the rate of anesthetic gas removal.

Following extubation, all animals should be placed in sternal recumbency with the neck extended. This position helps maintain a patent airway. Occasionally, fluid or mucus may accumulate in the pharynx or trachea and should be removed by suction.

Extubation. The endotracheal tube must be removed when the patient shows signs of imminent arousal. In dogs the appearance of the swallowing reflex (signaled by swallowing movements observed in the throat region) is most often cited as the appropriate time to remove the tube because the returning swallowing reflex will help protect the animal from aspiration if vomiting occurs. Animals that show voluntary limb or head movement or spastic movement of the tongue, or animals that attempt to chew the endotracheal tube are close to consciousness and should be extubated even if swallowing has not been observed. One exception to this general rule is brachycephalic dogs: many anesthetists prefer to delay extubation in brachycephalic dogs until the dog is able to lift its head unassisted. This is because early extubation may lead to significant respiratory distress in these animals. It is wise to prepare for possible respiratory distress in a brachycephalic dog by setting out a laryngoscope, an endotracheal tube, and the appropriate dose of thiopental or another inducing agent near the recovery cage of the animal in case reintubation becomes necessary.

In cats the endotracheal tube may be removed when signs of impending arousal are observed. These include swallowing, an active palpebral reflex, and voluntary limb, tail, or head movements. Delaying extubation is not advisable in cats because it may predispose the patient to laryngospasm.

In all patients, it is necessary to deflate the endotracheal tube cuff and untie any restraining gauze before removing the tube. Some anesthetists prefer to deflate the cuff and untie the gauze before signs of arousal are seen so that the tube can be quickly removed when swallowing occurs. When removing an endotracheal tube after a dental surgery or prophylaxis, or after any procedure in which blood or other fluid is present in the oral cavity, the cuff should be left partially inflated to prevent these fluids from entering the air passages.

Stimulation of the patient. In some cases patient recovery may be hastened by gentle stimulation. This may include talking to the patient, pinching the toes, opening the mouth, gently moving the limbs, or rubbing the chest. Stimulation of this type increases the flow of information to the reticular activation center (RAC) of the brain, which is the area responsible for maintaining consciousness in the awake animal. A lack of stimulation to the RAC may cause drowsiness in the conscious animal, and it is therefore speculated that stimulation of this area may help the animal to awaken. It is also advisable to turn the patient every 10 to 15 minutes to prevent pooling of blood in the dependent parts of the body, including the lungs. This condition is called *hypostatic congestion.*

Reassuring the patient.   During the recovery period, the anesthetist should take every possible step to comfort and reassure the awakening patient. The anesthetist should bear in mind that the animal has no means of understanding the events that have led to its present disoriented state. Quiet, calm handling and reassurance are therefore essential.

The anesthetist can take several steps to minimize patient discomfort during recovery. All ties restraining the animal to the surgery table should be removed before the animal regains consciousness. The anesthetist should ensure that all accessory procedures such as bandaging, chest tube placement, and urinary catheterization, have been completed; and that the esophageal stethoscope, ECG leads, and thermometer are removed before the patient returns to consciousness. As previously mentioned, it is advisable to leave venous access (that is, indwelling catheter or butterfly) in place until the endotracheal tube has been removed and patient recovery is seen to be uneventful.

Postoperative analgesics should be administered as requested by the veterinarian, preferably before the animal experiences postoperative pain. (See Chapter 8.) If the animal has received appropriate analgesic administration, it should be able to sleep comfortably and demonstrate minimal signs of pain after the surgery. A change in analgesic dose or frequency or a switch to another analgesic may be necessary if postoperative pain is apparent despite the administration of medication.

Nursing care.   Nursing care of the recovering animal should include the application of heat to all hypothermic animals. This can be achieved by various means, including the use of warm towels, hot water bottles wrapped in towels, infrared heat lamps placed approximately 1 meter (3 feet) from the patient, hot air dryers, or circulating warm water heating pads. The patient often is unable to move voluntarily at this point, and the anesthetist must ensure that the patient is not burned by prolonged contact with an external heat source. Gradual rewarming is preferred to rapid rewarming because the latter may cause dilation of cutaneous vessels, leading to hypotension. The patient should be provided with ample bedding or padded material to prevent heat loss and increase patient comfort.

Anesthetized or recovering animals must never be left alone on a table or in a cage with the door open because of the danger of falling. Food and water should not be left in the animal's cage during recovery because it is not unknown for recovering animals to drown in water bowls or suffocate in food bowls. Some patients may be able to drink soon after standing; however, most have little appetite for food for several hours after recovery. Vomiting during the recovery period is common, but provided the patient is conscious, this is seldom dangerous.

Preventing patient self-injury.   Some animals may pass through a period of excitement (similar to stage II anesthesia) before completely regaining consciousness. As in induction, stage II recovery is characterized by vocalization, delirium, hyperventilation, head thrashing, and rapid paddling movements of the front legs. Occasionally an animal may appear to hallucinate or suffer from disorientation during anesthetic recovery, and patients (particularly those recovering from ketamine anesthesia) may chew at their paws or claw their faces. Animals showing these or similar signs of a "stormy recovery" usually return to normal within a short time, but close observation is necessary to prevent self-trauma and hyperthermia. Any animal that is thrashing or making ineffectual attempts to right itself may disrupt the surgical repair and seriously injure itself.

Summary. The importance of nursing care during the recovery period cannot be overemphasized. Postoperative problems such as hemorrhage, the removal of sutures by the animal, vomiting and subsequent inhalation pneumonia, and burns from electric heating pads may be prevented if the animal is closely monitored. The anesthetist's duty toward the patient does not end until the patient is awake and standing, fully recovered from the anesthesia.

✔ KEY POINTS

1. General anesthesia is a state of controlled and reversible unconsciousness accompanied by analgesia, amnesia, and depressed reflex responses. Ideally, respiration and circulation are not affected; however, in practice they may be impaired to a greater or lesser extent.

2. General anesthetic agents may be administered by injection or inhalation. Inhalation anesthesia is generally considered to have a greater margin of safety than injectable anesthesia.

3. The anesthetic period can be divided into preanesthesia, induction, maintenance, and recovery. Traditionally, anesthetic depth has been described in terms of stages and planes of anesthesia, with stage III, plane 2 being suitable for most surgical procedures.

4. Anesthetic safety is improved through the use of preanesthetic agents, use of the minimum effective dosages, and by close monitoring of the patient.

5. Induction of anesthesia may be achieved by intravenous or intramuscular administration of an injectable agent or by mask or chamber administration of an inhalation agent. Regardless of the method used, the patient is often intubated immediately after induction and maintained on an inhalation agent.

6. Intubation improves the safety and efficiency of anesthesia; however, it may be associated with problems such as vagal nerve stimulation, laryngospasm, airway obstruction, and pressure necrosis of the trachea.

7. During the maintenance period, the anesthetist must monitor the animal closely to ensure that vital signs remain within acceptable limits. The anesthetist also must monitor reflex activity and other parameters to ensure that the anesthetic depth is appropriate.

8. Vital signs that should be monitored by the anesthetist include heart rate and rhythm, pulse strength, capillary refill time, mucous membrane color, respiration rate and depth, and temperature.

9. Through the use of monitoring instruments, it is possible to gain accurate knowledge of the patient's blood gas levels, oxygen saturation, exhaled carbon dioxide levels, ECG, central venous pressure, and blood pressure.

10. Indicators of anesthetic depth include reflexes (particularly the palpebral reflex), muscle tone, eye position, pupil size, and response to surgical stimulation. Heart rate and respiratory rate also may change as anesthetic depth is altered. The anesthetist should assess depth after considering several parameters because no single indicator is unfailingly accurate.

11. The anesthetist must keep accurate medical records, the nature of which will vary depending on the clinical situation.
12. Patient comfort must be ensured throughout the procedure. This is accomplished by the use of correct positioning and gentle handling procedures.
13. The length of the recovery period depends on many factors, including the anesthetic protocol and the patient's condition. Return to consciousness is accompanied by increasing heart and respiratory rates, increased reflex responses, and voluntary movement.
14. During the recovery period, the anesthetist must continue to monitor the patient's vital signs, particularly temperature. It is often helpful to administer oxygen for several minutes after the anesthetic has been discontinued.
15. In dogs extubation should occur when the swallowing reflex returns. In cats extubation should occur when the patient shows signs of impending arousal, such as voluntary movements, swallowing, or active reflexes.
16. Other recovery duties may include stimulation of the patient, administration of postoperative analgesics, and general nursing care.

 ## REVIEW QUESTIONS

1. As the depth of anesthesia increases, there will be a continued depression of the vital centers of the body.
   True   False
2. The surgical plane of anesthesia is generally considered to be:
   a. Stage III, plane 1
   b. Stage III, plane 2
   c. Stage III, plane 3
   d. Stage III, plane 4
   e. Stage IV
3. Breath holding, vocalization, and movement of the limbs are most likely an indication that the animal is in what stage/plane of anesthesia?
   a. Stage III, plane 1
   b. Stage I
   c. Stage II
   d. Stage IV
4. Anatomic dead space is considered to be the:
   a. Air within the circuit
   b. Air within the mouth and nose
   c. Air within the mouth, nose, and all airways except the alveoli
   d. Air within the alveoli
5. The minimum acceptable heart rate for an anesthetized large breed dog is ___ beats per minute.
   a. 60
   b. 70

    c. 80

    d. 90

    e. 100

6. A heartbeat that is audible through a stethoscope is a good indicator that there must also be a strong pulse.

    True   False

7. In general, a respiratory rate of less than ___ breaths per minute for an anesthetized patient should be reported to the veterinarian.

    a. 4

    b. 8

    c. 12

    d. 16

8. Tachypnea is:

    a. An increase in respiratory depth (tidal volume)

    b. An increase in respiratory rate

    c. A decrease in respiratory depth (tidal volume)

    d. A decrease in respiratory rate

9. The term atelectasis refers to:

    a. Increased fluid in the alveoli

    b. Hyperinflation of the alveoli

    c. Collapsed alveoli

    d. A decrease in the perfusion of blood around the alveoli

10. A patient that has been anesthetized usually will have a:

    a. Mild metabolic acidosis

    b. Mild metabolic alkalosis

    c. Mild respiratory acidosis

    d. Mild respiratory alkalosis

11. An animal that is in a surgical plane of anesthesia should not respond in any way to any procedure that is being done to it (for example, pulling on viscera should not change heart rate).

    True   False

12. A 15-year-old dog has been anesthetized by mask induction with isoflurane and after intubation is maintained on 2% isoflurane with a flow rate of 2 liters of oxygen per minute. The heart rate is 80 bpm, respiratory rate is 8 breaths per minute and shallow, the jaw tone is relaxed, and all reflexes are absent. This animal is most likely in what stage of anesthesia?

    a. Stage III, plane 1

    b. Stage III, plane 2

    c. Stage III, plane 3

    d. Stage III, plane 4

    e. Stage IV

13. After an anesthetic procedure, when is it best to extubate a dog?

    a. Right after you turn off the vaporizer

    b. About 10 minutes after turning off the vaporizer

    c. When the animal begins to swallow

    d. Any time that is convenient

14. *Hypostatic congestion* may be present at the end of the anesthetic protocol. This term refers to the:
    a. Accumulation of mucus in the trachea
    b. Pooling of blood in the lungs
    c. Build-up of bile in the biliary tract
    d. Pooling of ingesta in one area of the gastrointestinal tract
15. Pulse oximetry allows accurate determination of:
    a. Arterial blood pressure
    b. Pulse pressure
    c. Pao_2
    d. Percent saturation of hemoglobin
    e. Blood gas values

For the following questions, more than one answer may be correct.

16. Pale mucous membranes may be an indication of:
    a. Blood loss
    b. Anemia
    c. Decreased perfusion
    d. Hypertension
17. An endotracheal tube is used to:
    a. Decrease dead space
    b. Allow for a patent airway
    c. Protect the patient from aspiration of vomitus
    d. Allow the anesthetist to ventilate the patient
18. Possible complications of endotracheal intubation include:
    a. Decreased dead space
    b. Pressure necrosis of the tracheal mucosa
    c. Intubation of a bronchus
    d. Obstruction of the endotracheal tube
    e. Spread of infectious disease
19. An animal under stage III, plane 2 anesthesia would exhibit which of the following signs?
    a. Very brisk palpebral reflex
    b. Regular respiration
    c. Relaxed skeletal muscle tone
    d. Very dilated pupils
20. As you intubate an endotracheal tube into an animal, what clinical signs will indicate to you that the endotracheal tube is in the trachea?
    a. The animal may cough as you insert the tube down the trachea.
    b. You can feel only one tube in the neck region.
    c. The reservoir bag of the anesthetic machine moves as the patient breathes.
    d. When you compress the reservoir bag, the stomach rises.

Answers for Chapter 2

1. True   2. b   3. c   4. c   5. a   6. False   7. b   8. b
9. c   10. c   11. False   12. c   13. c   14. b   15. d
16. a, b, c   17. a, b, c, d   18. b, c, d, e   19. b, c   20. a, b, c

Selected Readings

EDWARDS NJ: *ECG manual for the veterinary technician*, Philadelphia, 1993, WB Saunders.

HASKINS SC: General guidelines for judging anesthetic depth, *Vet Clin North Am Small Anim Pract* 22(2):432-434, 1992.

HASKINS SC: Opinions in small animal anesthesia, *Vet Clin North Am Small Anim Pract* 22(2): 326-469, 1992.

LEE L: Recovery complications in small animal anesthesia, *Vet Tech* 13(5):327-335, 1992.

MUIR WW III, HUBBELL JAE: *Handbook of veterinary anesthesia*, St Louis, 1989, Mosby.

PADDLEFORD RR: *Manual of small animal anesthesia*, New York, 1988, Churchill Livingstone.

RIVERA A, RUDLOFF E, KIRBY R: Monitoring in the intensive care unit, *Vet Tech* 17(1): 27-43.

SHORT CE: *Principles and practice of veterinary anesthesia*, Baltimore, 1987, Williams & Wilkins.

WRIGHT B, HELLYER P: Respiratory monitoring during anesthesia: pulse oximetry and capnography, *Compendium* 18(10):1083-1097, 1996.

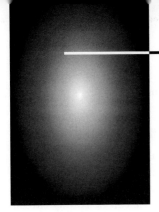

CHAPTER **3**

Anesthetic Agents and Techniques

PERFORMANCE OBJECTIVES

After completion of this chapter, the reader will be able to:

- Describe the advantages and disadvantages associated with the use of injectable anesthetic agents.
- Describe the advantages and disadvantages associated with the use of inhalation anesthetic agents.
- List the injectable anesthetic drugs that may be used as general anesthetics and be familiar with the following information regarding each agent: mode of action, effect on the heart and respiration, route of elimination from the body, and adverse side effects.
- List the various inhalation anesthetic agents that are available for use and the advantages and disadvantages of each agent.
- Describe the pharmacologic properties of halothane, isoflurane, methoxyflurane, and nitrous oxide.
- Describe the uptake, distribution, and elimination of the commonly used inhalation anesthetic agents.
- Define and explain the significance of minimum alveolar concentration, vapor pressure, solubility (partition) coefficient, and rubber solubility.
- Describe the use of nitrous oxide with oxygen and the potential dangers associated with nitrous oxide anesthesia.

A s described in Chapter 2, general anesthesia may be achieved through the administration of one (or more) potent anesthetic agents. These agents can be divided into two broad classes: injectable drugs (including barbiturates, cyclohexamines, neuroleptanalgesics, propofol, and etomidate) and inhalation agents (including halothane, isoflurane, methoxyflurane, and nitrous oxide). (See Fig. 2-1.) The pharmacology and physiologic effect of general anesthetics is one of the most fascinating areas in the field of anesthesiology and is described in detail in this chapter.

■ COMPARISON OF INHALATION AND INJECTABLE ANESTHESIA

Although both inhalation and injectable agents are commonly used in veterinary practice, inhalation anesthesia is considered to have a greater margin of safety. The advantages of inhalation anesthesia include the following:

- When an inhalation agent is used, the depth of anesthesia can be readily altered by the anesthetist. Inhalation agents continuously enter and leave the body via the respiratory system; this allows the concentration of anesthetic in the blood or brain to be changed rapidly. If the patient appears too awake, the concentration of anesthetic delivered by the anesthetic machine to the animal can be increased, resulting in a deeper level of anesthesia. If the anesthetist wishes to bring the patient to a lighter depth of anesthesia or to initiate recovery, the administration of the inhalation agent can be discontinued by turning off the anesthetic vaporizer. In contrast, the depth of the anesthesia produced by an injectable agent cannot be readily altered except by injection of additional drug to increase anesthetic depth.

- The elimination of inhalation agents, particularly isoflurane, occurs mainly through the lungs. This is in contrast to the elimination of injectable agents, which is achieved by redistribution of the drug within the body, by liver metabolism, and by renal excretion. Patient recovery from an injectable agent is generally more dependent on the patient's hepatic and renal functions than is the case with an inhalation anesthetic. These factors are not always significant in a young, healthy patient; however, they are often of concern to the veterinarian choosing an anesthetic protocol for a patient with preexisting problems. A geriatric cat with chronic renal failure is likely to be anesthetized more safely with isoflurane than with most injectable agents.

- Inhalation anesthesia allows the constant delivery of a high concentration of oxygen (close to 100%) to the patient. In contrast, animals under injectable anesthesia are often not intubated, and therefore breathe room air containing approximately 20% oxygen.

- Most patients under inhalation anesthesia are intubated, and mechanical ventilation using the anesthetic machine is relatively easy. This increases the safety of the anesthetic procedure because the anesthetist can respond promptly in case of hypoventilation or respiratory arrest.

The disadvantages of inhalation anesthesia compared with injectable anesthesia are the following:

- Inhalation anesthesia requires an anesthetic machine for delivery of anesthetic and oxygen to the patient. Injectable anesthetics do not require the use of this equipment and, in the short run, may be more economical to use. Once the equipment has been purchased, however, the cost of using an inhalation agent is comparable to that of injectable agents.

- Inhalation anesthesia has the potential for the escape of waste anesthetic gas into room air. Waste gas exhaled by the patient or leaked from anesthetic equipment results in operating room pollution. Personnel inhaling high levels of waste gas may be at increased risk for reproductive disorders and other health problems. (See Chapter 5.)

Many years of experience in veterinary anesthesia have shown that both injectable and inhalation anesthetics are effective and can be used with a wide margin of safety. It should be emphasized, however, that both injectable and inhalation agents have an overall depressant effect on the cardiovascular, respiratory, and thermoregulatory systems. Constant vigilance on the part of the anesthetist is necessary to prevent and to respond to anesthetic complications that may arise from the use of any agent.

■ INJECTABLE ANESTHETICS

The following injectable anesthetics are used in small animal anesthesia:
1. Barbiturates (including thiopental sodium, methohexital, and pentobarbital)
2. Cyclohexamines (including ketamine and tiletamine)
3. Neuroleptanalgesic agents (the combination of an opioid, such as morphine, meperidine, or oxymorphone, with a tranquilizing agent)
4. Propofol
5. Etomidate

Recommended dosages for these agents are given in Table 3-1. Dosages are approximate and should be adjusted according to the patient's age, physical status, and the veterinarian's recommendations.

Barbiturates

Classes of barbiturates.   All barbiturates in clinical use are derivatives of barbituric acid. Three classes of barbiturates are used in veterinary anesthesia: oxybarbiturates, thiobarbiturates, and methylated oxybarbiturates. Other classes of barbiturates, including long-acting barbiturates such as phenobarbital, are used as anticonvulsants but not as anesthetics.
- **Oxybarbiturates** (also called short-acting barbiturates). The only member of this class of drugs that is used for anesthesia is pentobarbital (Nembutal, Somnotol).
- **Thiobarbiturates** (also called ultrashort-acting barbiturates). Of this class of drugs, only thiopental (Pentothal) is currently available in North America.
- **Methylated oxybarbiturates.** Methohexital (Brevital) is the only methylated oxybarbiturate commonly used in small animal practice.

The three classes of barbiturate drugs vary in lipid solubility, distribution within the body, rapidity of action, and length of effect. Oxybarbiturates, such as pentobarbital, have low lipid solubility and are relatively slow to take effect. Oxybarbiturates rely on liver metabolism for the termination of their effects (which is relatively slow), and therefore the length of anesthesia and the recovery time are greater than for other barbiturate agents. In contrast, thiobarbiturates (such as thiopental) and methylated oxybarbiturates (such as methohexital) have a rapid effect and short duration of action, and recovery time is relatively brief. These agents are highly lipid soluble, and the termination of their effects is achieved by redistribution of the drug from the brain to muscle and fat.

Distribution and elimination of barbiturates.   To understand the mode of action of specific barbiturate agents, it is necessary to have some knowledge of the distribution and elimination of these drugs within the body. Thiopental, the most commonly used barbiturate agent, is always given by IV injection. Within seconds of injection it is dispersed throughout the body via the bloodstream. Large amounts of the drug rapidly enter the brain, partly because of the excellent blood supply this

TABLE 3-1

Suggested Dosage Ranges of Injectable Anesthetic Agents

Drug	Purpose	Dose (in mg/kg* IV)
Thiopental sodium	Intravenous induction	Dog: 10-12.5 mg/kg with premedication
	2% solution (20 mg/ml)	15-20 mg/kg without premedication
Methohexital	Intravenous induction 1% solution (10 mg/ml)	5 mg/kg with premedication
Pentobarbital	Intravenous anesthesia	15-20 mg/kg with premedication
		22-33 mg/kg without premedication
Ketamine/diazepam (a 50-50 mixture of 5 mg/ml diazepam and 100 mg/ml ketamine)	Intravenous induction (cats and dogs)	0.1-0.14 **ml**/kg with premedication
Ketamine/xylazine	Intramuscular (cats)	1 mg/kg xylazine, followed by 5-10 mg/kg ketamine
Ketamine (following acepromazine and atropine premedication)	Cats only: Intramuscular (minor procedures)	10-30 mg/kg
	Intramuscular (major procedures)	30-45 mg/kg
Propofol	Intravenous induction	3-8 mg/kg
	Maintenance of anesthesia	0.5-1 mg/kg every 3-5 minutes or continuous infusion 0.3-0.5 mg/kg/min
Etomidate	Intravenous induction	0.5-1.0 mg/kg

Modified from: *Veterinary teaching hospital undergraduate manual*, Guelph, 1992, Ontario Veterinary College.
*Except ketamine/diazepam

organ receives. Thiopental is highly lipid soluble, and the high lipid content of the brain also enhances its entry into brain tissue. The rapid penetration of thiopental into the brain explains why anesthesia is usually seen within 1 minute of injection. Pentobarbital is less lipid soluble and requires several minutes to reach its full effect.

All barbiturate agents produce their effects by depressing the reticular activating center of the brain, causing a loss of consciousness. This effect is terminated when the agent leaves the brain and is redistributed elsewhere in the body.

Tissues such as muscle and fat have proportionately less blood flow than the brain, and barbiturate levels in these tissues rise more slowly (Fig. 3-1). Gradually, the drug enters muscle and fat, and this causes the level of thiopental in the blood to fall. Once thiopental concentration in the blood falls below that in the brain tissue, the drug begins to leave the brain and reenter the circulation, where it continues to be redistributed to muscle, fat, and other body tissues. (The drug leaves the brain because barbiturates, like all drugs, diffuse from areas of high concentration to areas of low concentration.) The animal will show signs of recovery as the concen-

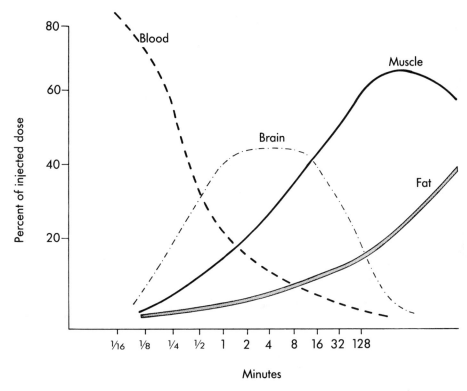

FIG. 3-1   Tissue levels of thiopental.

tration of thiopental in the brain decreases, although the drug is still present in other tissues. Over the next few hours, the barbiturate is gradually released from the muscle and fat and is eliminated from the body by liver metabolism and excretion of the metabolites in urine.

Because barbiturates are stored in the body and then slowly metabolized over time, it is inadvisable to administer these drugs on a continuous or repeated basis during the course of a surgical procedure because this could lead to an overdose or prolonged recovery.

The variation in lipid solubility of various barbiturate agents helps to explain differences in the duration of anesthesia for these agents. The rapid recovery of healthy animals from anesthesia with thiopental or methohexital is the result of the high lipid solubility and rapid redistribution of these agents into muscle and body fat. Pentobarbital is less soluble in lipids and, as a result, remains in circulation rather than being redistributed to body fat. Sustained blood levels of pentobarbital result in a sustained high concentration of the drug in the brain and a long duration of action.

Because of the high lipid solubility of thiopental, this agent has increased potency and duration of action in very thin animals, including sighthounds (Afghan hounds, whippets, salukis, borzoi, and greyhounds). Distribution of thiopental into body fat cannot readily occur in such lean animals, and therefore drug levels in the brain remain high. Hepatic metabolism of barbiturates may also be slow in sighthounds, further delaying clearance from the body. For these reasons, thiopental and pento-barbital are not recommended for use in lean animals, although another barbiturate agent, methohexital, is considered to be relatively safe.

Animals with hepatic or renal disease and animals suffering from hypothermia may exhibit prolonged recovery or "hangover" from thiopental because metabolism and excretion are delayed. Barbiturates also show greater potency in animals suffer-ing from hypotension or shock. The body responds to lowered blood pressure by re-ducing the blood flow to nonessential tissues (such as fat) and increasing blood flow to the brain and heart. Animals in shock can be expected to show greatly increased sensitivity to barbiturates because the normal redistribution of these agents from the brain to body fat stores does not occur. Metabolic acidosis is also present in most animals in shock, and this condition further increases the potency of barbiturates. (See the section on acidotic animals that follows.)

Use in practice.   The relative safety and low cost of barbiturates, and the rapid patient recovery observed, have led to the extensive use of barbiturates (particularly thiopental) in small animal anesthesia. Thiopental and methohexital are used as in-duction agents to allow endotracheal intubation. After intubation, anesthesia is usu-ally maintained with an inhalation anesthetic such as halothane or isoflurane. Thiopental may also be used as the sole agent of anesthesia for short procedures. En-dotracheal intubation is strongly advised for all patients anesthetized with barbitu-rates, even for brief periods, to prevent aspiration of fluid or vomitus and to allow the anesthetist to support ventilation if necessary.

Because of the potential toxicity of barbiturates to the cardiovascular and respi-ratory systems, and because of the variation in dose requirements among individual patients, these drugs are normally administered "to effect" (that is, only the amount necessary to induce anesthesia is given). Most commonly, half of the calculated dosage is given (as a bolus), and the effect of this bolus is observed before additional drug is administered. (This is described in more detail in Procedure 2-1.)

Effect on vital systems.   Barbiturates may have significant adverse effects on respiration and cardiovascular function. In fact, concentrated barbiturate solutions are commonly used as euthanasia agents, a fact that illustrates the potential toxicity of these drugs. Once injected into an animal, there is no way to retrieve or chemi-cally reverse a barbiturate drug. The most important adverse effects of barbiturates are respiratory depression and cardiac toxicity.

Respiratory depression.   Barbiturates may profoundly depress respiration. This effect is evident immediately after IV administration of thiopental for anesthetic in-duction, when a short period of apnea (cessation of breathing) is commonly seen. This results from direct depression of the respiratory center in the medulla, which is the area of the brain that controls respiration. In the awake animal, the respiratory center responds to rising levels of carbon dioxide in the blood by sending out im-pulses to the muscles that initiate inspiration. Barbiturates cause the respiratory cen-ter to become relatively insensitive to blood CO_2 levels, and as a result fewer nerv-ous impulses are sent to the respiratory muscles. Respiratory rate decreases and, in some cases, respiration may cease for a short time. The patient's mucous membrane color and heart rate should be closely monitored throughout the induction period to ensure that circulation is maintained during this period of apnea. Mucous mem-branes should remain pink, the heartbeat should be regular, and the pulse should be strong throughout the induction period. A pulse oximeter can also be used to monitor oxygenation levels. If spontaneous respiration does not resume within a few minutes, or if cardiovascular function appears to be threatened, ventilatory support may be necessary. This can be provided by periodic bagging or through the use of a mechanical ventilator. (See Chapter 7.) It should be noted that other induction agents (ketamine, propofol) can cause respiratory depression following IV injection and have the same requirement for close monitoring.

During anesthesia induced with a longer-acting agent such as pentobarbital, the most common effect on respiration is a persistent reduction in tidal volume (that is, shallow breaths). The effect may be short-lived, or the patient's respirations may appear shallow throughout the anesthetic period. Patients with reduced tidal volume are predisposed to respiratory acidosis and poor tissue oxygenation, particularly if barbiturates are used as the sole agent of anesthesia and oxygen delivery via an anesthetic machine is not available.

Respiratory depression is also a potential problem when barbiturates are used in cesarean surgeries. Barbiturates, like most anesthetic agents, readily cross the placenta and enter the fetal circulation. Thus they may interfere with the puppy or kitten's ability to breathe immediately after delivery. In fact, the fetus is more susceptible than the mother to the effect of barbiturates, and fetal respiration may be completely inhibited by doses of barbiturates that do not even cause anesthesia in the mother. Neonatal survival rates are particularly poor when a long-acting barbiturate, such as pentobarbital, is part of the anesthetic protocol for a cesarean.

Respiratory depression is not the only effect of barbiturates on the respiratory system: coughing and laryngospasm are also seen. These effects are thought to result from excessive salivation and may be minimized by the preanesthetic use of an anticholinergic such as atropine.

Cardiac toxicity.   Although less commonly seen than respiratory depression, cardiac toxicity may be significant in barbiturate anesthesia, particularly in the first 10 minutes after IV injection. It has been shown in the dog that barbiturates may directly depress myocardial cells, reducing cardiac output. The decline in cardiac function may cause blood pressure to fall immediately after barbiturate injection.

Thiopental and other anesthetics (particularly halothane) increase the heart's sensitivity to the action of epinephrine. This hormone is released by the adrenal gland, particularly in patients that are excited or stressed. Circulating epinephrine may have profound effects on the heart, causing potentially dangerous arrhythmias. It is not uncommon for cardiac arrhythmias such as ventricular premature contractions (VPCs) to occur during the induction period as a result of the combined effect of barbiturates, epinephrine, and hypoxia. These cardiac arrhythmias are not clinically significant in most patients; however, cardiac arrest has been reported in animals that are stressed during induction.

Toxic side effects on the heart can be minimized by ensuring that barbiturates are given slowly (over 10 to 15 seconds in the case of thiopental) and that dilute concentrations are used (for example, 2% or 2.5%). Barbiturate anesthesia should be avoided in animals with known cardiac disease because a dose of barbiturate that is well tolerated by a healthy heart may severely stress a diseased heart.

Other adverse side effects.   In addition to the cardiovascular and respiratory problems previously outlined, barbiturates may exhibit exaggerated and potentially dangerous potency in certain animals. Classes of patients that are particularly sensitive to barbiturates include hypoproteinemic animals, acidotic animals, and very lean animals.

Effect on hypoproteinemic animals.   Barbiturates are normally found in the blood both free and bound to plasma proteins. Only the free (unbound) molecules of barbiturate are able to enter the brain to induce the anesthetic effect because the molecules bound to proteins are unable to cross cell membranes. In hypoproteinemic animals (that is, those with total plasma protein less than 3 g/dl, often as a result of renal, hepatic, or intestinal disease) there is less plasma protein to bind barbiturate molecules. Consequently, there is relatively more barbiturate in the active, unbound form. The potency of barbiturates within the body is therefore increased in animals with low plasma protein levels. Dosages of barbiturates suitable for healthy animals may cause prolonged unconsciousness or death in these patients.

Effect on acidotic animals.   The potency of barbiturates depends on blood pH, and these drugs have greater effect if blood pH is low (acidosis). Therefore extreme care should be used when administering barbiturates to animals with metabolic or respiratory acidosis. A normal dose of barbiturates can produce high drug levels in the brain and an exaggerated response in these animals.

The effect of pH on the potency of barbiturates is significant in many patients. Metabolic acidosis is often encountered in small animal practice. It may be present in animals suffering from urinary obstruction, diabetic ketoacidosis, antifreeze poisoning, chronic renal failure, shock, and many other conditions. The dose of barbiturates required to anesthetize animals suffering from acidosis may be significantly less than that required to anesthetize healthy animals.

Tissue irritation.   Barbiturate solutions are strongly alkaline (pH 9.5 to 10.5) and may cause significant tissue damage if injected perivascularly, particularly if the concentration of barbiturate exceeds 2.5%. Perivascular injection of concentrated barbiturate solutions may be followed in 24 to 48 hours by local swelling, pain, necrosis, and even tissue sloughing. The irritation caused by perivascular barbiturate injections may cause the animal to chew at the area, thereby increasing tissue damage. Tissue sloughs are slow to heal and usually result in permanent scarring.

To avoid perivascular injections, a dilute solution of barbiturate should be used (in the case of thiopental, 2 to 2.5%). As an additional precaution, barbiturates are often administered through an IV catheter or butterfly. If perivascular injection occurs, the area should be immediately infiltrated with saline (in a volume equal to the volume of barbiturate injected) to dilute the barbiturate and reduce its irritating effect. Many veterinarians prefer to add 2% lidocaine without epinephrine to the saline to give a local analgesic effect.

Excitement during induction or recovery.   Perivascular injection or administration of a small dose of barbiturates may result in stage II excitement during induction. This occurs if the amount of barbiturate injected intravenously (that is, the amount reaching the brain) is insufficient to produce a deeper level of anesthesia. If excitement is exhibited, it is necessary to immediately administer more barbiturate to induce stage III anesthesia.

The use of barbiturates, particularly pentobarbital, is also associated with a high incidence of excitement during the recovery period. Paddling and vocalization are commonly seen but may be relieved by administration of IV diazepam.

Drug dependence.   Prolonged use of barbiturates is associated with drug dependence in humans, and for this reason most countries have enacted laws regulating the purchase, storage, and use of these agents. Careful record keeping is essential to comply with these regulations.

Loss of potency.   Thiobarbiturate agents are unstable in solution. These drugs are purchased in powdered form and are reconstituted by adding sterile saline or water. Once reconstituted, thiopental has a short shelf life (that is, a maximum of 2 weeks if refrigerated, less at room temperature). A solution should not be used if a precipitate is present.

Commonly used barbiturate drugs.   The characteristics of commonly used barbiturate agents are summarized in Table 3-2.

Thiopental.   Thiopental is among the most commonly used induction agents in small animal anesthesia and has also found widespread use as the sole anesthetic for brief procedures. The onset of action after injection is rapid (30 to 60 seconds) and duration is short (10 to 20 minutes). Complete recovery usually occurs within 1 to 2 hours. Thiopental has a wide margin of safety in healthy patients.

Thiopental is supplied as crystalline powder in multidose vials. Sterile water or saline is added to the vial, making a 2% or 2.5% (20 mg/ml or 25 mg/ml) or more concentrated solution. All vials should be labeled with the percent concentration and date of reconstitution because solutions remain stable for a limited time. Care should be taken to avoid injecting air into prepared solutions because this may cause premature precipitation of the barbiturate.

The dosage used varies from 6 to 20 mg/kg, depending on concurrent use of other agents and the depth of anesthesia required. Dosages are commonly reduced by up to 80% in debilitated animals or in animals that have been heavily sedated. As with other barbiturates, thiobarbiturates are given to effect. One method for IV induction using a thiobarbiturate is given in Procedure 2-1.

Although relatively safe, anesthetic induction using thiobarbiturates requires care.

- Perivascular infiltration should be avoided because local necrosis may result.
- Too-rapid infusion of barbiturate must be avoided during bolus induction because apnea or a dramatic drop in blood pressure may result.
- Transient apnea is commonly seen during induction, particularly if a concentrated thiobarbiturate solution is given rapidly IV. If apnea is prolonged, or if cyanosis or bradycardia is observed, it may be necessary to support ventilation by inserting an endotracheal tube and administering oxygen.
- Transient arrhythmias are commonly observed during induction, particularly if the drug is given rapidly. Cardiac arrhythmias may be successfully treated in most cases by the administration of two to three breaths of oxygen (performed by squeezing the reservoir bag of the anesthetic machine). Because of their arrhythmogenic tendency, thiobarbiturates are not well suited for induction of animals with heart disease.
- Thiobarbiturates should be avoided in sighthounds, since recovery in these breeds may be prolonged (for example, 2 to 4 times that of a normal animal).
- Muscle relaxation and analgesia are poor when a thiobarbiturate is used as the sole anesthetic agent.
- Repeated administration is cumulative, and recovery can be greatly prolonged if anesthesia is maintained for more than 30 minutes. For this reason it is not advisable to maintain anesthesia with repeated injections.

TABLE 3-2

Characteristics of Commonly Used Barbiturate Agents

Generic Name	Trade Name	Classification	Time to Onset of Anesthesia	Duration of Action	Recovery Time	Method of Elimination
Pentobarbital	Nembutal Sommotol	Short-acting	30-60 seconds	30 minutes-2 hours	6-24 hours	Liver metabolism
Thiopental sodium	Pentothal	Ultrashort-acting	30-60 seconds	10-20 minutes	1-2 hours	Redistribution followed by liver metabolism
Methohexital	Brevital	Ultrashort-acting	15-60 seconds	5-10 minutes	30 minutes	Redistribution followed by rapid liver metabolism

Methohexital.   Methohexital is a methylated oxybarbiturate similar to thiopental in that the onset of action is rapid (15 to 60 seconds), duration of anesthesia is short (5 to 10 minutes), and recovery is usually prompt. In fact, animals induced with methohexital and subsequently connected to an anesthetic machine may show signs of recovery before the inhalation anesthetic has had time to take effect. The rapid induction achieved with this agent is useful when anesthetizing a patient with a full stomach, because the anesthetist can intubate rapidly, decreasing the risk of aspiration of vomitus.

As with thiobarbiturates, methohexital is provided as a powder that must be reconstituted. The reconstituted drug has a shelf life of 6 weeks and does not require refrigeration.

Methohexital is administered in a manner similar to that of thiobarbiturates. One half to three fourths of the calculated dose is given intravenously over 10 seconds. One injection is usually sufficient to allow intubation, but additional drug should be given in 30 seconds if an adequate plane is not reached. Delay will result in a poor induction because of the rapid redistribution of the drug.

Methohexital is used most commonly in sighthounds because it produces faster recoveries and less hangover than thiopental. Liver metabolism of methohexital is much faster than the other barbiturates and therefore repeated administration is not cumulative.

Despite these useful applications in veterinary anesthesia, methohexital should be used with caution. Methohexital can cause profound respiratory depression, and the lethal dose is only 2 to 3 times the anesthetic dose. Methohexital is also associated with excitement during recovery, particularly if it is used as the sole anesthetic agent. For this reason, premedication is always recommended. Postoperative seizures that are sometimes seen with this agent may be controlled with IV diazepam.

Pentobarbital.   Pentobarbital is classified as a short-acting barbiturate. The onset of action is 30 to 60 seconds after IV injection, and the anesthetic effect lasts 30 minutes to 2 hours, depending on dosage and species.

Pentobarbital is supplied as a 6% or 6.5% solution (60 mg/ml and 65 mg/ml, respectively). It is commonly diluted with sterile water or saline to a 2% or 3% solution for use in dogs. The dosage used in dogs varies from 5 to 30 mg/kg, depending on concurrent use of other general anesthetic agents or preanesthetics. This agent must be used with caution because it has a narrow margin of safety: the euthanasia dose in healthy animals is only 40 to 60 mg/kg, approximately double the dose used for surgical anesthesia.

Pentobarbital, like all barbiturates, is given to effect. One third of the calculated dose is given over 3 to 5 seconds, and the animal is observed for at least 1 minute before additional drug is given. Small increments can be given until surgical anesthesia is achieved (usually 5 to 10 minutes after the initial injection). The animal should be intubated to preserve a patent airway and to allow oxygen administration if necessary. Additional drug can be given to prolong anesthesia; however, repeated dosages may be associated with excitement during the recovery period and with an extended recovery time.

Although pentobarbital is most commonly administered intravenously, intramuscular pentobarbital has been used as a premedication or sedative. It is also administered by intraperitoneal injection (particularly to rodents); however, its potency and duration of effect is variable when given by this route.

There are many problems associated with the use of pentobarbital in small animal anesthesia:

- Pentobarbital provides minimal muscle relaxation or analgesia
- Recovery from this agent is prolonged, particularly in cats, which lack the necessary liver enzymes to metabolize the drug quickly. Excitement during recovery is common in both cats and dogs anesthetized with pentobarbital.
- If pentobarbital anesthesia is performed without the benefit of intubation and the administration of oxygen, the patient may suffer from significant respiratory depression resulting in hypercapnia (that is, elevated blood CO_2) and respiratory acidosis.
- Anesthetic depth is difficult to control, except by injecting more agent.
- Recovery depends on adequate liver and kidney function.

Because of these disadvantages, the use of this agent for major surgical procedures is now uncommon in veterinary practice. It is still used occasionally in research, either as a sole anesthetic or in combination with nitrous oxide and a neuroleptanalgesic as part of a balanced anesthesia technique. Pentobarbital is also commonly used in the treatment of seizures arising from epilepsy, strychnine poisoning, and other causes.

Cyclohexamines

With the introduction of the injectable anesthetic phencyclidine in the late 1950s, a new class of injectable anesthetic drugs, the cyclohexamines, became available to veterinarians. Although phencyclidine is not used in veterinary medicine because of its tendency to cause hallucinations, its derivatives, ketamine hydrochloride and tiletamine hydrochloride, are used to induce anesthesia in many species.

Mechanism of action.   The mechanism of action of the cyclohexamines appears to be a disruption of nervous system pathways within the cerebrum and stimulation of the reticular activating center of the brain. Unlike most general anesthetics, which cause central nervous system (CNS) depression, cyclohexamines cause selective CNS stimulation. CNS stimulation may result from a suppression of inhibitory neurons by these drugs. This results in a distinctive type of anesthesia termed *dissociative anesthesia* or *catalepsy*, in which the animal appears awake but unaware of its surroundings (Fig. 3-2). Characteristics of dissociative anesthesia include the following:

- Reflex responses are exaggerated rather than depressed. For example, animals under dissociative anesthesia usually have a brisk palpebral reflex. Because reflex activity is preserved, it may be difficult to determine the level of anesthetic depth in patients under cyclohexamine anesthesia. Patients that show signs of purposeful movement are likely too light, whereas those with very depressed respiration are too deep. The anesthetist may have some difficulty in determining where an individual patient lies between these two extremes.
- Pharyngeal and laryngeal reflexes, although weak, may persist throughout anesthesia. The presence of these reflexes makes endotracheal intubation more difficult; however, the use of an endotracheal tube is still advisable to ensure patient safety. This is particularly true if a dental prophylaxis or other oral procedure is planned because blood, saliva, irrigating solutions, and other liquids present in the oral cavity may be easily aspirated if an endotracheal tube is not in place.

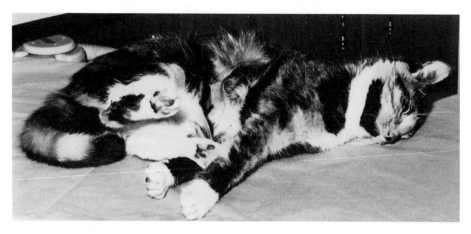

FIG. 3-2   Catalepsy induced by cyclohexamine agents.

- Animals anesthetized with these agents may show marked sensitivity to sound, light, and other sensory stimuli.
- Muscle tone is increased, almost to the point of rigidity. The animal assumes a stiff posture, with outstretched front limbs and extended neck. Spontaneous, random movements of the head and neck may be seen even when the animal is deeply anesthetized. This is in marked contrast to the muscle relaxation that is seen with inhalation agents. The concurrent use of a tranquilizing agent such as diazepam, acepromazine, or xylazine helps prevent excessive muscle rigidity, improves ease of intubation, and produces a more sleep-like state.
- Although dissociative anesthetics provide significant analgesia to the skin and limbs, visceral analgesia is poor. Because the analgesia provided by these agents is not adequate to relieve visceral pain, they should not be used as the sole anesthetic agent for abdominal surgery (including ovariohysterectomy), thoracic surgery, or orthopedic manipulations. A patient in dissociative anesthesia may be able to perceive pain but is unable to visibly respond to it, although growling may be heard if an endotracheal tube is not in place. It is the anesthetist's obligation to ensure that pain is not perceived, through the use of supplementary anesthetic agents and/or analgesics (for example, opioids or inhalation anesthetics) for all major surgical procedures.
- Dissociative agents are eliminated by metabolism in the liver or by renal excretion. These drugs may have an exaggerated effect on animals with liver or kidney dysfunction.

Use in practice.   Unlike thiopental, cyclohexamines may be given by either the IM or IV routes in some species. This versatility, plus the wide margin of safety of cyclohexamine drugs, has led to their widespread acceptance in veterinary anesthesia, particularly for use in cats. When given in combination with a tranquilizer (for example, diazepam, xylazine, acepromazine, or zolazepam) they are useful for short procedures, such as feline castrations, or as a means of induction before intubation and inhalation anesthesia. They are also useful for chemical restraint of intractable cats, allowing examinations and minor treatments without endangering hospital personnel. In dogs, cyclohexamine-tranquilizer combinations (usually ketamine and diazepam) are also commonly used as induction agents.

One limitation of cyclohexamine use in veterinary practice is the lack of an effective reversing agent. Such an agent would be helpful in speeding recovery and controlling postanesthesia excitement.

Effect on vital systems.   Dissociative anesthetics, such as ketamine and tiletamine, have some effect on the vital functions of anesthetized animals, but severe complications are rare.

Cardiac effects.   Unlike most anesthetics, ketamine does not decrease heart rate or depress myocardial function. In fact, most animals exhibit tachycardia, and blood pressure is often increased. These cardiovascular effects are not usually harmful to the animal; however, cyclohexamines should be used with caution in animals with cardiac arrhythmias or preexisting cardiac disease (for example, cats with hyperthyroidism or cardiomyopathy). Since ketamine and atropine both may induce tachycardia, some anesthetists prefer to use glycopyrrolate rather than atropine if an anticholinergic is required.

Effect on respiration.   Animals anesthetized with cyclohexamines exhibit *apneustic respiration,* a peculiar type of breathing pattern in which inspiration is followed by a prolonged pause and expiration is short. Respiratory rate and tidal volume may be reduced, although tissue oxygenation is usually adequate. Some animals appear to "hold their breath" when anesthetized with ketamine, but they often can be stimulated to exhale by tapping the nose or gently stroking the chest.

Other effects

Tissue irritation.   Ketamine and tiletamine are irritating to tissues, and many animals show transitory signs of discomfort when these drugs are given IM. However, tissue necrosis and sloughing do not occur with these agents.

Effect on salivation.   Cyclohexamine agents may cause increased salivation. A low dose of anticholinergic, such as glycopyrrolate or atropine, may be given before use of a cyclohexamine agent to prevent profuse salivation and the resultant risk of aspiration.

Effect on CSF pressure.   Ketamine may increase cerebral spinal fluid (CSF) pressure, and although this effect is not hazardous to most patients, the drug is contraindicated in cases of cranial trauma.

Effect on the eyes.   Unlike conventional anesthesia, the dissociative state produced by cyclohexamine agents does not result in closure of the eyelids or eyeball rotation. The eye normally remains open, with a central and dilated pupil. The use of ophthalmic lubricant is advised to prevent corneal drying. Another unusual characteristic of dissociative anesthetics is their tendency to induce nystagmus, a repetitive side-to-side motion of the eyeball. Ketamine-induced nystagmus is more commonly seen in cats than in dogs. This condition is harmless and resolves upon recovery from anesthesia.

CNS activity.   Animals recovering from cyclohexamine anesthesia often show an exaggerated response to touch, light, or sound, and seizure-like activity may be observed. Diazepam may be given IV (or, if IV injection is impossible, by the IM or rectal route) to reduce seizure activity. Reduction of light, sound, and other stimuli is also helpful. Some animals recovering from dissociative anesthesia may attempt to paw their faces or demonstrate other bizarre behavior, possibly a result of hallucinations induced by cyclohexamine agents. Because of the high incidence of excited recoveries seen with dissociative anesthesia, recovering patients should be closely monitored to prevent self-injury. It is advisable that recovery takes place in a hospital cage rather than in the owner's home.

Personality changes have been reported in animals following recovery from ketamine anesthesia. Fortunately, these usually resolve spontaneously after a few days or weeks.

Because CNS stimulation is seen with cyclohexamine agents, these drugs are contraindicated in animals with a history of epilepsy or other seizure disorders. Cyclohexamines should be avoided in animals that have ingested strychnine, metaldehyde, marijuana or other street drugs, organophosphates, and other toxins that affect the CNS. Cyclohexamines should also be used with caution in animals undergoing procedures involving the neurologic system, including CSF taps and myelograms, because the animal is at increased risk for postoperative seizures immediately following these procedures.

Cyclohexamine agents

Ketamine. Ketamine (Ketaset, Ketalean, Vetalar) is the most commonly used cyclohexamine agent and can be used to anesthetize not only cats and dogs but also birds, horses, and exotic species. At present ketamine is licensed only for use in cats. It is most commonly supplied as a 100 mg/ml solution.

Ketamine has a rapid onset of action after IV or IM administration. This is a result of its high lipid solubility, which allows quick entry into brain tissue. Cats may lose their righting reflex within 90 seconds of IV administration and within 2 to 4 minutes of an IM injection of ketamine.

IV administration has several advantages over IM administration; induction and recovery are more rapid and the dose is much less if the IV route is used. The anesthetist must ensure that the dose of ketamine is correct for the route of administration used: if the IM dose is inadvertently given by the IV route, death may result. Ketamine is given only by the IV route in dogs because IM ketamine may cause excitement and seizure activity.

Although ketamine can be administered repeatedly to maintain anesthesia, this should be done with caution. After repeated injections, large amounts of the drug accumulate in the tissues, increasing the risk of seizure activity during recovery and significantly prolonging the recovery period.

Recovery from ketamine anesthesia normally occurs within 2 to 6 hours in healthy patients, depending on the dosage given and the administration route. Unlike barbiturates, redistribution to body fat does not occur with cyclohexamines: recovery occurs as the drug gradually leaves the brain and is metabolized and excreted. Dogs appear to have faster recoveries than cats, probably because of differences in the method of ketamine excretion. Elimination of ketamine depends on hepatic metabolism in the dog, but in the cat it is primarily excreted through the kidney. Ketamine should be used with caution in dogs with hepatic disease and in cats with compromised renal function or urinary obstruction.

Ketamine is usually administered in combination with a tranquilizer, such as diazepam, xylazine, or acepromazine. The tranquilizer may be given as a premedication or mixed with ketamine and administered simultaneously. The use of a tranquilizer aids muscle relaxation and allows smoother recovery than the use of ketamine alone. As previously mentioned, administration of an anticholinergic is also suggested when ketamine is used, to prevent excessive salivation.

Ketamine-diazepam mixtures are popular for IV induction of cats and dogs and are formulated by combining equal volumes of diazepam (5 mg/ml) and ketamine (100 mg/ml). The resulting mixture may show precipitation if stored for a prolonged period. When ketamine-diazepam is given by IV administration at a dosage rate of 1 ml/7 kg, the animal loses consciousness within 30 to 90 seconds.

The combination of ketamine and diazepam has several advantages, including minimal toxicity to the heart. Respiratory depression, however, may be greater than that seen with ketamine alone. Muscle relaxation and anesthetic recovery are superior to that seen with the use of ketamine as the sole agent of anesthesia.

Ketamine-diazepam does not work well when given by the IM route because diazepam is poorly absorbed after IM injection. However, another benzodiazepine agent, midazolam, is water soluble and may be combined with ketamine in a manner similar to diazepam. The midazolam-ketamine mixture is well absorbed after IM administration in cats.

Ketamine-xylazine mixtures are also used for feline anesthesia, although the combination is associated with significant cardiovascular and respiratory side effects. Ketamine-xylazine may be given either IM or IV, a significant advantage of this combination. IM ketamine-xylazine is a particularly convenient anesthetic combination for use in uncooperative cats. The combination induces profound catalepsy with excellent muscle relaxation and some analgesia (although the analgesia is considered inadequate for major surgery and probably lasts only 15 minutes or less).

Because of the potentially adverse effect of xylazine on the cardiovascular and respiratory systems, this anesthetic combination does not offer the safety of ketamine-diazepam mixtures. Patients recovering from ketamine-xylazine anesthesia should be closely monitored because anesthetic complications and even death may result from cardiovascular collapse and respiratory depression long after the surgical procedure is finished. The combination of ketamine and xylazine is also associated with an increased risk of aspiration of vomitus because xylazine acts as an emetic in cats, and the swallowing reflexes may not be maintained adequately. This risk may be alleviated somewhat by premedicating the patient with atropine and xylazine and allowing 10 or 15 minutes for emesis to occur before anesthesia is achieved by the administration of ketamine.

Ketamine-acepromazine combinations are used commonly in cats for IV or IM administration. Acepromazine (and atropine, to reduce salivation) may be given as a premedication, followed 15 minutes later by ketamine; or the three drugs can be mixed together in a syringe. There is less respiratory depression and fewer cardiovascular side effects with this combination than with ketamine-xylazine. Muscle relaxation, however, is limited. As with other ketamine-tranquilizer combinations, the anesthesia produced is not sufficient for major surgery unless supplemented with an opioid agent or inhalation anesthetic.

Tiletamine.   Tiletamine is a newer dissociative agent with effects similar to ketamine. Tiletamine is sold only in combination with zolazepam, which is a benzodiazepine agent closely related to diazepam. The use of zolazepam in combination with tiletamine reduces the risk of seizures during recovery and helps promote skeletal muscle relaxation. The product is sold as a powder, which when reconstituted, has a pH of 2 to 3 and is stable for 4 days at room temperature or 14 days if refrigerated. Telazol is a class III controlled substance in the United States. It is currently unavailable in Canada.

The combination of tiletamine and zolazepam (Telazol) is similar in effect to ketamine-diazepam but offers the following advantages:

- Tiletamine appears to cause less pronounced apneustic respiration than ketamine. However, respiratory depression may be present, particularly if tiletamine is used in combination with other sedatives or anesthetics.
- Tiletamine-zolazepam may be administered by the IM, IV, or SC route.
- Telazol is approved in the United States for use in both dogs and cats, although at present it is approved for IM use only.
- Because of the IM route of administration, Telazol is particularly useful for chemical restraint of aggressive dogs and cats. A mixture of 3 mg/kg tiletamine and 0.4 mg/kg butorphanol given IM provides adequate restraint for examination and minor procedures in dogs. In fractious cats, a dose of 2.5 mg/kg tiletamine can be given subcutaneously.
- Tiletamine can be given orally to dogs at a dose of 20 mg/kg. It is usually combined with acepromazine to enhance sedation.

Onset of anesthesia is 2 to 5 minutes after IM injection, and duration of anesthesia is 20 to 30 minutes. As with ketamine, intramuscular injection may be painful.

Many reflexes are maintained throughout tiletamine-zolazepam anesthesia (including the palpebral, corneal, laryngeal, pedal, and pinna reflexes), and depth of anesthesia may be difficult to judge. As with ketamine, there is some analgesia, but visceral analgesia is probably inadequate for major abdominal surgery unless supplemented with other agents. Cardiac arrhythmias may be present in light anesthesia, but may be prevented by atropine premedication. Like ketamine, tiletamine induces marked salivation unless the patient is premedicated with an anticholinergic agent.

Tiletamine has been associated with tremors, seizure activity, and hyperthermia during anesthetic recovery. As with ketamine, ataxia and increased sensitivity to stimuli are commonly observed during the recovery period. Recovery may be prolonged (up to 5 hours after IM injection), particularly if high doses are administered. Because the drug is excreted via the kidneys, prolonged recovery may also be seen if the animal has kidney dysfunction.

Neuroleptanalgesia

As outlined in Chapter 1, the combination of an opioid and a tranquilizing agent can be used to induce the state of profound sedation termed *neuroleptanalgesia*. The same combination of drugs can be used to induce general anesthesia of dogs when given by IV injection (IV use of potent opioids should be avoided in cats because they may induce excitement). The opioid agents most commonly used for neuroleptanalgesia are morphine, meperidine, and oxymorphone. These are combined with a tranquilizer such as acepromazine, diazepam, or droperidol.

Neuroleptanalgesia combinations (with the exception of oxymorphone/acepromazine) are not suitable for routine induction of anesthesia in healthy young animals. This is because true anesthesia is unlikely to occur in these patients unless nitrous oxide or another anesthetic agent is given as well. However, neuroleptanalgesics may have a profound effect in high-risk or debilitated patients and are a useful and safe alternative to barbiturates or ketamine induction in these animals.

Induction with opioid-tranquilizer combinations provides a wide margin of safety in most patients, although care must be taken to administer the drugs slowly. If opioid-tranquilizer combinations are rapidly injected, CNS stimulation may be seen. The anesthetist using neuroleptanalgesia agents must also be prepared to intubate and ventilate the patient if necessary because profound respiratory depression may occur (as with any opioid agent).

Several procedures have been described for induction of anesthesia using neuroleptanalgesics. These include:

1. Administration of atropine and acepromazine 15 minutes before slow IV injection of the opioid.
2. Administration of atropine, followed 15 minutes later by slow IV administration of a tranquilizer-opioid mixture. If diazepam is selected as the tranquilizing agent, the opioid should be given first, followed 1 to 2 minutes later by diazepam. If diazepam is given before the opioid agent has taken effect, excitement may be seen (especially in spaniel and setter breeds). In young dogs, acepromazine offers more reliable sedation than diazepam and can be given at the same time as the opioid.
3. Administration of atropine and acepromazine, followed 15 minutes later by rapid administration of IV fluids containing the opioid agent. Administration of the fluids may be discontinued when the desired level of anesthesia is reached.
4. IM administration of a mixture of acepromazine and an opioid (usually oxymorphone or meperidine).

The above regimens can be safely carried out without atropine, provided the heart rate is carefully monitored. If bradycardia is noted, atropine or glycopyrrolate should be administered.

Propofol

Propofol (Diprivan, Rapinovet) is a recently introduced anesthetic induction agent that may be used as the sole agent for short procedures or for anesthetic induction before inhalant anesthesia. It is a substituted phenol with a chemical structure unlike that of other anesthetic or preanesthetic agents. Propofol has a neutral pH and is provided as an oil-in-water emulsion with a concentration of 10 mg/ml. Although this agent has a milky appearance, it can be safely administered intravenously.

Injections should be given by the IV route only, over a period of 20 to 60 seconds until the desired anesthetic depth is reached. One effective induction method is to give one third to one half of the calculated dose as an initial bolus. Smaller amounts can be administered every 30 seconds until the desired plane of anesthesia is reached. The dose of propofol needed for a patient and the duration of anesthesia is dependent upon the type of premedication used (Table 3-3). When given at a dose rate of 6 mg/kg IV, onset of anesthesia is less than 60 seconds and duration of anesthesia is 5 to 10 minutes.

Anesthesia may be maintained for longer periods by administering additional drug. Unlike cyclohexamines or barbiturates, propofol can be given repeatedly to a canine patient without concern that a poor recovery will occur. Injections can be repeated every 3 to 5 minutes or as required, depending on the status of the patient. Alternatively, propofol can be delivered by continuous infusion. In this procedure, a small dose of propofol (0.4 mg/kg/min) is continuously administered to the patient by a syringe pump, syringe driver, or intravenous line. This method allows the anesthetist to precisely control the depth of anesthesia at a stable plane for up to several hours.

In dogs, recovery is rapid and smooth, even after multiple injections. Dogs that have received propofol usually wake up rapidly, and may appear completely recovered within 20 minutes of injection. Cats recover quickly from single injections but may experience longer recoveries after multiple injections.

TABLE 3-3

Influence of Premedication Drugs on the Dose of Propofol Required for Anesthesia

Preanesthetic	Mg/kg IV Administered	Time Interval Before Next Dose (min:sec)
None	6.6 mg/kg over 60 sec	6:52
Tranquilizer (for example, acepromazine)	3.3-4.4 mg/kg	5:38
Alpha-2 agonist (for example, xylazine)	1.1-3.3 mg/kg	10:30
Analgesic (for example, oxymorphone)	2.2-4.4 mg/kg	6:49
Neuroleptanalgesia (tranquilizer and opioid)	1.1-2.2 mg/kg	

Modified from Franks PT: Proceedings of a roundtable discussion. Supplement to *Compendium Small Animal*, Trenton, NJ, 1997, Veterinary Learning Systems.

Propofol has a rapid onset and short duration of action because it is very lipophilic, similar to the thiobarbiturates. It is rapidly taken up by vessel-rich groups such as the brain, heart, liver, and kidneys; but then propofol, like thiopental, rapidly leaves these areas and is redistributed to muscle and fat. Dogs have the ability to metabolize propofol much more rapidly than thiopental. This helps to account for the ability to give repeated propofol injections with minimal hangover effects.

Propofol has several advantages over other injectable agents, including a wide margin of safety in both the dog and cat. Other characteristics include the following:

- Transient excitement and muscle tremors are seen occasionally during induction.
- Overall effects on the cardiovascular system are minimal, although episodes of tachycardia or bradycardia may occur. Although propofol may cause transient arterial and venous dilation and depress cardiac contractility, it is considered safe for use on most cardiac patients. Hypotension has been seen in some patients immediately after injection; however, this is usually corrected rapidly in animals with normal cardiovascular function. Animals with preexisting hypotension are less able to respond and, for this reason, propofol is not recommended in animals in shock or those suffering from blood loss or dehydration. Propofol should be used with caution in animals that have suffered recent trauma or severe illness.
- Propofol has the potential to depress respiration, particularly after rapid IV injection. Apnea is seldom a problem if the drug is given by titration rather than as a single bolus. Given the potential respiratory depression associated with the use of propofol, the anesthetist should monitor respiratory rate and depth carefully during the first 1 to 2 minutes after injection. If apnea lasts more than 1 minute, or if pulse oximetry shows oxygen saturation to be less than 90%, the patient should be intubated and ventilated with oxygen.
- Atropine premedication is not necessary. However, preanesthetic tranquilizers are useful since they decrease the dose of propofol required (See Table 3-3) and facilitate intravenous injection in fractious animals.
- Propofol appears to be safe for use in sighthounds, and recovery is rapid.
- Some muscle relaxation occurs with this agent, although analgesia is poor.

- Propofol can be diluted with 5% dextrose (D5W) or saline for use in small dogs and cats. Dilution allows more accurate dosing and helps to prevent respiratory and cardiovascular side effects. The manufacturer recommends that propofol not be diluted to a concentration less than 0.2% (2 mg/ml). It should not be mixed with other fluids or drugs.

One significant disadvantage of propofol is the poor storage characteristics of this agent. Because the product contains soybean oil, egg lecithin, and glycerol, it will support bacterial growth. Ampules and bottles should be handled in a strict aseptic manner, and any unused product should be discarded within 6 hours of opening to avoid contamination. (Unopened, the shelf life is approximately 3 years.) Life-threatening infections have been reported in human patients who received injections of propofol from syringes left for several hours at room temperatures.

Etomidate

Etomidate (Amidate) is a sedative-hypnotic imidazole drug that is occasionally used for induction of anesthesia in cats and dogs, often in conjunction with diazepam. It is always administered intravenously and has a short duration of effect. Like propofol, it can be administered in repeated boluses or as an infusion. It has minimal effect on cardiovascular function (including blood pressure and heart rate) but is a mild respiratory depressant. Metabolism in the liver is rapid.

Although etomidate has a wide margin of safety, it has several potential adverse side effects. Intravenous injection is reported to be painful and may cause phlebitis, especially when injected into small veins. Retching, apnea, and excitement may occur during induction or recovery, particularly in patients that have not been adequately premedicated. Etomidate is also significantly more expensive than other intravenous induction agents.

■ INHALATION ANESTHETICS

Inhalation anesthesia has become so commonplace in veterinary and human anesthesia that it is difficult to imagine the impact that the introduction of the first inhalation anesthetic had on surgical practice. Before the introduction of anesthesia, every surgical procedure was associated with pain, and it was usually necessary for surgeons to work at breakneck speed while the patients were manually restrained by attendants. The introduction of diethyl ether in 1842 and nitrous oxide in 1844 allowed the performance of safe and humane surgery, marking one of the most significant advances of medical science. Indeed, inhalation anesthesia continues to be the safest and most commonly used form of surgical anesthesia.

The inhalation anesthetics in common use in small animal practice at the present time are halothane and isoflurane. Of the many inhalation agents available, these two have proven to be the best suited to veterinary patients based on their convenience, cost, safety, and effectiveness. Methoxyflurane, enflurane, sevoflurane, desflurane, and nitrous oxide are occasionally used in some practices and referral institutions. Many other inhalation agents that were used in the past (including diethyl ether, chloroform, divinyl ether, and trichloroethylene) are now of historical interest only.

Characteristics of an Ideal Agent

Although each inhalation agent has desirable properties, the "ideal" inhalation agent does not exist. The characteristics of such an agent would include:

1. Minimal toxicity to the patient, particularly to the cardiovascular, respiratory, hepatic, renal, and nervous systems
2. Minimal toxicity of waste gas vapors to anesthetists and other operating room personnel
3. Ease of administration, even to fractious animals
4. Rapid and gentle induction and recovery
5. Anesthetic depth easily controlled and altered
6. Good muscle relaxation
7. Adequate postoperative analgesia
8. Low cost
9. Adequate potency to achieve surgical anesthesia
10. Handling safety (that is, agent should be nonflammable and nonexplosive)
11. No requirement for expensive equipment

Both halothane and isoflurane approach this standard in several respects and are safe for most veterinary patients.

In choosing an inhalation agent to be used for a particular procedure, the veterinarian must consider several factors, including the availability of each agent, the special needs of the patient, the preference of the anesthetist and surgeon, and cost.

Classes of Inhalation Agents

Diethyl ether.   Diethyl ether ("ether") was for many years the most widely used anesthetic. Animals anesthetized with this agent normally maintain a relatively stable cardiac output and blood pressure, although heart rate may be slightly elevated. Ether does not sensitize the heart to epinephrine, and thus there is little risk of cardiac arrhythmias. It also produces good muscle relaxation and analgesia.

Despite these advantages, ether has significant drawbacks that have greatly limited its use in contemporary anesthesia. One major problem is the irritating effect of this agent on the tracheal and bronchial mucosa. This results in increased salivation and mucous secretions and an increased risk of laryngospasm and airway blockage. Recovery from ether anesthesia may be prolonged, and postoperative nausea is common. In addition, ether is flammable and explosive and requires an explosion-proof refrigerator for safe storage.

Nitrous oxide.   Nitrous oxide, introduced as an anesthetic more than 150 years ago, is still used extensively in human anesthesia and, to a lesser extent, in veterinary anesthesia as well. In contrast to the other inhalation agents (which are liquids), nitrous oxide is a gas. As such, it is delivered directly from compressed air tanks and does not require a vaporizer for administration.

Chlorofluorocarbons.   The two most commonly used inhalation agents, halothane and isoflurane, are chemically similar and are classified as halogenated organic compounds (chlorofluorocarbons). Other chlorofluorocarbon agents include methoxyflurane, enflurane, sevoflurane, and desflurane. Each of the six agents is a liquid at room temperature but vaporizes readily within an anesthetic machine. It is the vaporized anesthetic, mixed with oxygen, that is administered to the patient to achieve and maintain general anesthesia.

The physical properties and pharmacology of the most commonly used chlorofluorocarbon agents are summarized in Tables 3-4 and 3-5.

TABLE 3-4

Physical Properties of the Common Inhalation Anesthetics

	Nitrous oxide	Halothane	Methoxyflurane	Isoflurane	Sevoflurane
Formula	N_2O	$CF_3CHClBr$	$CH_3OCF_2CHCl_2$	$CF_3CHClOCHF_2$	$CFH_2COCF_3CF_3$
Molecular weight	44	197	165	184	200
Date of first clinical use	1845	1956	1959	1981	
Trade name	—	Fluothane	Metofane Penthrane	Forane AErrane	
Saturated vapor pressure (mm Hg)	800 (psi)	243	22.5	261	160
Solubility					
Blood	0.47	2.4	13	1.4	0.6
Oil	1.4	224	825	60	53
Rubber	1.2	120	635	62	
MAC in dogs (%)	188	0.87	0.23	1.2	2.1-2.3

Modified from Warren RG: *Small animal anesthesia*, St Louis, 1989, Mosby.

TABLE 3-5

Pharmacologic Properties of Selected Agents

Property	Methoxyflurane	Halothane	Isoflurane	Sevoflurane
Muscle relaxation	Excellent	Fair	Good	
Effect on nondepolarizing muscle relaxants	None	Increased	Greatly increased	Probably increased
Analgesia	Excellent	Slight	Slight	Slight
Effect on respiration	Marked depression of rate and depth	Some depression	Depression	Depression
Effect on heart	Mild depression	Severe depression	Slight	Slight
Potential for causing cardiac arrhythmias	Some	Very common	None reported	None reported
Effect on blood pressure	May decrease	Decreases	Decreases	Decreases
Elimination from the body	Metabolism 50% Respiration 50%	Metabolism 20% Respiration 80%	Respiration 99%	Respiration 97%
Effect on the liver	Rare toxicity reported in humans	May rarely cause hepatitis in humans	None reported	Possible risk of toxicity
Effect on the kidneys	Toxicity reported in humans and animals	None reported	None reported	
Lipid solubility	High	Moderate	Low	Low
Maintenance range	0.25%-1%	0.5%-2%	1%-3%	

Modified from McKelvey D: Halothane, isoflurane and methoxyflurane, *Vet Tech* 12(1):25, 1991.

Mechanism of Action of Inhalation Agents

The mechanism of action of anesthetic molecules within the brain is poorly understood. It has been suggested that anesthetics exert their effects by inhibiting the breakdown of gamma-aminobutyric acid (GABA), an inhibitory neurotransmitter. According to this theory, this results in an increased level of GABA in the anesthetized patient's brain, inhibiting nerve function. Another theory suggests that anesthetics dissolve in nerve cell membranes and cause the membrane to lose its ability to conduct nerve impulses. This theory suggests that anesthetics with greater lipid solubility will have a more potent effect than will those with minimal lipid solubility. This observation holds true for the inhalants in common use. Methoxyflurane, the most lipid soluble, is the most potent. Halothane has moderate lipid solubility and moderate potency. Isoflurane is the least lipid soluble and is the least potent of the three agents.

Distribution and Elimination of Inhalation Agents

To understand the properties of the inhalation agents, it is necessary to briefly discuss their intake into, distribution within, and elimination from the body. Liquid anesthetic in the anesthetic machine is vaporized, mixed with oxygen, and delivered to the patient by mask or endotracheal tube. The anesthetic travels via the air passages to the lung alveoli, where it diffuses across the alveolar cells and enters the bloodstream. The rate of diffusion is controlled by the concentration gradient between the alveolus and the bloodstream, as well as the lipid solubility of the drug. During the induction period, the concentration of the agent in the alveolus is high, and the concentration in the blood is low. This creates a steep concentration gradient, and diffusion of anesthetic from the alveolus into the blood is rapid during this period.

Because of their relatively high lipid solubility, inhalation agents readily leave the circulation and enter the brain, inducing anesthesia. Anesthesia is maintained as long as sufficient quantities of inhalation agent are delivered to the alveoli so that the blood, alveolar, and brain concentrations are maintained.

When the concentration of the inhalation agent administered is reduced or discontinued by adjusting the anesthetic machine vaporizer, the amount of anesthetic in the alveolus is reduced. Since the blood level is still high, the concentration gradient now favors the diffusion of anesthetic from the blood into the alveoli. The blood levels of the anesthetic are quickly reduced, provided the animal continues to breathe and eliminate anesthetic from the alveoli. The anesthetist can hasten the elimination of anesthetic by periodically bagging the animal with 100% oxygen. This removes anesthetic from the alveoli and reestablishes a steep concentration gradient between the alveoli and the blood. As the concentration of the anesthetic in the blood falls, the agent leaves the brain and recovery from the anesthetic is achieved.

Some anesthetic agents (in particular, methoxyflurane) have high lipid solubility and may accumulate in body fat stores, thereby escaping elimination through the lungs at the end of anesthesia. These agents rely on liver metabolism and renal excretion for their complete elimination from the body. Slower recovery and prolonged anesthetic hangover occur routinely with these agents.

Properties of Inhalation Agents

Isoflurane, halothane, methoxyflurane, and nitrous oxide differ considerably in their anesthetic effects, in part, because of differences in their physical and chemical properties. The properties of chief importance to the anesthetist include vapor pressure, solubility coefficient, minimum alveolar concentration (MAC), and rubber solubility. These agents also vary in their pharmacologic properties, including their effects on the cardiovascular, respiratory, and other vital systems. The physical properties and pharmacology of commonly used inhalation anesthetic agents are summarized in Tables 3-4 and 3-5.

Vapor pressure.   The vapor pressure of an inhalation anesthetic is a measure of the amount of liquid anesthetic that will evaporate at 20° C. Agents with a high vapor pressure, such as halothane or isoflurane, are termed *volatile* because they evaporate easily. In fact, both isoflurane and halothane evaporate so readily that they may reach a concentration of over 30% in the oxygen delivered to the patient, a level which could cause a fatal anesthetic overdose. The *precision vaporizer*, a special type of vaporizer, limits the evaporation of these agents and allows their safe use for anesthesia. Precision vaporizers allow a maximum concentration of 5%, a level that is sufficient for all practical uses. The use of these volatile inhalation agents in a simple, nonprecision vaporizer is difficult because of the lack of control over the evaporation of the anesthetic and the increased risk of overdose. A skilled anesthetist and very close monitoring of the patient and anesthetic machine are required.

Some agents, such as methoxyflurane, have relatively low vapor pressure and do not require the use of a precision vaporizer. At 20° C the maximum methoxyflurane concentration attainable in the anesthetic circuit is 4%. A simple, inexpensive, nonprecision vaporizer, such as a glass jar with a wick, is adequate for methoxyflurane anesthesia. Precision vaporizers for methoxyflurane are available on some machines; however, they are not a requirement for safe anesthesia.

Because each type of vaporizer is designed for use with a particular agent and its specific vapor pressure, it is theoretically necessary to use a different vaporizer for each agent. In practice, the similar vapor pressures of isoflurane and halothane result in similar evaporation rates, and isoflurane may be used safely in many vaporizers designed for halothane use. A new or recently serviced halothane vaporizer should deliver predictable levels of isoflurane within 10% of the dial setting, which is considered acceptable for anesthesia. Before use with isoflurane, a halothane vaporizer should be completely drained and the residual halothane evacuated by allowing oxygen to flow through the vaporizer for several hours. The use of halothane vaporizers for isoflurane is not recommended by anesthetic or vaporizer manufacturers for litigation reasons because mistakes involving confusion of agents can occur if the anesthetic currently in the vaporizer is not clearly labeled.

Although it is inadvisable to combine halothane and isoflurane together in the same vaporizer, it is acceptable to switch from one anesthetic to another during the course of surgery if the patient demonstrates an adverse reaction to the first anesthetic. In this case, separate vaporizers must be available for each anesthetic because time would not allow evacuation of the first anesthetic from the vaporizer.

Because of significant differences in vapor pressure, methoxyflurane should not be used in a vaporizer designed for halothane or isoflurane.

Solubility coefficient.   The blood-to-gas solubility coefficient (or partition coefficient) is a measure of the distribution of the inhalation agent between the blood and gas phases in the body. It is therefore a measure of the tendency of an anesthetic agent to exist as a gas or, alternatively, to dissolve in the blood. An inhalation anesthetic with a low solubility coefficient tends to remain in the gas phase in the pulmonary alveoli rather than dissolving into the tissues and blood. This phenomenon produces a high concentration of the agent in the alveoli and a steep diffusion gradient between the alveoli and the blood. As a result, an agent with a low solubility coefficient, although not intrinsically soluble in the blood, will quickly enter the circulation and escape into the brain, resulting in rapid induction and recovery. An example of such an agent is isoflurane, which has an extremely low blood-to-gas solubility coefficient and demonstrates rapid induction and recovery. Halothane has a slightly higher solubility coefficient and is therefore less rapid in its effect.

In contrast, an agent with a high solubility coefficient will be extremely soluble in the blood and tissues. Because the anesthetic is rapidly absorbed into the tissues (called the "sponge effect"), high levels of the anesthetic do not build up within the alveoli, and a concentration gradient is not established. Additionally, the highly soluble agents are trapped in the blood and tissues to a greater extent, resulting in less escape into brain tissue and wider distribution throughout the body. Therefore agents with high solubility coefficients induce anesthesia less rapidly than do agents with low solubility coefficients. Methoxyflurane is an example of an agent with a high solubility coefficient and, as expected, demonstrates relatively slow induction and recovery rates.

The solubility coefficient of an inhalant agent has a significant effect on the clinical use of the agent. The rapid induction possible with isoflurane and halothane allows the use of these agents for mask or chamber induction, whereas methoxyflurane is not well suited to these induction methods. Agents with low solubility coefficients (such as isoflurane) also have the advantage of allowing a rapid patient response to changes in anesthetic concentration during anesthesia. Patients anesthetized with isoflurane may respond within 1 minute to changes in the vaporizer setting. If an agent with a higher solubility coefficient is used (such as halothane), the anesthetist will observe a slower response to changes in the vaporizer setting.

Minimum alveolar concentration.   The minimum alveolar concentration (MAC) of an anesthetic agent is the lowest concentration that produces no response in 50% of the patients exposed to a painful stimulus (for example, a clamp applied to the base of the tail). The MAC thus indicates the strength of an inhalation anesthetic: an agent with a low MAC is a more potent anesthetic than an agent with a high MAC. For example, halothane has a lower MAC than isoflurane and is, therefore, more potent; a higher concentration of isoflurane will be necessary to maintain a similar anesthetic depth.

For a given inhalation anesthetic, a vaporizer setting of approximately $1 \times$ MAC will produce light anesthesia in most patients, $1.5 \times$ MAC will produce a surgical depth of anesthesia, and $2 \times$ MAC will produce deep anesthesia. These figures are useful only as a rough guide: MAC varies with the species, age, and body temperature of the patient. Factors such as disease, pregnancy, obesity, and treatment with other drugs may also alter the potency of an anesthetic agent in a given patient. The anesthetist should also be aware that the response to an anesthetic depends on the concentration of the anesthetic in the patient's brain, which is not necessarily the same as that indicated by the vaporizer, particularly early in the induction period. (See Chapter 4.)

Halothane

Halothane is one of the most commonly used inhalation agents in veterinary anesthesia.

Physical and chemical properties.   The chief physical and chemical properties of halothane are as follows:

- Halothane has a relatively high vapor pressure and, as such, normally requires a precision vaporizer for its safe use. Halothane delivered through a nonprecision vaporizer may readily achieve a concentration over 30%, which dangerously exceeds the normal concentration required for anesthesia (1% to 2%). Special techniques are required for use of halothane in a nonprecision vaporizer.
- Halothane has a moderately low solubility coefficient and moderate fat solubility, allowing fairly rapid induction and recovery. Delivery of halothane by mask usually results in unconsciousness and stage III anesthesia in a tranquilized animal within 10 minutes. Recovery time from anesthesia varies with length of anesthesia, patient condition, and the concurrent use of other agents; however, sternal recumbency is usually achieved in less than 1 hour after the anesthetic is discontinued. Because of its moderate lipid solubility, a portion of the anesthetic is retained within body fat stores rather than being eliminated by the lungs during recovery. The stored halothane is subsequently metabolized by the liver, with elimination of the metabolites by the kidney.
- Halothane has a moderate MAC and, in terms of anesthetic potency, is midway between methoxyflurane and isoflurane.
- Halothane has moderate rubber solubility. This is of concern to the anesthetist because hoses, reservoir bags, and other anesthetic machine parts contain rubber and may absorb halothane during the course of anesthesia. Release of the agent from machine parts may delay patient recovery after the vaporizer has been turned off.
- Halothane is somewhat unstable, and for commercial use is mixed with the preservative thymol. The presence of a preservative may cause a build-up of residue within the vaporizer, turning the liquid in the vaporizer yellow. Ultimately, the residue build-up will cause a malfunction unless the vaporizer is periodically serviced.

Pharmacologic effects.   Halothane is a relatively safe agent for veterinary use; however, it does have some adverse effects on organ function:

- Halothane sensitizes the heart to the action of catecholamines (such as epinephrine) and thus may induce arrhythmias. Arrhythmias may be treated by increasing patient ventilation and ensuring that anesthetic depth is adequate. If this does not alleviate the arrhythmia, the patient may be given IV lidocaine or switched to another anesthetic, if available.
- Halothane increases vagal tone, and bradycardia may result.
- Halothane has a mild depressant effect on myocardial cells, decreasing myocardial contraction and cardiac output.
- Halothane decreases peripheral resistance of the blood vessels by causing vasodilation. Vasodilation predisposes the animal to excessive heat loss and, therefore, hypothermia. Vasodilation also may cause a fall in blood pressure that is roughly parallel to anesthetic depth. For this reason, halothane anesthesia should be used with caution in hypovolemic or hypotensive patients.
- Halothane causes some depression of respiration, and respiratory rate and tidal volume usually fall if anesthesia is prolonged. Halothane and all other inhalation anesthetics readily cross the placenta and may depress respiration in the newborn.
- Halothane is moderately lipid soluble. A portion of the administered dose is retained in body fat stores and, subsequently, metabolized in the liver. It has been

associated with hepatotoxicity and liver necrosis in human patients. There is no clear evidence at present that hepatotoxicity occurs with halothane use in veterinary patients; however, the use of alternative inhalation agents is probably advisable for patients with hepatic disease.

- Halothane produces adequate muscle relaxation but only slight analgesia. Halothane and nitrous oxide may be used in combination to achieve even greater muscle relaxation and significant analgesia.
- Halothane use is associated with malignant hyperthermia, a rare but often fatal disorder of thermoregulation. Affected animals show increased temperature, muscle rigidity, and cardiac arrhythmias, and may die. Treatment consists of removal from halothane, cooling, and administration of oxygen and specific drugs such as dantrolene.

Isoflurane

Physical and chemical properties.   Isoflurane is closely related chemically to methoxyflurane, but its properties are more similar to those of halothane. The margin of safety of this agent is apparently greater than that of halothane or methoxyflurane, which has led to its wide acceptance in veterinary anesthesia despite its considerable cost (at present, approximately 4 times the cost of halothane). Isoflurane is licensed for use only in dogs and horses, although it has gained widespread use in other species.

The chief physical and chemical properties of isoflurane are as follows:
- The vapor pressure of isoflurane is almost identical to that of halothane. Because of its volatile nature, isoflurane is normally used in a precision vaporizer. Some halothane vaporizers have been adapted successfully for isoflurane administration, although this practice is discouraged by manufacturers.
- The solubility coefficient of isoflurane is extremely low. This, combined with the relatively low lipid solubility of this agent, results in extremely rapid induction and recovery. Isoflurane is better suited to mask or chamber induction than are slower-acting agents such as methoxyflurane. It is important that the anesthetist refrain from turning off the anesthetic machine vaporizer until the end of surgery because return of consciousness may occur as rapidly as 1 to 2 minutes after isoflurane administration is discontinued. The low solubility coefficient of isoflurane also allows the anesthetist to change the patient's depth of anesthesia rapidly during the course of anesthesia. An animal that appears too deep or too light usually responds rapidly (within 1 or 2 minutes) after adjustment of the anesthetic level.
- The MAC of isoflurane is higher than that of halothane and thus it is less potent. Anesthesia is maintained in most patients at a concentration of 1.5% to 2.5% isoflurane in oxygen.
- The rubber solubility of isoflurane is very low, and there is little absorption of this anesthetic by rubber-containing components.
- Isoflurane is stable at room temperature, and no preservative is necessary. This is an advantage because there is no preservative residue to accumulate in isoflurane vaporizers. (These vaporizers, however, still require periodic maintenance.)

Pharmacologic effects.   Of all the volatile anesthetics commonly used in veterinary anesthesia, isoflurane is considered to have the fewest adverse effects on the heart and other vital systems.

- When used at normal anesthetic levels, isoflurane maintains cardiac performance close to that of preanesthetic levels. It causes only a small decrease in cardiac output, with little or no depression of myocardial cells and little effect on heart rate. Isoflurane does not sensitize the myocardium to the effects of epinephrine and is therefore not arrhythmogenic. Because of its minimal effect on the heart, isoflurane is considered to be the inhalation agent of choice for patients with cardiac disease. As with halothane, however, vasodilation and decreased blood pressure may be observed, particularly at deeper levels of anesthesia.
- Isoflurane depresses respiration. The effect of isoflurane on respiration is greater than that of halothane.
- Nearly all of the isoflurane administered to a patient is exhaled quickly once the vaporizer is turned off. Isoflurane has low fat solubility; consequently, there is little retention of isoflurane in body fat stores, little hepatic metabolism, and very little renal excretion of metabolites. For this reason isoflurane is well suited to animals with liver or kidney disease. Isoflurane is also the preferred anesthetic for use in neonatal and geriatric animals, in which hepatic metabolism and renal excretion mechanisms may be less efficient than in the healthy adult animal.
- Animals anesthetized with isoflurane show good muscle relaxation.
- Isoflurane has little or no analgesic effect in the postanesthetic period. The use of postoperative analgesics is advisable because this lack of analgesic effect, combined with the rapid recoveries experienced with this agent, may lead to pain and excitement during recovery.

Methoxyflurane

Although difficult to obtain in some countries because of limited production, methoxyflurane is a useful anesthetic agent in small animal patients.

Physical and chemical properties

- The vapor pressure of methoxyflurane is significantly lower than that of halothane or isoflurane, and as a result methoxyflurane may be safely used in a nonprecision vaporizer. Since an anesthetic machine with a nonprecision vaporizer is considerably less expensive than one with a precision vaporizer, the initial equipment costs are less for methoxyflurane anesthesia than they are for halothane or isoflurane.
- The solubility coefficient of methoxyflurane is considerably higher than that of halothane or isoflurane, as is the lipid solubility. These two factors combine to produce slow induction and recovery rates in animals anesthetized with methoxyflurane. Because of the slow induction rates, it is not generally advocated that this agent be used for mask induction or chamber induction because stage II of general anesthesia (excitement stage) may be prolonged.
- Methoxyflurane is the most potent inhalation anesthetic in common use because the MAC of methoxyflurane is considerably lower than that of the other volatile inhalation anesthetics. Methoxyflurane is approximately twice as potent as halothane.
- Methoxyflurane has considerable solubility in rubber or plastics and readily dissolves in reservoir bags, hoses, and endotracheal tubes. This may lead to deterioration of these products unless they are rinsed out immediately after use.

The solubility of methoxyflurane in rubber or plastic anesthetic machine parts may also result in considerable release of methoxyflurane gas into the anesthetic circuit after the vaporizer has been turned off.

- As with halothane, methoxyflurane requires the addition of a preservative to extend its shelf life. The accumulation of preservative may interfere with vaporizer function; however, cleaning and maintenance procedures for nonprecision vaporizers are much easier than those for precision vaporizers.

Pharmacologic effects.   Methoxyflurane has a good margin of safety in both the dog and cat.

- Methoxyflurane, unlike halothane, does not sensitize the myocardium to the arrhythmogenic effects of catecholamines.
- Methoxyflurane is the most potent respiratory depressant of all the inhalation anesthetics. Both the respiratory rate and the tidal volume are decreased, and it is important to monitor anesthetized animals to ensure adequate ventilation. The use of a ventilator or periodic bagging by hand will help expand lung alveoli and prevent hypercapnia (elevated levels of carbon dioxide in the blood). However, the anesthetist should avoid continuous bagging of a patient under methoxyflurane anesthesia unless the vaporizer setting is reduced. Failure to reduce the setting may lead to excessive anesthetic being delivered to the patient because the concentration of anesthetic increases as oxygen is forced through a nonprecision vaporizer by the bagging procedure.
- Because of its high lipid solubility, methoxyflurane is retained in body fat stores such that over half of the anesthetic delivered to the animal is eventually metabolized and excreted by the liver and kidney. The presence within the kidney of toxic metabolites, such as fluoride ions, may lead to renal damage, particularly if flunixin (Banamine) or other potentially nephrotoxic drugs are administered concurrently. This effect has been well documented in human anesthesia, although its occurrence in veterinary anesthesia seems limited to dehydrated animals with preexisting renal damage. Urine concentrating ability may be impaired for up to 3 days after methoxyflurane use, even in healthy patients. From the standpoint of operating room personnel, the persistence of methoxyflurane within body fat raises some concern about long-term deleterious effects. (See Chapter 5.)
- Methoxyflurane causes marked skeletal muscle relaxation and has considerable analgesic effect. This allows surgery to proceed at relatively light planes of anesthesia, minimizing cardiovascular depression. The analgesic effect of this agent and the relatively slow recovery rate also ensure that recovery from methoxyflurane anesthesia is generally smooth, and patient distress seldom occurs.

Other Chlorofluorocarbon Agents

Enflurane, a volatile gaseous anesthetic used in human medicine, has not found wide acceptance in veterinary anesthesia. Induction and recovery are relatively rapid and smooth, with minimal effects on heart rate and no sensitization of the myocardium to catecholamines. However, enflurane causes profound depression of respiration, and spontaneous ventilation of the patient is poor under this anesthetic. In the dog, enflurane also induces significant muscle hyperactivity, and seizure-like muscle spasms may result.

Sevoflurane and desflurane are recently introduced volatile anesthetic agents that are occasionally used in human medicine. Both agents have a low solubility coefficient and allow rapid induction and recovery. They undergo minimal biotransformation in the liver and are excreted unchanged by the lungs. Both desflurane and sevoflurane are significantly less potent than isoflurane or halothane, with a MAC in dogs of 7.2% and 2.1%, respectively. The cardiovascular and respiratory effects of these agents are similar to those of isoflurane. Unfortunately, both sevoflurane and desflurane have vapor pressures significantly different from those of isoflurane or halothane (160 for sevoflurane and 664 for desflurane, compared with 243 for halothane and 261 for isoflurane), and neither agent can be used in an isoflurane or halothane vaporizer. Sevoflurane can be used in adapted enflurane vaporizers, but desflurane requires its own vaporizer, which is significantly more expensive than vaporizers for halothane or isoflurane. Sevoflurane is also somewhat chemically unstable and reacts with soda lime within the anesthetic machine.

Nitrous Oxide

Physical and pharmacologic properties.   Nitrous oxide (N_2O) is an odorless gas that can be used as an adjunct to anesthesia with other inhalation agents, particularly halothane and methoxyflurane. It is seldom used as the sole anesthetic agent in domestic animals.

The property that limits the use of nitrous oxide in veterinary anesthesia is its lack of potency (that is, a high MAC) in domestic species. The MAC of nitrous oxide in humans is approximately 100%, whereas the MAC in the dog and horse is close to 200% and in the cat is approximately 250%. As these figures demonstrate, it is impossible to achieve a surgical plane of anesthesia in a healthy dog or cat using nitrous oxide alone.

Other properties of nitrous oxide can be summarized as follows:

- The use of nitrous oxide with another inhalation anesthetic (such as halothane) usually allows the anesthetist to lower the concentration of the other agent being administered. Nitrous oxide reduces the MAC (and therefore the vaporizer setting) of other anesthetics by 20% to 30%. This reduces the toxicity of the anesthetic agents and allows faster recoveries. Nitrous oxide also has been shown to speed the uptake of other anesthetic gases into the bloodstream by the "second gas effect" when used at high concentrations (50% to 70% of the total gas flow).
- Nitrous oxide has an extremely low solubility coefficient and is associated with rapid induction and recovery rates. It is therefore a helpful addition to slow-acting agents such as methoxyflurane. It does little to enhance anesthesia with rapid-acting agents such as isoflurane.
- Nitrous oxide has little effect on the cardiovascular, respiratory, hepatic, or urinary systems and is considered to have a wide margin of safety. Nitrous oxide offers good analgesia and excellent muscle relaxation.

Despite these advantages, the use of nitrous oxide in veterinary anesthesia has declined in recent years. One reason is the increased cost of N_2O anesthesia, compared with anesthesia using an inhalation agent alone. Another reason is the increased use of isoflurane, which provides rapid induction and recovery even without the concurrent use of nitrous oxide.

Special precautions.   The use of nitrous oxide is associated with several potential problems, including the following:

Risk of hypoxia.   The use of nitrous oxide in an anesthetic machine limits the amount of oxygen that is delivered to the patient to the extent that nitrous oxide replaces oxygen in the circuit. Since the minimal amount of nitrous oxide necessary to achieve analgesic effects is 50% (and values of 60% to 66% are recommended), the use of this agent decreases the amount of oxygen delivered to the patient by 50% to 66%. The anesthetist must ensure at all times that at least 30 ml/kg/minute of oxygen is delivered to the patient and that the oxygen content of the inspired gases is at least 33%. This can be achieved by ensuring that the nitrous oxide flow (in liters per minute) is no more than twice the oxygen flow and that oxygen flow rates less than 300 ml/minute are avoided.

The patient breathing nitrous oxide is at increased risk of hypoxia and should be monitored closely for cyanosis, cardiac arrhythmias, and other indications of hypoxia. Because of the risk of hypoxia, animals with preexisting lung disease are poor candidates for N_2O anesthesia. For all patients, care should also be taken when adjusting the flowmeters of the anesthetic machine so that the oxygen controls are not confused with those for nitrous oxide.

Diffusion into air pockets.   Because of its low solubility coefficient, nitrous oxide is able to diffuse into trapped air pockets within the body. This diffusion may result in an increase in the amount of gas within an organ and consequent distension of the organ containing trapped gas. For this reason, the use of nitrous oxide is contraindicated in animals with intestinal obstruction, gastric torsion, pneumothorax, or diaphragmatic hernia.

Use in closed anesthesia systems.   Nitrous oxide should never be used in a closed anesthetic circuit. (That is, one with low oxygen flow rates and no pop-off or other waste gas exhaust; see Chapter 4.) As oxygen is removed from a closed system by the animal, the level of nitrous oxide in the circuit may increase to dangerous levels, resulting in hypoxia.

Diffusion hypoxia.   During recovery from anesthesia, nitrous oxide will readily exit from the body via the respiratory system. Because of the rapid outpouring of nitrous oxide into the lungs, a state of "diffusion hypoxia" may be created. In this condition, oxygen molecules normally found in the alveoli are displaced by the large numbers of nitrous oxide molecules exiting from the body. Diffusion hypoxia can be prevented by keeping the animal on high oxygen flow rates for at least 5 minutes after the nitrous oxide has been turned off and ensuring that the animal is frequently bagged with pure oxygen.

Waste anesthetic gas hazards.   Exposure of operating room personnel to waste nitrous oxide has been linked to several health disorders. (See Chapter 5.)

■ AGENTS USED IN THE POSTANESTHETIC PERIOD

Two classes of drugs, reversing agents and analeptics, are available to hasten recovery after anesthesia. An *analeptic agent* is a drug that causes general CNS stimulation. The most commonly used analeptic agent is doxapram. A *reversing agent* is a drug that negates the effect of a specific anesthetic or preanesthetic agent (usually by competing with the anesthetic for specific receptor sites). Several reversing agents are discussed in Chapter 1.

Although useful, these drugs should not be substituted for careful anesthetic technique. The anesthetist should rely primarily on precise control of anesthetic depth to ensure rapid and smooth patient recovery. However, the use of reversing agents and analeptics in selected patients may be a valuable addition to an anesthetic protocol.

Doxapram

Doxapram (Dopram) is a respiratory stimulant and analeptic agent. When given intravenously, doxapram will increase respiratory rate and depth and may accelerate arousal from barbiturate or inhalation anesthesia. The required dose is much greater for patients that have undergone injectable anesthesia than it is for patients recovering from inhalation anesthesia. Although doxapram has a wide margin of safety, it may cause tachycardia and arrhythmias in some patients and should be used with caution in animals with cardiac disease. Doxapram must be used only in the presence of adequate oxygen levels in the brain; otherwise CNS damage may result.

Doxapram is particularly useful for stimulating respiration in newborn puppies and kittens delivered by cesarean section: two or three drops placed under the tongue may greatly increase respiration rate and depth.

✔ **KEY POINTS**

1. Injectable anesthetics are eliminated by redistribution, liver metabolism, and renal excretion. Inhalation anesthetics are eliminated primarily by exhalation from the lungs. Some inhalation anesthetics are also subject to liver metabolism and renal excretion.
2. Both injectable and inhalation anesthetics have a wide margin of safety; however, most agents have depressant effects on the cardiovascular, respiratory, and thermoregulatory systems.
3. Injectable anesthetics include barbiturates, cyclohexamines, neuroleptanalgesic agents, propofol, and etomidate.
4. Several classes of barbiturates are available for veterinary anesthesia, including short-acting barbiturates such as pentobarbital, ultrashort-acting barbiturates such as thiopental, and methylated oxybarbiturates such as methohexital. These classes differ in their lipid solubility, duration of effect, and distribution within the body.
5. Barbiturates are used most commonly as induction agents and are normally administered by titration to achieve the minimum effective dose.
6. Barbiturates may cause respiratory depression and respiratory acidosis. Other adverse side effects include tissue necrosis (when injected perivascularly), cardiac arrhythmias, and excitement during anesthetic induction and/or recovery.
7. Barbiturates show unusual potency in patients that are acidotic, hypoproteinemic, or hypotensive. They may cause prolonged sleeping times in sighthounds.
8. Pentobarbital can be given intravenously or intramuscularly to achieve anesthesia, but it is seldom recommended because poor muscle relaxation, lack of analgesia, respiratory depression, and prolonged recoveries are associated with its use.

9. Thiobarbiturates have a rapid onset of action and short duration and are well suited as induction agents for dogs and cats. Transient apnea may be seen during induction. Methohexital is an alternative agent for use in sighthounds.

10. Cyclohexamine agents such as ketamine and tiletamine produce a state of dissociative anesthesia characterized by exaggerated reflex responses, central nervous system excitement, apneustic respiration, tachycardia, and increased muscle tone. These agents may be given by intramuscular injection in cats or intravenous injection in cats or dogs. Concurrent use of a tranquilizer (such as diazepam, zolazepam, acepromazine, or xylazine) is recommended to promote muscle relaxation and to prevent excitement during recovery. Anticholinergic agents commonly are used to prevent excessive salivation.

11. Neuroleptanalgesia is a profound hypnotic state produced by the administration of an opioid and a tranquilizing agent. These agents provide safe induction in debilitated patients.

12. Propofol is a recently introduced induction agent that has a wide margin of safety and can be given by repeat injection to maintain anesthesia.

13. The four inhalation agents in common use are halothane, isoflurane, methoxyflurane, and nitrous oxide. Each of these agents is administered by means of an anesthetic machine and either a mask or an endotracheal tube. These agents enter the body by absorption through the alveolus, at a rate that depends on the solubility coefficient of the agent and the concentration gradient between the alveolar air and the blood.

14. Anesthetic agents vary in their solubility coefficient, vapor pressure, and minimum alveolar concentration (MAC). These physical properties affect the speed of induction and recovery, the type of vaporizer that should be used, and the vaporizer setting that is required for anesthesia.

15. All inhalation anesthetics may cause respiratory depression and decrease blood pressure. In addition, halothane may potentiate cardiac arrhythmias. Of the commonly used chlorofluorocarbon agents, isoflurane is considered to have the greatest margin of safety and the shortest induction and recovery times.

16. Isoflurane is eliminated almost entirely through respiration. Halothane and methoxyflurane undergo some hepatic metabolism and renal excretion as well as respiratory elimination.

17. Methoxyflurane has some analgesic properties and usually produces slow, uneventful recoveries. Its high degree of lipid retention (and subsequent metabolism and excretion) has raised some concerns regarding the toxicity of waste gas vapors to health care personnel.

18. Nitrous oxide has few cardiovascular or respiratory side effects and is a useful adjunct to halothane or methoxyflurane anesthesia. It is too weak to be used as a sole anesthetic agent in animals. The anesthetist must be aware of the risk of hypoxia associated with this agent, particularly in the period immediately after discontinuation of the agent.

19. Reversing agents and analeptics may be given after anesthesia to hasten anesthetic recovery. Doxapram is a nonspecific respiratory stimulant that may accelerate arousal from barbiturate or inhalation anesthesia.

REVIEW QUESTIONS

1. Barbiturate drugs have a pH that is:
   a. Strongly alkaline (>9.5)
   b. Strongly acidic (<2)
   c. Close to normal body pH
2. Drugs that are highly fat soluble are likely to be taken up by the brain more quickly than drugs that are not fat soluble.
   True   False
3. Which of the following is an example of a dissociative anesthetic?
   a. Thiopental sodium
   b. Pentobarbital sodium
   c. Ketamine hydrochloride
   d. Propofol
4. One of the disadvantages of the drug methohexital is that animals that are anesthetized with it often may demonstrate excitement during recovery.
   True   False
5. Metabolism and elimination of ketamine hydrochloride are the same in the dog as they are in the cat.
   True   False
6. Compared with methoxyflurane, halothane is considered to have a:
   a. Higher vapor pressure
   b. Similar vapor pressure
   c. Lower vapor pressure
7. Halothane may sensitize the heart to catecholamines.
   True   False
8. Halothane is moderately soluble in rubber, which may result in release of this gas from anesthetic equipment.
   True   False
9. An anesthetic agent that has a low solubility coefficient will result in _____ induction and recovery time.
   a. Slow
   b. Moderate
   c. Fast
10. An example of a volatile anesthetic with a high solubility coefficient is:
    a. Halothane
    b. Isoflurane
    c. Enflurane
    d. Methoxyflurane
11. As a rough guideline, to safely maintain a surgical plane of anesthesia, the vaporizer should be set at _____ × MAC.
    a. 0.5
    b. 1
    c. 1.5
    d. 2
    e. 2.5

12. Isoflurane is a more potent cardiac depressant than halothane.

    True   False

13. A patient known to have pulmonary dysfunction would be considered a (an) _____ candidate to receive nitrous oxide.

    a. Excellent
    b. Good
    c. Fair
    d. Poor

14. To be considered effective, nitrous oxide should be used in concentrations of:

    a. 20%
    b. 40%
    c. 60%
    d. 90%
    e. None of the above percentages are correct

For the following questions, more than one answer may be correct.

15. The depressant effects that barbiturates have on the vital centers of the body are less likely to occur if:

    a. Only a dilute (for example, 2%) solution is used
    b. Injection of the drug is not too rapid (greater than 10 seconds)
    c. Only a concentrated solution (4% or greater) is used
    d. None of the above are correct

16. Effects that halothane may have on the body include:

    a. Vasodilation
    b. Nystagmus
    c. Sensitization of myocardium to catecholamines
    d. Depression of myocardial cells
    e. Respiratory depression

17. Effects that barbiturates may have on the body include:

    a. Reduction of respiratory rate
    b. Tachycardia
    c. Cardiac arrhythmias
    d. Decreased blood pressure

18. The concentration of barbiturate entering the brain is affected by a variety of factors such as:

    a. Perfusion of the brain
    b. Lipid solubility of the drug
    c. Plasma protein levels
    d. Blood pH of the animal

19. Effects that are commonly seen after administration of a cyclohexamine drug include:

    a. Increased blood pressure
    b. Increased heart rate
    c. Increased CSF pressure
    d. Increased ocular pressure

20. Effects that isoflurane may have on the body include:
    a. Hepatic toxicity
    b. Accumulation in body fat stores
    c. Depression of respiration
    d. Convulsions during recovery
21. MAC will vary with:
    a. Temperature of the patient
    b. Age of the patient
    c. Species
    d. Anesthetic agent
22. Factors that may affect the speed of the induction process with a volatile gaseous anesthetic include:
    a. Solubility coefficient of the agent
    b. Concentration of the agent
    c. MAC of the agent
    d. Concurrent use of atropine
23. Nitrous oxide may be included as part of an anesthetic protocol because it:
    a. Has good analgesic properties
    b. Will reduce the amount of volatile anesthetic needed
    c. Has minimal depressant effects on the respiratory or cardiovascular centers
    d. Can replace oxygen in the anesthetic circuit
24. When pentobarbital sodium is used as an anesthetic, which of the following may be noted:
    a. Relatively slow onset of action
    b. Respiratory depression
    c. Poor analgesia
    d. Slow recovery
    e. Easily reversed
25. Which of the following drugs may be safely given IM or IV in a cat?
    a. Thiopental sodium
    b. Telazol
    c. Ketamine hydrochloride
    d. Methohexital sodium

Answers for Chapter 3

1. a	**2.** True	**3.** c	**4.** True	**5.** False	**6.** a	**7.** True
8. True	**9.** c	**10.** d	**11.** c	**12.** False	**13.** d	**14.** c
15. a, b	**16.** a, c, d, e	**17.** a, c, d	**18.** a, b, c, d	**19.** a, b, c, d		
20. c	**21.** a, b, c, d	**22.** a, b	**23.** a, b, c	**24.** a, b, c, d	**25.** b, c	

Selected Readings

HASKINS SC: Opinions in small animal anesthesia, *Vet Clin North Am Small Anim Pract* 22(2): 326-469, 1992.

MAMA K: New drugs in feline anesthesia, Compendium Small Animal 20(2):125-138, 1998.

McKELVEY D: Halothane, isoflurane, and methoxyflurane: physical properties and pharmacology, *Vet Tech* 12(1):21-28, 1991.

MUIR WW III, HUBBELL JAE: *Handbook of veterinary anesthesia*, ed 2, St Louis, 1995, Mosby.

PADDLEFORD RR: *Manual of small animal anesthesia*, New York, 1988, Churchill Livingstone.

SHORT CE: *Principles and practice of veterinary anesthesia*, Baltimore, 1987, Williams & Wilkins.

STEFFEY EP, WOLINER MJ, HOWLAND D: Accuracy of isoflurane delivery by halothane-specific vaporizers, *Am J Vet Res* 44(6):1072-1078, 1983.

WARREN RG: *Small animal anesthesia*, St Louis, 1983, Mosby.

WEAVER BM, RAPTOPOULOS D: Induction of anesthesia in dogs and cats with propofol, *Vet Rec* 126(25):617-620, 1990.

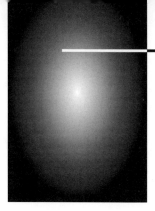

CHAPTER 4

Anesthetic Equipment

PERFORMANCE OBJECTIVES

After completion of this chapter, the reader will be able to:

- Identify equipment that is used for the induction and maintenance of general anesthesia in the dog or cat.
- Differentiate among the various types of endotracheal tubes and list the advantages and disadvantages of each.
- List the advantages and disadvantages of cuffed versus noncuffed tubes.
- Describe the functions and components of an anesthetic machine.
- Trace the flow of oxygen through an anesthetic machine and patient breathing circuit.
- State the difference between a rebreathing and a nonrebreathing system with regard to equipment, airflow pattern, and indications for use.
- Understand the advantages and disadvantages of both rebreathing and nonrebreathing systems.
- Differentiate between a precision and nonprecision vaporizer, and recognize the advantages and disadvantages of each.
- Understand the importance of flow rates as they relate to anesthetic concentration within the breathing circuit, type of circuit created (that is, closed versus open), safety for the patient, and waste gas production.
- Understand the advantages and disadvantages of low-flow anesthesia and how it differs from conventional anesthesia.
- Explain the procedure that should be followed in preparing an anesthetic machine for use.
- Describe the proper maintenance procedures for anesthetic machines and associated equipment.

B efore the introduction of anesthetic machines, administration of anesthesia was a relatively hazardous undertaking. Anesthetic liquids such as ether or chloroform were poured onto a cloth that was then held over the patient's nose and mouth until the desired depth of anesthesia was achieved. Alternatively, the patient was sometimes required to inhale vapors rising from a jar of liquid anesthetic. The development of modern anesthetic equipment allowed the administration of precise amounts of anesthetic under controlled conditions, greatly increasing the safety and convenience of inhalation anesthesia.

This chapter describes the function and use of anesthetic equipment as well as the maintenance procedures that are likely to be the responsibility of the veterinary technician in practice.

■ EQUIPMENT NEEDED FOR ANESTHESIA

Useful equipment for routine intravenous (IV) induction and inhalation anesthesia includes the following:

- Syringes and needles for administering preanesthetic and induction agents
- Alcohol and absorbent cotton
- Plain (nonstretch) gauze for tying endotracheal tube
- Syringe for inflating endotracheal tube cuff
- Laryngoscope
- Endotracheal tubes
- Stylet for small endotracheal tubes
- Electric clipper
- Intravenous catheter, administration set, and IV fluid bag
- Lubricating gel for endotracheal tubes (gel containing a local analgesic may be preferred for use in cats)
- Lidocaine spray (for use in cats)
- Ophthalmic ointment or drops
- Face mask
- Inhalation anesthesia machine with oxygen (O_2) and nitrous oxide (N_2O) tanks
- Machine connections, including hoses, Y piece, nonrebreathing circuit
- Reservoir bag
- Cylinder wrench
- Ventilator (if controlled ventilation is required)
- Emergency drugs (contained in crash kit)
- Towels, blankets, or other means of conserving patient's body heat
- Stethoscope, thermometer, penlight, and other monitoring devices
- Scavenging system
- Form for anesthesia record (if required)

Of the many types of equipment listed above, only two will be discussed in detail in this chapter: endotracheal tubes and the anesthetic machine.

Endotracheal Tubes

Many types of endotracheal tubes are available for veterinary anesthesia. Tubes used in small animal practice are usually made of rubber, vinyl plastic, or silicone rubber. *Rubber* endotracheal tubes (which are red) are relatively inexpensive and common in veterinary practice. The technician should be aware of some potential problems associated with their use, including the following:

- Rubber tubes may absorb disinfectant solutions, causing the outer surface of the tube to become dry and cracked after prolonged use.

Murphy eye

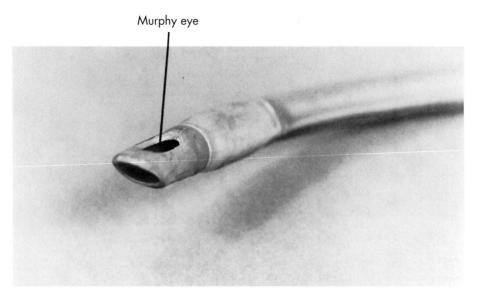

FIG. 4-1   Close-up of a Murphy endotracheal tube showing eye. (From Warren RG: *Small animal anesthesia,* St Louis, 1983, Mosby.)

- Rubber tubes are extremely flexible, and kinking or collapse of the tube is a potential hazard, particularly for small tubes. Specialized rubber tubes, called spiral or anode tubes, contain a coil of metal or nylon embedded in the rubber. These tubes are flexible but resist kinking or collapse from external pressure.

Tubes made of transparent *vinyl plastic* are also used in veterinary anesthesia. These tubes are less porous than rubber and resist cracking. But because they are less flexible than rubber, they tend to become stiff with age.

Silicone rubber tubes, although expensive, are well suited to veterinary anesthesia. They are smooth, flexible, and less irritating to tissues than either rubber or vinyl plastic tubes.

Whether manufactured from rubber, silicone rubber, or vinyl plastic, endotracheal tubes are available in several shapes and sizes. Two types of tubes are used in veterinary practice, the Murphy tube and the Magill tube. Both have a beveled (slanted) end, but they differ in that the Murphy tube has an eye near the bevel whereas the Magill tube does not (Fig. 4-1). The eye helps prevent complete obstruction of the tube if the bevel is plugged by mucus or by the tracheal wall.

Unfortunately, several different systems of size classification have been used in the past, and this has led to some confusion when selecting tubes (Table 4-1). The classification used most commonly is based on the internal diameter of the tube as expressed in millimeters. The internal diameter of each tube is written on its surface (Fig. 4-2). Endotracheal tubes ranging from 5 to 18 mm are suitable for use in dogs (Table 4-2). The endotracheal tubes used most commonly in cats are those with

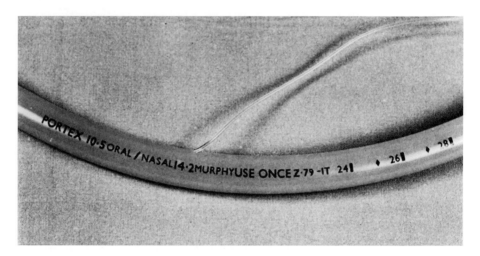

FIG. 4-2   Detail of endotracheal tube with internal diameter of 10.5 mm. (From Warren RG: *Small animal anesthesia,* St Louis, 1983, Mosby.)

TABLE 4-1

A Comparison of Three Systems Used to Classify Endotracheal Tubes

Magill Scale	French Scale	Internal Diameter Scale (mm)
00	13	4
0	16	5
	18	
1	20	
2	22	6
3	24	7
4	26	8
5	28	
6		9
7	30	10
8	32	11
9	34	12
10	36	

Modified from Warren RG: *Small animal anesthesia,* St Louis, 1989, Mosby.

internal diameters of 3, 3.5, 4, and 4.5 mm. Very small animals may be more easily intubated with a special type of tube called a Cole catheter.

Tubes may be labeled *oral* or *nasal* according to their intended use in humans; however, endotracheal tubes are almost always passed orally in small animals to avoid damage to the sensitive nasal turbinates (the scroll-shaped passages within the nose).

Endotracheal tubes may be obtained with or without cuffs. By inflating a cuff with air, the anesthetist can obtain an airtight seal between the endotracheal tube and the trachea. The use of cuffed tubes offers three advantages over tubes without cuffs:

TABLE 4-2

Guide for Selection of Veterinary Endotracheal Tubes According to Body Weight

Body Weight (kg)	Internal Diameter (mm)
CATS	
2	3
4	4
6	4.5
DOGS	
2	5
4	6
7	7
9	7-8
12	8
14	9-10
16-20	10-11
30	12
40	14-16

Modified from Warren RG: *Small animal anesthesia,* St Louis, 1989, Mosby.

1. The airtight cuff helps prevent leakage of waste gas around the tube and therefore reduces operating room pollution.
2. Use of cuffed tubes reduces the risk of aspiration of blood, saliva, vomitus, and other material into the lungs.
3. Animals intubated with cuffed tubes are prevented from breathing room air, which may otherwise enter the breathing passages by flowing around the outside of the tube. Animals breathing significant amounts of room air are difficult to maintain at adequate anesthetic depth because room air dilutes the anesthetic vapor.

Despite these advantages, cuffed tubes should be used with caution, especially in small patients. The cuff of the tube may exert significant pressure on the tracheal mucosa and cause local necrosis, particularly after prolonged use.

The use of endotracheal tubes is outlined in detail in Chapter 2.

Anesthetic Machines

Function.   The anesthetic machine (Fig. 4-3) is designed to deliver a volatile gaseous anesthetic (usually halothane, isoflurane, or methoxyflurane) to and from a patient by means of a circuit of corrugated tubing. The anesthetic is contained within a carrier gas, which is either oxygen alone or oxygen in combination with nitrous oxide.

To achieve this result, the anesthetic machine must perform several important functions, including the following:

- It must deliver oxygen (with or without nitrous oxide) at a controlled flow rate.
- It must vaporize a designated concentration of liquid anesthetic (usually isoflurane, halothane, or methoxyflurane), mix it with oxygen (and nitrous oxide, if used), and deliver the resulting mixture to the patient.

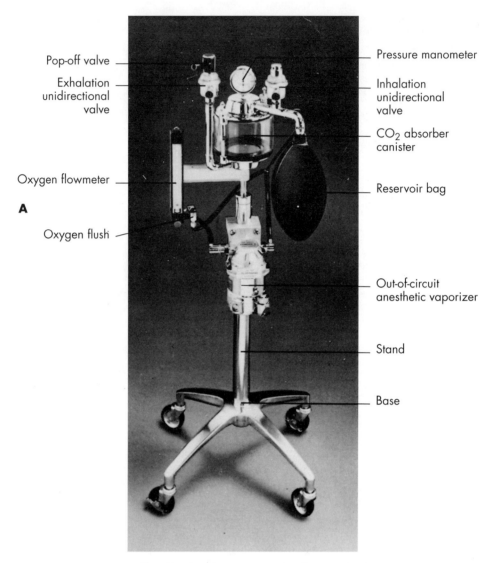

Pop-off valve

Exhalation
unidirectional
valve

Oxygen flowmeter

A

Oxygen flush

Pressure manometer

Inhalation
unidirectional
valve

CO₂ absorber
canister

Reservoir bag

Out-of-circuit
anesthetic vaporizer

Stand

Base

FIG. 4-3   A, Basic inhalation anesthesia machine with an out-of-circuit precision vaporizer.
A, B, and **C** from Warren RG: *Small animal anesthesia,* St Louis, 1983, Mosby.)

- It must move exhaled gases away from the patient and either dispose of them through a scavenging system or recirculate them to the patient. If the exhaled gases are recirculated, the machine must remove carbon dioxide before returning the gases to the patient.

Anesthetic machines are used not only for inhalation anesthesia but also as a means of delivering oxygen to critical patients. In these situations, the machine is used with the vaporizer (that is, the anesthetic source) turned off, and the hoses deliver oxygen to a mask held over the patient's face (or to an endotracheal tube, if the patient has been intubated).

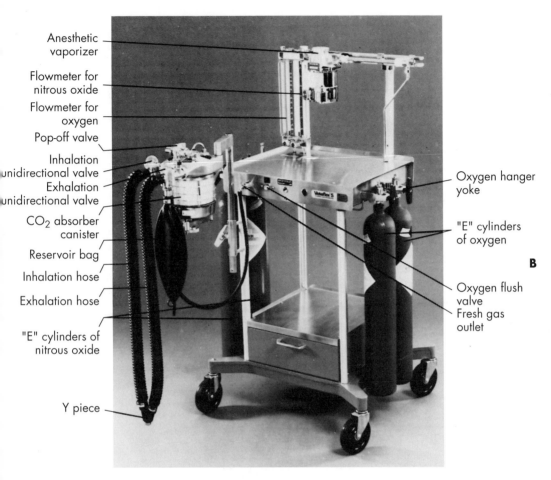

Anesthetic vaporizer

Flowmeter for nitrous oxide

Flowmeter for oxygen

Pop-off valve

Inhalation unidirectional valve

Exhalation unidirectional valve

CO$_2$ absorber canister

Reservoir bag

Inhalation hose

Exhalation hose

"E" cylinders of nitrous oxide

Y piece

Oxygen hanger yoke

"E" cylinders of oxygen

B

Oxygen flush valve

Fresh gas outlet

FIG. 4-3 cont'd   **B,** Two-gas inhalation anesthesia machine with out-of-circuit precision vaporizer for methoxyflurane.

Components.   The components of an anesthetic machine and the way in which an anesthetic machine works can best be understood by following the path of oxygen starting with the oxygen tank, passing through the machine to the patient, and returning again to the machine. For the sake of clarity, one type of anesthetic setup (that is, the circle system using a precision vaporizer) will be described. This system is illustrated schematically in Fig. 4-4.

Gas cylinders.   Oxygen must be continuously supplied to every patient throughout anesthesia. Anesthetic machines provide up to 100% oxygen (compared with room air, which contains approximately 20% oxygen). The high concentration of oxygen is desirable for two reasons:

1. The anesthetized patient has a higher metabolic requirement for oxygen than the normal awake animal.
2. The anesthetized patient has a reduced tidal volume compared with the awake animal, and the amount of air taken in with each breath is therefore smaller.

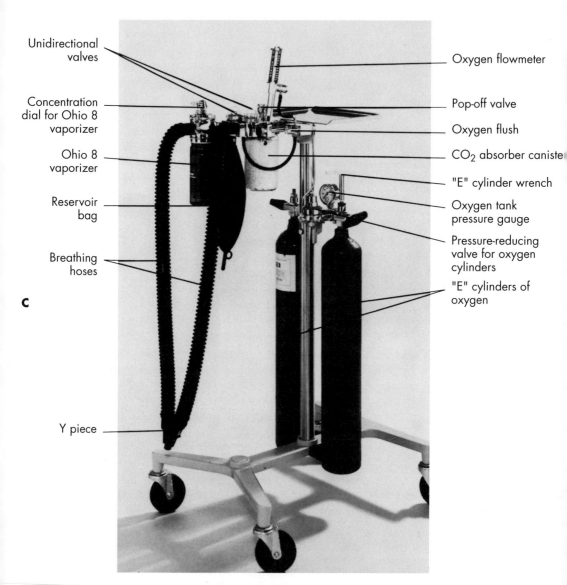

Unidirectional valves

Concentration dial for Ohio 8 vaporizer

Ohio 8 vaporizer

Reservoir bag

Breathing hoses

Oxygen flowmeter

Pop-off valve

Oxygen flush

CO$_2$ absorber canister

"E" cylinder wrench

Oxygen tank pressure gauge

Pressure-reducing valve for oxygen cylinders

"E" cylinders of oxygen

C

Y piece

FIG. 4-3 cont'd   C, Inhalation anesthesia machine with an Ohio No. 8 glass jar vaporizer for methoxyflurane.

This combination of increased oxygen requirement and decreased tidal volume may result in hypoxia if high concentrations of oxygen are not provided, using either 100% oxygen or a mixture of oxygen and nitrous oxide.

Oxygen flow from the machine to the patient not only meets the metabolic requirements of the animal but also carries the anesthetic to the patient. Anesthetic machines are designed so that no liquid anesthetic can be delivered to the patient unless oxygen is present to act as a carrier gas.

Oxygen used for anesthesia is obtained as a compressed gas contained in metal cylinders. The gas is held under pressure in the cylinder (tank) in order that a large

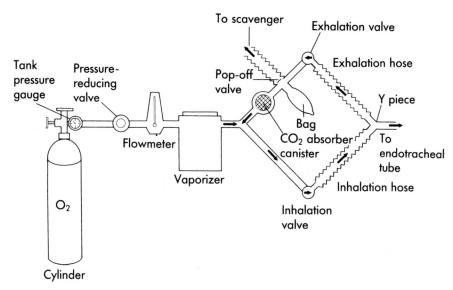

FIG. 4-4   Schematic of anesthetic machine (circle system, vaporizer out of circle). (Redrawn from Hartsfield SN: Machines and breathing systems for administration of inhalation anesthetics. In Short CE [editor]: *Principles and practice of veterinary anesthesia,* Baltimore, 1987, Williams & Wilkins.)

TABLE 4-3			
Capacity of Compressed Gas Cylinders			
Cylinder Dimensions	**Empty Weight (kg)**	**Capacity (Liters of Oxygen)**	**Capacity (Liters of Nitrous Oxide)**
E Cylinder	5.9	659	1590
4.25 inches OD* × 26 inches			
G Cylinder	50	5331	13,836
8.5 inches OD × 51 inches			
H Cylinder	59	5570-7500	15,899
9.25 inches OD × 51 inches			

Modified from Warren RG: *Small animal anesthesia,* St Louis, 1989, Mosby.
*Outside diameter.

amount of gas may be stored in a relatively small container. These cylinders may be small, in which case they are usually attached to the anesthetic machine (E cylinders are illustrated in Fig. 4-3). Large cylinders, which stand separately from the machine (Fig. 4-5), are also available. The capacities of several types of cylinders are given in Table 4-3.

Oxygen flow into the machine occurs when the outlet valve on the top of the gas cylinder is opened in a counterclockwise direction (that is, to the left). The flow is discontinued when the valve is turned completely clockwise (that is, to the right). The mnemonic "left loose, right tight" has been used by several generations of anesthesia students as an aid in remembering these facts.

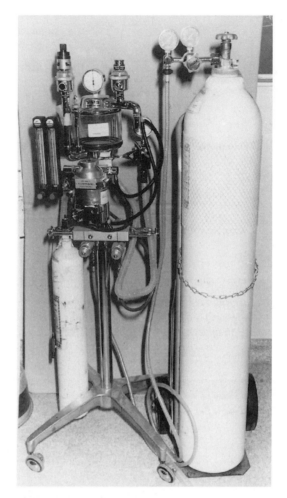

FIG. 4-5   Large cylinder connected to anesthetic machine.

Many anesthetic machines are designed to provide not only oxygen but also nitrous oxide gas. Like oxygen, nitrous oxide is contained in a compressed gas cylinder. This may be a large freestanding tank or a smaller tank attached to the machine. Some machines have a device that discontinues nitrous oxide administration to the patient if the oxygen flow is cut off. This mechanism prevents inadvertent asphyxiation of the patient, which could occur if the patient breathed nitrous oxide in the absence of oxygen.

Gas cylinders that are part of the anesthetic machine are attached to it by a yoke (Fig. 4-6), whereas freestanding cylinders are connected to the machine by gas lines. Gas lines may take the form of flexible hose, or gas may be carried in pipes mounted within a wall.

Anesthetic machines are designed so that it is difficult or impossible to attach the wrong type of gas cylinder to the machine connections. The yokes for each gas are

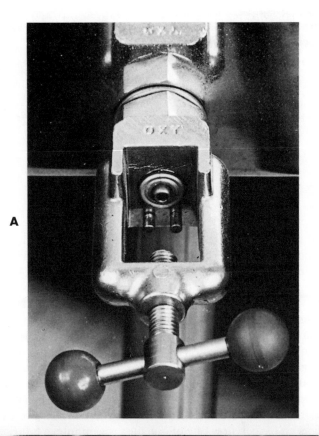

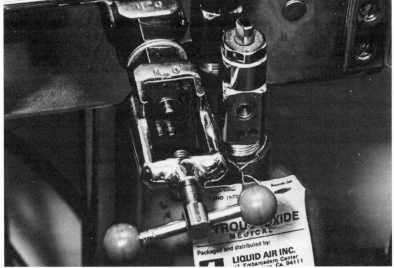

FIG. 4-6   Yokes, showing pin indexing. **A,** Pins for oxygen tank. **B,** Pins for nitrous oxide tank. (From Warren RG: *Small animal anesthesia,* St Louis, 1983, Mosby.)

TABLE 4-4

Characteristics of Compressed Gas Cylinders

Gas	Formula	Color	Full Tank Pressure psi and kPa @ 21°C	Pressure (psi and kPa) at Which Tank Should Be Changed	State Within Cylinder
Oxygen	O_2	White or Green	2200-2650 psi 15,000-18,000 kPa	100-200 psi 680-1360 kPa	Gas
Nitrous oxide	N_2O	Blue	760 psi 5170 kPa	500 psi 3400 kPa	Liquid/Gas

Modified from Warren RG: *Small animal anesthesia,* St Louis, 1989, Mosby.

equipped with a pin system so that an oxygen cylinder, for example, cannot be put on a nitrous oxide yoke. (See Fig. 4-6.) In addition, cylinders and gas lines are color–coded to prevent inadvertent delivery of an incorrect gas. Oxygen cylinders are white or green and nitrous oxide cylinders are blue (Table 4-4).

Cylinders are designed to store large quantities of gas under pressure. The volume (in liters) of oxygen present in any E cylinder can be calculated by multiplying the pressure (in pounds per square inch [psi]) by 0.3. For a full cylinder of oxygen, the pressure is approximately 2200 psi (15,000 kilopascals [kPa]) indicating that 660 liters of oxygen gas (that is, 0.3×2200 psi) is contained in the tank. A reading of 1100 psi (7500 kPa) indicates the tank is approximately half full and therefore contains approximately 330 liters of oxygen. The volume of the oxygen in the tank indicates to the anesthetist how much longer the tank can be used. For example, if the anesthetist selects an oxygen flow rate of one liter per minute, a full E tank containing 660 liters of oxygen will last approximately 11 hours (that is, 660 minutes), and a half-full tank will last approximately 5½ hours (that is, 330 minutes).

The pressure of oxygen being delivered by any given tank is indicated by a pressure gauge attached to the cylinder (Fig. 4-7, *A* and *B*). The pressure gauge will read zero when the tank is empty. It also reads zero when the tank is turned off and the remaining gas in the line has been evacuated (that is, "bled off"). When the tank valve is opened (that is, the tank is turned on), the gauge reading rises to indicate the pressure of gas remaining in the tank.

During use, oxygen is gradually released from the tank; the pressure within the tank falls, as indicated by the reading on the pressure gauge. The anesthetist may notice a considerable drop in indicated pressure during a lengthy anesthesia. The anesthetist must, of course, periodically monitor the oxygen tank pressure gauge during each procedure and change the tank when the valve indicates the tank is close to empty. Because of the gradual way in which oxygen tank pressure falls, the anesthetist can rely on the gauge to roughly indicate the amount of oxygen remaining. Usually it is not necessary to change oxygen tanks until the pressure drops below 100 to 200 psi (680 to 1360 kPa), indicating only 30 to 60 liters of oxygen remaining in the tank. Tanks should be changed between procedures (not during) if possible.

Nitrous oxide is also stored in compressed air tanks, although at considerably less pressure than oxygen. The normal pressure for a full nitrous oxide tank is 770 psi

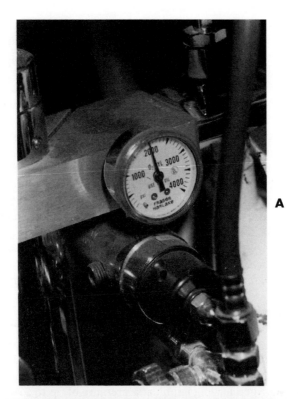

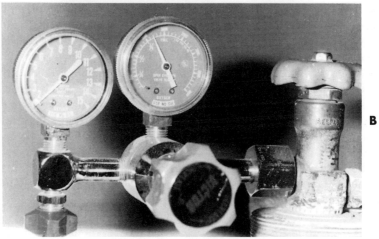

FIG. 4-7   Tank pressure gauges. **A,** Tank pressure gauge for E tank attached to anesthetic machine. **B,** Flowmeter (left) and tank pressure gauge (right) for freestanding oxygen tank.

(5170 kPa). Unlike oxygen, nitrous oxide is present in both the liquid and gas states within the pressurized tank. The pressure gauge reads only the pressure of the gas within the tank and not that of the liquid. As the gas leaves the tank, more liquid evaporates and enters the gas state. As a result, the pressure of the gas within the tank will not change until all of the liquid has evaporated. The anesthetist therefore should not expect the nitrous oxide tank gauge reading to change—even after several hours of anesthesia—unless the tank is close to empty. It follows that the pressure gauge reading on a nitrous oxide tank will not tell the anesthetist how full the tank is. This information can only be determined by weighing the tank before use. An E cylinder of nitrous oxide weighs approximately 8 kg (18 lb) when full and about 5.9 kg (13 lb) when empty. The full and empty weights are normally stamped on the outside of each cylinder.

The anesthetist is usually not concerned with the exact amount of nitrous oxide present in the tank. But the anesthetist must be aware when the tank is close to empty and a tank change is required. Because liquid nitrous oxide is continually evaporating and maintaining the pressure of gas in the tank, the gauge reading does not fall until the liquid nitrous oxide is exhausted and the tank is nearly empty. Therefore, nitrous oxide tanks should be changed as soon as the pressure gauge starts to drop below 500 psi (3400 kPa).

As a gas moves from a high-pressure tank into the anesthetic machine, the pressure is lowered by a pressure-reducing valve, also called a pressure regulator. The use of a pressure-reducing valve allows a constant flow of gas into the machine regardless of the pressure changes within the tank and provides a safe operating pressure for the machine. Oxygen leaving a tank at a pressure of up to 2200 psi (15,000 kPa) is reduced to a pressure of 50 psi (340 kPa) before entering the anesthetic machine.

Flowmeter.   From the cylinder, the pressure gauge, and the pressure-reducing valve, oxygen travels through a low-pressure hose to a flowmeter. (See Figs. 4-3 and 4-4.) The flowmeter allows the anesthetist to set the gas flow rate, which is the amount of oxygen that travels through the machine to be delivered to the patient. Flow rates are expressed in liters of gas per minute (L/minute). If a machine is set up to use both nitrous oxide and oxygen, it is necessary to have separate flowmeters so that the flow rates of the two gases can be monitored and adjusted separately. Some machines provide two flowmeters for oxygen: one for flow rates greater than 1 L/minute and one to accurately adjust flow rates less than 1 L/minute.

Each flowmeter consists of a dial attached to a glass cylinder of graduated diameter. Within the cylinder is a rotor or ball that indicates the gas flow rate (of either oxygen or nitrous oxide) on a scale that measures liters of gas per minute. Each gas enters the bottom of its respective flowmeter and exits at the top. When the dial is turned, a valve within the flowmeter opens and gas enters the cylinder. The ball or rotor rises, indicating the amount of gas flow. The anesthetist therefore can control the gas flow by adjusting the valve. For flowmeters that have a ball indicator, the center of the ball should be read to determine the flow rate. In the case of a rotor indicator, the reading should be taken at the top of the rotor.

It is the flowmeter, rather than the tank pressure gauge, that indicates the amount of oxygen or nitrous oxide being delivered to the patient. When the anesthetist opens the oxygen tank, the tank pressure gauge will indicate the pressure of gas being released from the tank; however, this does not necessarily mean that the patient receives any oxygen. Oxygen flow through the machine is indicated by the flowmeter. If it is set at zero flow, the patient does not receive any oxygen.

The flowmeters allow the anesthetist to accurately control the relative amounts of oxygen and nitrous oxide received by the animal. If the nitrous oxide flowmeter is set to deliver 2 L/minute of nitrous oxide to the patient and the oxygen flowmeter is adjusted to deliver 1 L/minute of oxygen to the patient, the resulting mixture will be a 2:1 ratio of nitrous oxide to oxygen. (This represents approximately 67% nitrous oxide and 33% oxygen.) Some machines automatically set the O_2 and N_2O proportions, and an adjustment of the flow rate of one gas will automatically change the flow rate of the other.

When using nitrous oxide, the anesthetist should ensure that the nitrous oxide/oxygen ratio never exceeds 3:1, or the patient will receive insufficient oxygen and asphyxiation may result. It is also imperative that a minimum of 30 ml/kg/minute of oxygen flow be delivered throughout anesthesia to any patient receiving a mixture of nitrous oxide and oxygen.

As oxygen or nitrous oxide passes through the flowmeter, the gas pressure is further reduced, from 50 psi (340 kPa) to 15 psi (100 kPa). This pressure is only slightly above atmospheric pressure and is the optimum pressure for passage of gas to the patient.

Vaporizer.   Oxygen gas exits at the top of the oxygen flowmeter and continues through a low-pressure hose to the vaporizer. (See Figs. 4-3 and 4-4.) The function of the vaporizer is to convert a liquid anesthetic such as halothane or isoflurane to a gas state and to add controlled amounts of the vaporized anesthetic to the carrier gases (O_2 and N_2O) flowing through the machine. The vaporized anesthetic can only be released from the vaporizer by dialing a flow of carrier gas, which moves the anesthetic from the vaporizer into the breathing circuit of the anesthetic machine. No anesthetic is delivered to the patient if the flowmeters read zero because there is no flow of carrier gases into the vaporizer. Anesthetic vaporizers are further discussed in a separate section on pages 165-171.

Fresh gas inlet.   After passing through the vaporizer, the oxygen (and nitrous oxide, if used) carrying the vaporized anesthetic enters a low-pressure hose. The anesthetic machine is constructed so that this mixture of gases, commonly known as fresh gas, is not able to return to the vaporizer but will be confined to a series of machine parts arranged in a roughly circular design. These machine parts, consisting of the flutter valves, hoses, CO_2 absorber canister, pop-off valve, and reservoir bag, together make up the anesthetic circuit.

Once fresh gas enters the anesthetic circuit, there are a variety of flow paths, depending on the type of machine used. Most commonly, fresh gas passes first through either the reservoir bag or the inhalation flutter valve.

Reservoir (rebreathing) bag.   Fresh gas entering the circuit is conveyed to an inflatable rubber bag called the reservoir bag or rebreathing bag. (See Figs. 4-3 and 4-4.) This bag is gradually filled as gases enter the circuit and is deflated when the patient breathes in. The bag therefore expands and contracts continuously, reflecting the patient's respirations.

The reservoir bag should have a minimum volume of 60 ml/kg of patient weight. Bags are available in various sizes, from 500 ml (for very small patients) to 30 liters (intended for use in horses). The most common sizes used for small animal anesthesia are 1 liter and 2 liters.

In addition to storing gas, the reservoir bag serves a number of functions including the following:

- It is easier for a patient to breathe from a reservoir bag than to rely solely on a continuous flow of air through a piece of tubing.
- The bag allows the anesthetist to observe the animal's respirations. Both the respiratory rate and the depth of respirations are indicated by the movement of the bag. Inadequate movement of the bag may indicate that the patient is breathing room air rather than gas from the machine. Often this occurs because the endotracheal tube is too small or because the cuff is inadequately inflated and air is passing around the tube. Alternatively, minimal movement of the reservoir bag may indicate that the patient's tidal volume is small, alerting the anesthetist to possible respiratory problems.
- Movement of the bag with the animal's respirations indicates to the anesthetist that the endotracheal tube is within the trachea and not the esophagus, and therefore is a useful check on the location of the endotracheal tube.
- The reservoir bag allows the anesthetist to deliver oxygen (with or without anesthetic) to the patient by means of "bagging." In this procedure the reservoir bag is gently squeezed, forcing oxygen and anesthetic into the patient's lungs and causing the patient's chest to rise slightly. It is advisable to periodically "bag" an anesthetized patient to gently inflate the lungs with fresh oxygen and anesthetic. Use of this technique to manually ventilate the patient is further described in Chapter 7.

There are three reasons why bagging may be beneficial to the anesthetized patient:

1. Bagging helps prevent a condition called *atelectasis,* in which the alveoli in certain sections of the lungs are collapsed and not useful for oxygen and anesthetic transfer to the patient. Bagging the patient helps reinflate the collapsed alveoli.
2. Anesthetized patients have a decreased ability to breathe, and the volume of air inhaled with each breath may be as little as 50% of normal. By bagging the animal, the anesthetist flushes the airways and alveoli with fresh gas, removing air that has increased CO_2 content and reduced anesthetic and oxygen concentration.
3. Bagging may be a lifesaving procedure if the patient is not breathing (a condition called respiratory arrest). Bagging allows the anesthetist to continue to deliver oxygen directly to the lungs and therefore is an effective means of artificial respiration.

The anesthetist should ensure that the reservoir bag is properly inflated during anesthesia. The bag should not be allowed to overfill (assuming the appearance of an inflated beach ball), because this will increase pressure in the breathing circuit (called "back pressure") and make it difficult for the animal to exhale. Additionally, it is difficult to monitor respiration using an overfilled bag. There is also some risk that the excessive pressure may rupture alveoli in the patient's lungs. On the other hand, the bag should not be allowed to empty completely when the animal inhales, because this defeats its purpose, which is to act as a reservoir. Complete emptying of the bag indicates that the amount of gas flow is inadequate, the bag is too small, or that the pop-off valve is open too widely.

Inhalation flutter valve, hoses, Y piece, and exhalation flutter valve.   Fresh gas entering the anesthetic circuit passes through a one-way valve, variously called an inhalation flutter valve or unidirectional valve. (See Figs. 4-3 and 4-4.) The inhalation flutter valve allows gases to flow in only one direction (in this case, toward the patient).

When the patient inhales, the inhalation flutter valve opens, allowing the oxygen and anesthetic to enter the hoses. The gases travel through the inspiratory hose to the Y piece and are directed into the endotracheal tube or mask. Upon reaching the patient's lungs, oxygen and anesthetic molecules are absorbed and enter the bloodstream. At the same time, carbon dioxide and anesthetic molecules are released from the bloodstream, enter the alveoli, and are exhaled on the next breath.

Exhaled gases leave the patient and travel through another hose to reenter the anesthetic machine. At the point at which the exhalation hose attaches to the machine, there is another flutter valve, commonly called the exhalation valve or expiratory unidirectional valve. (See Figs. 4-3 and 4-4.) As with the inhalation valve, this valve controls the direction of gas flow and only allows gases travelling back into the anesthetic machine to pass through. It is important that gas can flow in only one direction through the circuit because this prevents expired gases from returning to the patient without first passing through the CO_2 absorber canister.

Oxygen flush valve.   Many anesthetic machines have a valve marked "oxygen flush." This valve, if depressed, allows oxygen to bypass the flowmeter and vaporizer and enter the machine between the flutter valves, often at the carbon dioxide absorber. Pure oxygen is thereby delivered directly to the anesthetic circuit at a flow rate of 30 to 50 L/minute. This feature is particularly useful when delivering oxygen to a critical patient, and it also can be used to rapidly fill a depleted reservoir bag. The oxygen flush is also useful at the end of the anesthetic period when it allows the anesthetist to add pure oxygen to the system, thereby diluting the residual anesthetic being exhaled by the animal. The oxygen flush should not be used with certain nonrebreathing systems (such as the Bain system) because a high flow rate of oxygen into this type of circuit can seriously damage an animal's lungs.

Pop-off valve.   Almost all anesthetic machine circuits contain a pressure relief valve, usually in the form of a pop-off valve or overflow valve. (See Figs. 4-3 and 4-4.) This valve is similar to a tap in that it can be turned fully open, partly open, or closed off entirely, allowing varying amounts of gas to exit. The pop-off valve is usually kept partly open during anesthesia, allowing some gas to escape. It is closed or nearly closed when the anesthetist wishes to bag the patient or when very low gas flows are used.

The pop-off valve has several uses, including the following:

- Waste gases (for example, oxygen, nitrous oxide, inhalation anesthetic, and carbon dioxide) exit from the anesthetic circuit at this valve and enter the scavenging system.
- By venting excess gas, the pop-off valve prevents the build-up of excessive pressure or volume of gases within the circuit. If allowed to occur, this excess pressure would eventually reach the animal's lungs, causing the alveoli to distend and possibly rupture.
- If the pop-off valve is closed, the anesthetist can increase the pressure of gas present in the circuit, allowing the animal to be bagged.

Carbon dioxide absorber canister.   Any gases that do not exit from the system through the pop-off valve are directed to the carbon dioxide absorber canister before being returned to the patient. (See Figs. 4-3 and 4-4.) Gas may enter the canister through the bottom or the top, depending on the design. The canister contains an absorbing chemical, either soda lime or barium hydroxide lime. In both cases, the absorbing ingredient is calcium hydroxide, $Ca(OH)_2$, which removes carbon dioxide from the gases that percolate through the canister. The chemical reaction that takes place within the canister is as follows:

$$2 CO_2 + Ca(OH)_2 + 2 NaOH \rightarrow Na_2CO_3 + CaCO_3 + 2 H_2O + heat$$

The heat released by this reaction is sufficient to raise the temperature of the carbon dioxide absorber canister, and it may become warm to the touch during use. The water produced by this reaction is captured in a trap that lies immediately below the absorbing granules.

Soda lime and barium hydroxide lime granules do not last indefinitely: after several hours of use the granules become exhausted and will no longer absorb carbon dioxide molecules. The use of depleted granules is not advised because this may result in the delivery of excessive amounts of carbon dioxide to the patient, leading to hypercapnia. There are several ways in which the anesthetist may become aware of granules that are exhausted and must be replaced, including the following:

- Fresh granules, containing mainly $Ca(OH)_2$, can be chipped or crumbled with finger pressure, whereas granules saturated with carbon dioxide (containing mainly $CaCO_3$) become hard and brittle. This test can be used to determine the saturation of the granules before or after the anesthetic procedure.
- The color of the granules may indicate their degree of saturation. Absorber granules contain a pH indicator that causes the granules to change color when they are saturated with carbon dioxide. This color change will vary with the type of granules used: some granules become whiter in appearance when exhausted, whereas other granules are normally white or pink and turn blue when exhausted. The color reaction is time-limited, and granules that have changed color (indicating saturation with carbon dioxide) may return to the original color after a few hours although they are still saturated with carbon dioxide. Thus it is important that the anesthetist remove any granules that have changed color as soon as possible after using an anesthetic machine.

Pressure manometer.   Many machines have a pressure gauge (also called a pressure manometer) situated on top of the carbon dioxide absorber canister (Fig. 4-8). This gauge measures the pressure of the gases within the anesthetic system (expressed in centimeters of water or in millimeters of mercury [mm Hg]). This pressure, in turn, reflects the pressure of the gas in the animal's airway and lungs. Pressures over 15 cm of water (11 mm Hg) indicate a build-up of air within the machine, either because the pop-off valve is not sufficiently open or because the oxygen flow rate is too high.

The pressure manometer is a useful aid when bagging an animal because it indicates the approximate pressure being exerted on the animal's lungs when the anesthetist squeezes the reservoir bag. The pressure should not exceed 15 to 20 cm of water (11 to 15 mm Hg) during bagging.

Negative pressure relief valve.   Some machines have an additional valve called the negative pressure relief valve. This valve is designed to open and admit room air

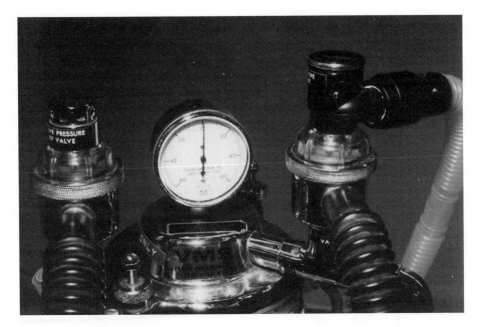

FIG. 4-8   Pressure manometer.

to the circuit if, for some reason, a negative pressure (partial vacuum) is detected in the circuit. This may happen when an active scavenging system is attached to the circuit, particularly if excessive suction is present.

Negative pressure may also develop in the circuit if the oxygen flow rate is too low or if the tank runs out of oxygen. By adding room air to the circuit, the negative pressure relief valve ensures that the patient always receives some oxygen. It is certainly preferable that the patient receive 21% oxygen in room air rather than none at all, as would otherwise be the case if the machine ran out of oxygen.

Vaporizers

Of all the components of the anesthetic machine, the vaporizer is the most complicated and often the most expensive to purchase and service. The function of the vaporizer is to add anesthetic to the carrier gases (that is, either oxygen alone or oxygen plus nitrous oxide) that flow to the patient. Regardless of the type of anesthetic used, it is purchased in liquid form and put into the vaporizer before use. When oxygen passes through the vaporizer, the anesthetic is evaporated and conveyed to the patient as a gas.

Almost all vaporizers have an indicator window at their base that allows the technician to inspect the amount of liquid anesthetic remaining in the vaporizer. This should be checked before the machine is used, and the vaporizer should be refilled if the level indicates that over half of the anesthetic has evaporated. The indicator window also allows the anesthetist to assess the color of the anesthetic. With prolonged use, excessive amounts of preservative may accumulate within a halothane vaporizer, resulting in a yellow discoloration of the liquid. Servicing or vaporizer flushing is recommended if this discoloration is apparent because vaporizer function may be impaired by high levels of preservative. (See pages 184-185.)

TABLE 4-5

Comparison of Precision and Nonprecision Vaporizers

Parameters	Precision Vaporizer	Nonprecision Vaporizer
Temperature compensation	Yes; output not affected by temperature in most models	No; output affected by temperature
Flow compensation	Yes; output not affected over a wide range of flow rates	No; output affected by flow rate
Back pressure compensation	Yes; changes in back pressure do not affect output	No; changes in back pressure affect output
Maintenance requirements	Requires periodic factory recalibration and cleaning	Minimal; can be done by hospital staff
Cost	High	Minimal
Anesthetics commonly used	Isoflurane, halothane (that is, those with high vapor pressure)	Methoxyflurane (that is, those with low vapor pressure); isoflurane and halothane with low-flow techniques
Control over anesthetic concentration	Precise; given as a percentage	Not precise; given as a control lever setting (1-10)
Position relative to anesthetic circuit	Out of circle (VOC)	In circle (VIC)

Anesthetic machines may be equipped with either a precision or nonprecision vaporizer. The characteristics of these two types of vaporizers are summarized in Table 4-5.

Precision vaporizers. A precision vaporizer is designed to deliver an exact concentration of anesthetic as selected by the anesthetist. The dial of a precision vaporizer (Fig. 4-9) is graduated in percent concentration (for example, 1%, 2%, etc.). For most patients, a concentration of 1.5 times the MAC (minimum alveolar concentration) of that anesthetic will result in a moderate depth of anesthesia. For example, the MAC of isoflurane in the dog is 1.2%. A concentration of approximately 2% isoflurane therefore can be expected to maintain surgical anesthesia in most dogs. Halothane has a slightly lower MAC (0.87%), and a vaporizer setting between 1% and 1.5% is often adequate to maintain anesthesia. This is only a rough guideline, and the anesthetist must, of course, monitor each animal's response to the anesthetic to determine the optimum setting for that individual.

Precision vaporizers are expensive, but they offer the advantage of closely controlling the delivery of anesthetic. This is of particular importance if the anesthetic used has a high vapor pressure (for example, halothane and isoflurane). Anesthetics with a high vapor pressure evaporate readily and may reach a concentration close to 30% within the anesthetic circuit if vaporization is not controlled. Since the maximum safe concentration of these agents is less than 5%, uncontrolled evaporation could be dangerous for the patient. It is therefore customary to use halothane and isoflurane in a

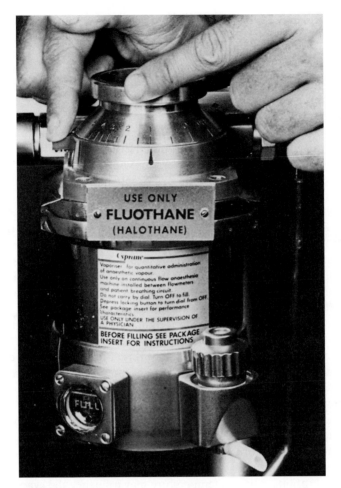

FIG. 4-9   Precision vaporizer. (From Warren RG: *Small animal anesthesia,* St Louis, 1983, Mosby.)

precision vaporizer, affording the anesthetist more exact control of the anesthetic concentration in the circuit. (For information on the use of halothane or isoflurane in a nonprecision vaporizer, see the section that follows on low-flow anesthesia.)

Not all anesthetics require this degree of control. For example, methoxyflurane has a low vapor pressure (that is, it does not evaporate readily) and will only produce a maximum of 4% concentration in the carrier gases. This is a safe level for anesthesia of most patients, so a nonprecision vaporizer is adequate for methoxyflurane delivery.

A variety of precision anesthetic vaporizers are available on the market. Each vaporizer is designed for use with an anesthetic of a particular vapor pressure; therefore vaporizers are labeled for use with one anesthetic only. There is one exception to this rule: halothane and isoflurane have similar vapor pressures and may be used interchangeably in some vaporizers, although this practice is not recommended by vaporizer manufacturers.

Most vaporizers have keyed filler systems that help prevent inadvertent introduction of the wrong anesthetic into the vaporizer. If the wrong anesthetic is accidentally put into a vaporizer (for example, halothane into a methoxyflurane vaporizer), the vaporizer should be drained, flushed with oxygen, and allowed to air overnight before use.

When using an anesthetic machine, it is easy to assume that the concentration of anesthetic delivered depends only on the vaporizer setting. However, the concentration delivered may be affected by three other factors: (1) temperature, (2) carrier gas flow rate, and (3) back pressure. Newer precision vaporizers are compensated for all three factors and can deliver the concentration indicated on their dials with little error or variation. However, technicians working with older precision vaporizers or nonprecision vaporizers such as the Ohio 8 or Stephens vaporizer should realize that these are not automatically compensated for all of these factors.

Temperature compensation.   Volatile anesthetics, like all liquids, evaporate more readily at a high temperature than at a low temperature. If a vaporizer is not constructed to compensate for temperature changes, the amount of anesthetic vaporized will vary with changes in room temperature. If a noncompensated vaporizer is used in a cold room, the amount of anesthetic vaporized may be considerably less than that indicated on the dial. Conversely, in a warm room, the amount vaporized may be greater than the reading on the dial.

Temperature compensation is also important because at high oxygen flow rates, the passage of oxygen will cause the temperature of the liquid anesthetic to fall. Unless the vaporizer has built-in compensation for this effect, this leads to decreased vaporization and a decreased concentration of anesthetic being delivered to the patient. The result is that at high flow rates, a noncompensated vaporizer may deliver less anesthetic than the amount indicated by the dial.

Most precision vaporizers are temperature-compensated to prevent variation of anesthetic output. Older models that are not temperature-compensated provide a thermometer and temperature adjustment scale that allow the anesthetist to adjust the vaporizer setting to account for room temperature.

Flow compensation.   Just as temperature may influence the evaporation rate of a volatile anesthetic, the amount of gas that flows over the liquid anesthetic (the carrier gas flow rate) will also affect the evaporation rate. In a vaporizer that is not flow-compensated, the concentration of anesthetic that is released at an oxygen flow rate of 3 L/minute may be different from that released at a flow rate of 500 ml/minute. Most modern precision vaporizers are compensated to prevent this variation and will vaporize the amount of anesthetic indicated on the vaporizer dial throughout a wide range of flow rates. Older halothane vaporizers are not flow-compensated, however, and provide a chart that estimates the dial setting required for a range of flow rates.

For any precision vaporizer, flow compensation is not unlimited. Flows that are very high (that is, in excess of 10 L/minute) or very low (that is, below 500 ml/minute) may affect the amount of anesthetic liquid that is vaporized even in a flowcompensated precision vaporizer. The vaporizer setting does not accurately reflect the concentration of anesthetic released at these extreme flow rates.

Although an exact percentage output is indicated by the dial or chart on the vaporizer, the amount of anesthetic received by the animal is somewhat affected by the flow of the carrier gas in the circuit, even in a compensated precision vaporizer. High flows allow the patient to achieve a percent concentration close to that dialed because a large amount of fresh gas is continuously delivered to the circuit. Lower flows result in more rebreathing of the patient's expired gases, which have had some anesthetic removed by the animal. This lowers the anesthetic concentration within the circuit. For example, if a 20-kg dog is connected to an anesthetic machine with a flow rate of 300 ml/kg/minute (in this case, 6 L/minute) and a vaporizer setting of 2%, the actual concentration of anesthetic being breathed by the animal is close to 2%. If the flow is reduced to 100 ml/kg/minute (in this case, 2 L/minute), then to 50 ml/kg/minute (1 L/minute), and finally to 10 ml/kg/minute (200 ml/minute), the percent concentration of anesthetic being inspired may drop to 1.8%, 1.2%, and 0.8%, respectively. In each case the vaporizer is producing a 2% concentration of anesthetic, but the lower the fresh gas flow, the more the expired gases dilute the anesthetic flowing into the machine. This is why precision vaporizer settings must be increased if low oxygen flow rates are used. (See page 182.)

Back pressure compensation.   A vaporizer that is not back pressure compensated will release additional anesthetic if gas from the circuit passes through it under pressure. This may occur, for example, when the animal is bagged. Precision vaporizers are normally back pressure compensated in that they are placed outside the anesthetic circuit and gas from the circuit cannot reenter the vaporizer and affect the evaporation of the anesthetic. Bagging therefore does not affect the amount of anesthetic released by these vaporizers.*

Nonprecision vaporizers.   Not all machines are equipped with precision vaporizers. Nonprecision vaporizers are available that are much simpler in design and much less expensive than precision vaporizers. They are acceptable for use with anesthetics that have a low vapor pressure (for example, methoxyflurane) and, under certain circumstances, with anesthetics that have a high vapor pressure (for example, isoflurane and halothane).

One example of a nonprecision vaporizer is the Ohio No. 8 vaporizer, which consists of a glass jar containing a wick. The wick absorbs anesthetic contained in the jar, and as oxygen gas flows past the wick, the anesthetic is vaporized. In a nonprecision vaporizer, the concentration of anesthetic delivered to the patient is not known exactly. It therefore cannot be given as a percentage and is indicated only by a control lever setting (Fig. 4-10). The anesthetist varies the amount of anesthetic delivered to the patient by opening or closing the control valve, basing this decision on the patient's depth of anesthesia. This type of control is adequate for methoxyflurane, which has a low vapor pressure and will only achieve a maximum of 4% concentration even if the vaporizer is fully open. However, many anesthetists have traditionally felt that this control is inadequate for more volatile anesthetics such as halothane or isoflurane, which can achieve very high concentrations in such a system and lead to a rapid increase in patient depth. Machines have recently become available that feature a nonprecision vaporizer that can be used with isoflurane or halothane (for example, Stephens Universal Vaporizer). The vaporizer of this machine is made inefficient by removal of the wick, allowing halothane or isoflurane to be delivered at a concentration suitable for anesthesia. The two advantages of this system are:

1. It can be used with low flow rates and is therefore economical.
2. The initial cost is somewhat less than that of a precision vaporizer.

Use of isoflurane or halothane in this type of vaporizer is discussed on pages 182–183.

---

*Despite back pressure compensation, an increased amount of anesthetic may be delivered to a patient that is bagged continuously. This occurs because the volume of gas entering the lungs in a bagged animal is greater than that breathed by an anesthetized patient on its own. It is therefore important to reduce the setting of a precision vaporizer when continuous bagging is administered, particularly if patient depth seems excessive.

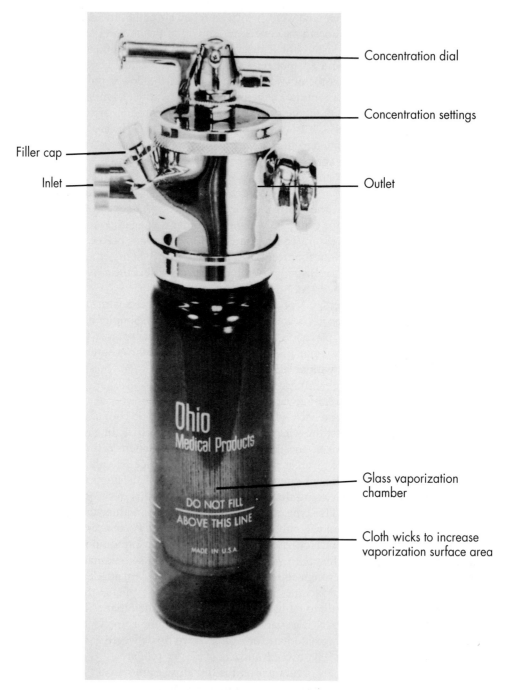

FIG. 4-10   Nonprecision vaporizer. (From Warren RG: *Small animal anesthesia,* St Louis, 1983, Mosby.)

The chief disadvantage of any nonprecision vaporizer is that it is not compensated for temperature, carrier gas flow rates, or back pressure. This has several serious implications that must be understood by the anesthetist using this type of vaporizer, particularly if isoflurane or halothane is to be administered.

Lack of temperature compensation.   At any given setting, the vaporizer will deliver a greater concentration of anesthetic in a warm room than in a cold room.

Lack of flow compensation.   The amount of anesthetic delivered to the patient will increase if the patient breathes more deeply. Increased respiration rate results in increased flow of gas through the vaporizer and thus will increase evaporation of the anesthetic. Eventually the high flow rates will cause the temperature of the anesthetic in the vaporizer to fall, and the concentration of anesthetic may decrease. The variation of anesthetic output with flow rate does not occur in a flow compensated precision vaporizer, in which anesthetic output will not vary despite changes in respiratory rate or depth or changes in oxygen flow rate.

Lack of back pressure compensation.   Most importantly, because nonprecision vaporizers are not back pressure compensated, a build-up of pressure within the circuit (as may occur when the patient is bagged or a ventilator is used) may result in increased evaporation of anesthetic. The increased delivery of anesthetic to the patient being bagged may result in excessive anesthetic depth. Controlled ventilation therefore is difficult with these vaporizers. The anesthetist must ensure that the vaporizer setting is greatly reduced (or the vaporizer is turned off) when bagging the animal or when delivering intermittent positive pressure ventilation by means of a ventilator. In contrast, it is not normally necessary to turn off a precision vaporizer when bagging because of the back pressure compensation of these vaporizers.

Monitoring.   The use of a nonprecision vaporizer with a volatile anesthetic such as isoflurane offers less precise control over anesthetic depth than does a standard precision vaporizer. Close monitoring of the patient is essential, particularly during the first 5 minutes of anesthesia, when patient depth increases rapidly.

Use with nonrebreathing systems.   Nonprecision vaporizers are difficult to adapt to nonrebreathing systems such as the Bain circuit.

VOC versus VIC.   The anesthetist may occasionally find an anesthetic machine referred to as VOC or VIC. The letters *VOC* are an abbreviation for *vaporizer out of circle* and indicate that the vaporizer is not placed within the anesthetic circle itself (Fig. 4-11, *A*). The "circle" referred to includes the flutter valves, hoses, carbon dioxide absorber canister, pop-off valve, and reservoir bag. This is the type of setup described earlier in this chapter and applies to all anesthetic machines with precision vaporizers. The letters *VIC* indicate a *vaporizer in circle* (Fig. 4-11, *B*). In this type of machine (for example, the Ohio No. 8) the carrier gases enter the circuit directly from the flowmeter. The vaporizer (which is nonprecision in this case) is part of the circuit, and exhaled gases reenter the vaporizer each time they flow through the circuit.

It is reasonable to ask at this point why precision vaporizers are found out of circle and nonprecision vaporizers are found in circle. The position of a vaporizer in circle or out of circle is governed by the resistance it offers to the passage of gases. Nonprecision vaporizers offer little resistance to gas flow and do not impede the passage of gases around the circuit. Precision vaporizers, however, offer a high resistance to gas flow and must be placed out of circle.

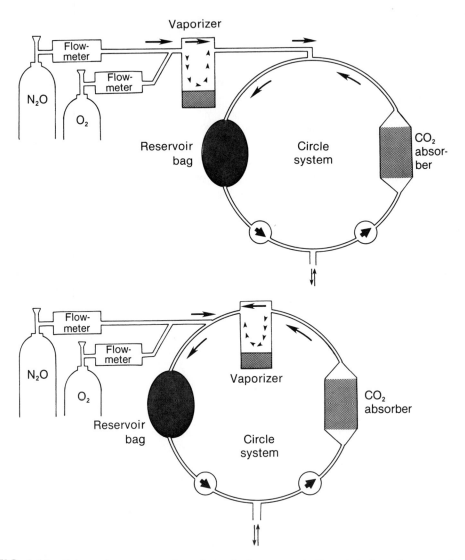

FIG. 4-11   Schematic representation of anesthetic system. **A,** Out of circle and **B,** in circle. (From Warren RG: *Small animal anesthesia,* St Louis, 1983, Mosby.)

■ OPERATION OF THE ANESTHETIC MACHINE

The anesthetist operating any anesthetic machine has a number of options regarding its use. The most important decision is the type of breathing system to be used. There are three systems in common use: total rebreathing (closed), partial rebreathing (semiclosed), and nonrebreathing (open). The choice of system to be used is important because it will determine the following:

- Whether the patient will breathe back in ("rebreathe") the gases that have been exhaled
- Oxygen and nitrous oxide flow rates

- Position of the pop-off valve (closed or open)
- Type of equipment used (for example, whether a Bain system will be required)

Rebreathing Systems

In the system described thus far in this chapter (a circle system with a VOC precision vaporizer), the gases exhaled by the patient travel through the expiratory hose and enter the carbon dioxide canister. They are then directed into the reservoir bag and back toward the patient through the inhalation flutter valve. At this point, fresh oxygen and anesthetic enter the circuit from the vaporizer and mix with the patient's exhaled gases. The flow of gas through the anesthetic machine therefore is circular (reservoir bag, inhalation flutter valve, inspiration hose, animal, expiration hose, exhalation flutter valve, carbon dioxide canister, back to the inhalation flutter valve). The machine adapts to the patient's ventilation patterns and maintains a constant flow of gas to the patient through the use of a reservoir bag, pop-off valve, and negative pressure relief valve.

This type of system allows recirculation of exhaled gases to the patient and therefore is called a *rebreathing system*. It is also sometimes referred to as a *circle system*. The patient rebreathes its own exhaled gases, from which carbon dioxide has been removed and a small amount of fresh oxygen and anesthetic are continuously added.

Rebreathing systems are further subdivided into *total rebreathing systems* (also called *closed systems*) and *partial rebreathing systems* (also called *semiclosed systems*). The main difference between these systems lies in the amount of oxygen that is delivered to the patient, called the oxygen flow rate. In a closed, total rebreathing system, the oxygen flow rate is relatively low, providing only the oxygen necessary to meet the patient's metabolic requirements. In this type of system, it may be necessary to turn the pop-off valve to the closed position to prevent gases from escaping, particularly if the suction from the scavenger is strong. A total rebreathing system recirculates all of the exhaled gases (with the exception of carbon dioxide, which is removed by the absorber), and only a small amount of fresh oxygen and anesthetic is added to the system. The amount of oxygen used by the patient is closely matched by the amount of oxygen entering the circuit from the vaporizer.

In the semiclosed, partial rebreathing system, the flow rate of fresh oxygen and anesthetic entering the system must be considerably higher than that for the closed, total rebreathing system. The pop-off valve is left partly open, allowing some exhaled gases to escape. Thus although some of the exhaled gases are recirculated to the patient, much of the exhaled gases exit via the scavenger. The exiting gases are replaced by fresh oxygen and anesthetic entering the circuit.

Nonrebreathing Systems

The total and partial rebreathing systems discussed above are well suited to many patients. However, in some circumstances the anesthetist may prefer to use a different type of anesthetic setup, called a *nonrebreathing system*. In a nonrebreathing system, little or no exhaled gases are returned to the patient; instead, they are evacuated by a scavenger connected to a pop-off valve or exit port. The characteristics of rebreathing and nonrebreathing systems are compared in Table 4-6.

As with the rebreathing system, the nonrebreathing system can best be understood by following the path of an oxygen molecule from the tank, to the patient, and finally to the scavenger. Just as in a rebreathing system, oxygen (and nitrous oxide

TABLE 4-6

Comparison of Rebreathing and Nonrebreathing Systems

Parameters	Nonrebreathing	Rebreathing (Semiclosed or Closed System)
CO_2 absorption	Not required	Must have CO_2 absorber canister
Changes in depth of anesthesia	Quickly	Slowly
Flow rates	High flow rates: must equal or exceed the respiratory minute volume	Low-flow rates: only to meet the metabolic oxygen requirement
Cost of operation	High because of the amount of oxygen and anesthetic used	Low, because less oxygen and anesthetic used
Amount of waste gas produced	High	Minimal
Pop-off position	Full open, or no pop-off	Closed (total rebreathing) or partly open (partial rebreathing)
Heat and moisture conservation (from exhaled gases)	Poor	Good
Vaporizer position	No circle, or VOC	VOC or VIC
Size of animal	Any size: limited only by the total gas flow that is delivered. Generally recommended for animal under 7kg.	Only for animals over 7 kg

gas, if used) flows from the tank, through a flowmeter, and into the vaporizer. At this point, however, gases exiting the vaporizer go directly into a hose for delivery to the patient, bypassing the inhalation flutter valve. Exhaled gases pass through another hose and may enter a reservoir bag, but do not enter a carbon dioxide canister. The gas is then released through a pop-off valve, pressure relief valve, or other mechanism connected to a scavenger. Since most of the gases exit through the scavenger and are not returned to the patient, the system is accurately described as nonrebreathing.

It is evident that several anesthetic machine parts that are used for a rebreathing system are not required in a nonrebreathing system. These include the carbon dioxide canister and the flutter valves.

Although most anesthetic machines are designed to be used as a rebreathing or partial rebreathing system, a conventional anesthetic machine (with a CO_2 absorber canister and flutter valves) can be converted to a nonrebreathing system by using a high oxygen flow rate (200 to 300 ml/kg/minute), which effectively flushes most of the exhaled gases through the pop-off valve. Alternatively, the anesthetic machine may be easily converted to a nonrebreathing system through the use of attachments, such as the Bain system (The Kendall Company, Boston, MA 02161) (Figs. 4-12 and 4-13

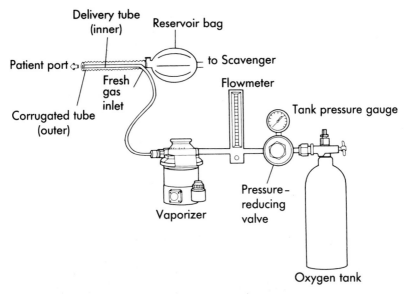

FIG. 4-12 Components of an anesthesia delivery system using a Bain circuit. (Redrawn from Hodgson DS: The case for nonrebreathing circuits for very small animals. In Haskins SC: Opinions in small animal anesthesia, *Vet Clin North Am Small Anim Pract* 22[2]:326–469,1992.)

A and *B*), the Ayres T piece, the Mapleson A system (Magill), the Kuhn circuit, the Norman mask elbow, an anesthetic chamber, or similar equipment. Each of these attachments delivers the fresh gas from the vaporizer to the animal and conducts the expired gases to a scavenger. Most systems have a fresh gas inlet, reservoir bag, tubing, scavenger outlet, and endotracheal tube connection but differ in the site of fresh gas inflow, the position of the reservoir bag, and the location of the exhalation port.

Because the Bain system is a commonly used nonrebreathing attachment, it will be discussed in more detail here. Readers are referred to more detailed reference texts or equipment manufacturers for information on other systems.

The Bain system consists of inner tubing (which conducts gas to the patient and corresponds to the inspiratory hose of a rebreathing system) surrounded by larger, corrugated tubing (which conducts gas away from the patient and corresponds to the expiratory hose in a rebreathing system). The arrangement of the tubing into an inner and outer hose makes the setup less cumbersome and allows the incoming gases to be warmed slightly by the exhaled gases that surround them, before reaching the patient. When using or cleaning a Bain circuit, care must be taken to ensure that the inner tubing does not detach from the rest of the circuit, or gas will not be delivered to the patient.

Gas from the outer, exhalation tubing enters a reservoir bag before exiting the system. Bain circuits are not equipped with an overflow valve or pop-off valve, and it may be necessary to cut the tail of the reservoir bag to allow the escape of waste gases. In this case, the tail of the reservoir bag should be connected to the scavenging system to allow proper disposal of the waste gas. It may be necessary to partially clamp the outlet of the reservoir bag with a paper clip or screw clamp to act as a pop-off valve and allow the anesthetist to control the rate at which the reservoir bag empties.

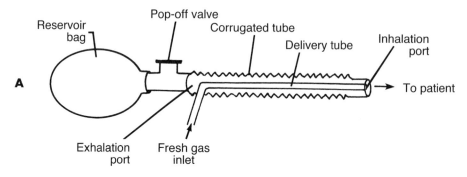

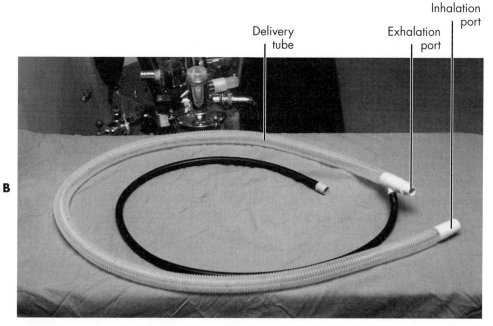

FIG. 4-13 A, Schematic of Bain system. **B,** Bain circuit.

Alternatively, a Bain mount is available that allows the use of an uncut bag. This mount features a pop-off valve, which allows easy scavenging and bagging.

When using a nonrebreathing system such as the Bain, the oxygen flow rate is normally high (usually at least 130 ml/kg/minute) and a large proportion of the exhaled gases enters the scavenger. Some rebreathing of gas can occur if a reservoir bag is present, particularly during peak inspiration or if the respiratory rate is rapid. The amount of rebreathing depends on the oxygen flow rate, and therefore can be controlled by the anesthetist. If the anesthetist selects a high oxygen flow rate (for example, 2 L/minute for a 5-kg cat), there is little return of exhaled gases to the patient. The system is therefore completely nonrebreathing, and the reservoir bag outlet is kept fully open. At lower flow rates (for example, 500 ml of oxygen/minute for a 5-kg cat), significant rebreathing of exhaled gases may occur even with a Bain circuit, and the setup would be more properly classified as a partial rebreathing system rather than a nonrebreathing system. Because the Bain system does not remove carbon dioxide from exhaled gases, low flow rates are contraindicated.

When using a Bain circuit, a rebreathing setup is more economical than a nonrebreathing setup because lower oxygen flow rates can be used and therefore the amount of anesthetic vaporized is less. However, significant rebreathing of gas is not advisable when using a nonrebreathing system such as the Bain circuit. There is some risk that CO_2 levels may become dangerously high in such a system because a CO_2 absorber is not used.

Choice of Rebreathing Versus Nonrebreathing System

The decision of whether to use a rebreathing system (such as the conventional anesthetic machine setup) or a nonrebreathing system (such as a Bain) is made on the basis of the following factors:

- *Patient size.* Nonrebreathing systems such as the Bain are most commonly used in patients weighing less than 7 kg (15 lb). Nonrebreathing systems offer little resistance to respiration, a significant advantage for small patients. If a rebreathing system is used, the flutter valves, carbon dioxide canister, and pop-off valve increase the resistance to air movement within the system. Small patients may have difficulty inhaling with enough force to draw air from such a circuit into their lungs.*
- *Convenience.* In addition to offering less resistance to breathing, nonrebreathing circuits are generally lighter than the Y piece and hose assembly of a rebreathing circuit and therefore cause less drag on the endotracheal tube.
- *Cost.* Total rebreathing (closed) systems are more economical than nonrebreathing (open) systems because gas flows are relatively low and less anesthetic and oxygen are used. Partial rebreathing (semiclosed) systems are not as economical as total rebreathing systems but require much less oxygen and anesthetic (on a per kg basis) than nonrebreathing systems such as the Bain. For this reason, rebreathing systems (either total or partial rebreathing) are commonly used in large patients, which would require prohibitively large amounts of anesthetic and oxygen in a nonrebreathing system.
- *Control.* The speed at which the anesthetist can change anesthetic depth depends, in part, on the type of system used. A rebreathing system has a relatively slow turnover of gases because the flow rate of fresh oxygen and anesthetic into the system is low. A nonrebreathing system allows a much faster turnover of gases because flow rates of fresh gas are higher and a large proportion of exhaled gases exit the system through the scavenger. This means that changes made in the (precision) vaporizer setting will result in rapid changes in anesthetic concentration within a nonrebreathing system, and the percentage of anesthetic breathed by the patient is very close to that indicated by the dial. Changes in anesthetic concentration within a rebreathing system, however, require a longer time, and the concentration of anesthetic inhaled by the patient may not be the same as that indicated on the dial for several minutes after the dial setting is changed.†

---

*The size of the endotracheal tube has a greater effect on resistance than does the type of circuit used. The use of an endotracheal tube that is too small results in far greater resistance to air passage than that offered by the remainder of the anesthetic circuit, even in a rebreathing setup.
†The type of volatile anesthetic used will also determine how quickly anesthetic depth can be changed, irrespective of oxygen flow rates or the type of circuit used. Anesthetics with high solubility coefficients (such as methoxyflurane) will allow only slow changes in anesthetic depth, whereas anesthetics that have a low tissue solubility (such as isoflurane and halothane) will pass quickly between the blood and the alveolus, allowing rapid changes in anesthetic depth. See discussion on pages 133-134.

- *Conservation of heat and moisture.* Rebreathing systems automatically warm and humidify inspired gases within the circle. Nonrebreathing systems may be associated with significant loss of heat and water from the patient because the warmed and humidified gases exhaled by the patient are not returned. In a nonrebreathing system, inspired fresh anesthetic gases have a relative humidity close to 0% and a temperature of approximately 16° C, whereas exhaled gases have a relative humidity of almost 100% and a temperature close to 25° C.
- *Production of waste gas.* Total rebreathing systems release little or no waste anesthetic gas because oxygen flow rates are low and exhaled gases are recirculated rather than vented through the pop-off valve.

Carrier Gas Flow Rates

For each anesthetic procedure, the anesthetist is faced with the problem of deciding how much flow (or volume) of carrier gas is required. Usually the carrier gas is oxygen alone, but if both oxygen and nitrous oxide are used, flow rate determinations must consider the total flow of gas as well as the individual flow rates of each gas. Thus it may be decided that for a particular patient and machine setup, a total flow of 1 L/minute is required. The 1 liter may consist of pure oxygen or some combination of nitrous oxide and oxygen (for example, 600 ml/minute of nitrous oxide and 400 ml/minute of oxygen). If nitrous oxide is used, the nitrous oxide flow should be 1.5 to 2 times the oxygen flow rate.

The calculation of the flow rate to be used for each anesthetic procedure is based on several factors, including the period of anesthesia (that is, either induction, maintenance, or recovery) and whether a rebreathing or nonrebreathing system is preferred. These factors are summarized in Box 4-1.

Flow rates during induction. It is customary to use higher flow rates during induction than during the maintenance period. This is particularly true if mask induction or chamber induction is used. Use of high flow rates in the induction period allows the anesthetist to saturate the anesthetic circuit with carrier gas and anesthetic and dilute the expired gases of the patient. Once the animal reaches the desired plane of anesthesia, flow rates are decreased.

- For mask induction it is generally agreed that a flow rate per minute should equal 30 times the tidal volume. Since the tidal volume of most animals is approximately 10 ml/kg/minute, the recommended flow rate is approximately 300 ml/kg/minute. For animals under 10 kg, 1 to 3 liters is usually adequate, and 3 to 5 L/minute is suggested for animals over 10 kg.
- A flow rate of 5 L/minute is recommended for chamber induction.
- For animals induced with an injectable anesthetic and subsequently intubated and connected to an anesthetic machine, the minimum flow rate during the initial anesthetic period is the respiratory minute volume, which is the tidal volume (10 ml/kg) times the number of breaths per minute. A figure of 200 ml/kg/minute is commonly used, which results in a flow rate between 500 ml and 5 L/minute, depending on the size of the animal and whether a rebreathing (low oxygen flow) or nonrebreathing (high oxygen flow) system is preferred.

Flow rates in the maintenance period. Once the animal achieves a satisfactory level of anesthetic depth, the flow rate may be safely reduced to a maintenance level. This value depends on the type of system used (total rebreathing, partial rebreathing, or nonrebreathing).

Box 4-1 Recommended Flow Rates

INDUCTION
Chamber Induction
- 5 L/minute

Face Mask Induction
- 300 ml/kg/minute, or 1-3 L/minute for animals under 10 kg, 3-5 L/minute for animals over 10 kg

Intravenous Induction
- 200 ml/kg/minute (500 ml to 5 L/minute depending on patient size)

MAINTENANCE
Nonrebreathing systems
- Bain: 130-200 ml/kg/minute
- Other systems: 200-300 ml/kg/minute

Rebreathing systems
- Total rebreathing (closed) system: minimum of 15 ml/kg/minute; use of N_2O is inadvisable at this flow rate
- Partial rebreathing (semiclosed system): 25-50 ml/kg/minute
- Semiclosed system with minimal rebreathing: 150-200 ml/kg/minute
  Flow rates in excess of 2 L/minute should be avoided when using nonprecision vaporizers.
  Many vaporizers deliver inaccurate amounts of anesthetic at flow rates less than 500 ml/minute or greater than 10 L/minute.
  When using nitrous oxide, a minimum oxygen flow of 30 ml/kg/minute must be provided.
  Nitrous oxide flow rate should be 1.5 to 2 times the oxygen flow rate.

Nonrebreathing systems require relatively high flow rates on a per kg basis because the expired gases are evacuated by the scavenger and, for the most part, are not returned to the patient. Fresh gas must be continuously provided because there is minimal rebreathing of exhaled gases. The recommended flow rate for a Bain circuit is 130 to 200 ml/kg/minute. For a 5-kg animal, this flow rate is 650 ml to 1 L/minute of pure oxygen. If nitrous oxide is used, flow rates of 600 ml nitrous oxide and 400 ml of oxygen per minute (a ratio of 1.5:1) would be appropriate.

For other types of nonrebreathing circuits, flow rates of 200 to 300 ml/kg/minute are generally accepted.

Rebreathing systems require relatively low flow rates compared with nonrebreathing systems because carbon dioxide absorption is available and the expired gases are returned to the patient. Provided the carbon dioxide absorber canister is effective, the carrier gas and anesthetic can be recycled continuously and only a small amount of fresh gas is required. For a total rebreathing (closed) system, the oxygen flow must only equal the oxygen requirements of the animal. The minimum oxygen requirement for an animal is 5 to 10 ml/kg/minute, although to account for leaks within the circuit, a value of 15 ml/kg/minute is usually recommended. (See the following section on low-flow anesthesia.) The anesthetist should be aware that flow rates less than 500 ml/minute will not allow most precision vaporizers to accurately deliver the dialed vaporizer concentration.

Flow rates of 25 to 50 ml/kg/minute are recommended for partial rebreathing systems.

Flow rates at the end of anesthesia.   It is recommended that the flow rates be increased immediately after the vaporizer is turned off. During this time, anesthetic gas is exhaled by the patient and may accumulate within the circuit, particularly if a rebreathing system is used. To evacuate this anesthetic and to allow the patient to breathe pure oxygen, a flow rate similar to that used during induction is recommended. The anesthetist should periodically remove expired gases from the circuit by opening the pop-off valve and evacuating the reservoir bag. The bag can be refilled using the oxygen flush control.

Summary.   Within the aforementioned guidelines, there is considerable leeway for the anesthetist's own judgment in determining the flow rate for any particular procedure. (See Box 4-1 and Box 4-2 for a summary of currently recommended flow rates and examples of flow rate calculations.) In many cases, the ultimate decision may be based on economic factors: high gas flow rates are less economical than low-flow rates because more oxygen, nitrous oxide, and anesthetic are used. It is evident, therefore, that nonrebreathing systems are less economical than rebreathing systems. If the patient is small, the flow rate, even with a nonrebreathing system, is likely to be less than 1.5 L/minute, and the cost of anesthetic and oxygen is relatively minor. Economic considerations are more important when considering whether to use a total or partial rebreathing system for a larger animal. Partial rebreathing systems use higher flow rates and, for this reason, may be considerably more expensive than total rebreathing systems.

Safety Concerns When Using a Total Rebreathing System

Most patients weighing over 7 kg are anesthetized using either a partial or total rebreathing system. Although total rebreathing systems are more economical than partial rebreathing systems, there are serious safety concerns that must be addressed when using a total rebreathing system:

- *Carbon dioxide accumulation.* If the carbon dioxide absorber in a closed system is not operating efficiently, exhaled carbon dioxide will build up within the circuit. This is less likely to happen in a semiclosed, partial rebreathing system, in which some CO_2 is vented to the scavenger.
- *Increased pressure in the anesthetic circuit.* In a total rebreathing system, the volume of gas in the system may increase as fresh gas enters the circuit, particularly if the pop-off valve is closed. Excessive pressure may build up in the circuit, making it difficult for the animal to exhale. In a partial rebreathing system, the pop-off valve is partly to fully open and excessive gas is vented.
- *Oxygen depletion and nitrous oxide accumulation.* In any anesthetic machine setup, oxygen is gradually depleted as the patient breathes the circulating gas. This is normally compensated by fresh oxygen entering the circuit. In a total rebreathing system, the oxygen flow rate is low and the amount of fresh oxygen added to the circuit may not entirely compensate for this loss. This is particularly serious if nitrous oxide is used in addition to oxygen, because the relative amount of nitrous oxide in the circuit may increase as the amount of oxygen decreases. As a result, the patient may breathe dangerously high levels of nitrous oxide gas. This effect is less likely to occur in a partial rebreathing system, in

Box 4-2 Examples of Flow Rates

1. Given a 5-kg cat and an anesthetic machine with a precision vaporizer, what type of circuit and flow rate would normally be used? Calculate the flow rates for oxygen alone and for oxygen and nitrous oxide used together (maintenance).
   Answer: Since the cat weighs less than 7 kg, a Bain or other nonrebreathing system is preferred. The flow rate recommended for the Bain system is 130 to 200 ml/kg/minute. Thus the anesthetist could select 200 ml × 5 kg = 1000 ml or 1 liter of gas flow per minute. Note that if nitrous oxide is used for this animal, a 2:1 ratio of N_2O/O_2 should be provided. For a 1-liter total flow of gas, this is equal to:
   Oxygen: ⅓ of 1 L/minute = 333 ml/minute
   Nitrous oxide: ⅔ of 1 L/minute = 667 ml/minute
      If nitrous oxide is used, the anesthetist must ensure that the animal receives adequate oxygen (30 ml/kg/minute). For this cat, the minimum is 30 ml oxygen/minute × 5 kg = 150 ml of oxygen/minute. (Therefore, 333 ml is safe.)
2. Given a 25-kg dog and a precision vaporizer, what type of circuit and flow rate would be preferred during the maintenance period?
   Answer: For economic reasons, the type of circuit used would probably be a circle system. If a total rebreathing system is used, the minimum oxygen flow rate is 15 ml × 25 kg/minute, which is 375 ml/minute. (For many vaporizers, this flow rate is too low and should be increased to a minimum of 500 ml/minute.) If, as is more common, a partial rebreathing system is used, the flow rate should be 25 to 50 ml/kg/minute. For this animal, the flow rate would therefore be 625 ml to 1.25 liters of oxygen per minute. If the anesthetist wishes to increase the flow rate to achieve a nonrebreathing system, the flow rate would be calculated as 150 to 200 ml/kg/minute, which is 3.75 to 5 L/minute in this patient.
      The oxygen flow rate therefore can be set at a minimum of 500 ml/minute and at a maximum of 5 L/minute (if the pop-off valve is completely open and the animal is not rebreathing any expired gases). Many anesthetists would choose a flow rate midway between these two extremes, approximately 1 to 1.5 L/minute.
3. Given a 15-kg dog anesthetized with a nonprecision methoxyflurane system, what would be the recommended flow rate during the maintenance period if:
   a. A semiclosed, partial rebreathing system is used?
   b. Minimal rebreathing is desired?
   Answer: If the dog is on a semiclosed system, the flow rate should be 25 to 50 ml/kg/minute. For this animal, the flow rate therefore would be 375 to 750 ml/minute.
      If minimal rebreathing is desired, the anesthetist should use a flow rate of 200 ml/kg/hr, which is 3 L/minute. However, since the vaporizer in this example is not compensated for flow rate, it would be inadvisable to use a flow rate over 2 L/minute.

which nitrous oxide escapes through the pop-off valve and oxygen flow rates are higher. The use of a minimum of 30 ml/kg/minute of oxygen in the presence of nitrous oxide prevents N_2O buildup, but this flow rate is not possible in a total rebreathing system. Total rebreathing (closed) systems therefore are not recommended if nitrous oxide is part of the anesthetic protocol.

These disadvantages must be balanced against the economic advantages of a low-flow system (that is, less oxygen and anesthetic used) and the fact that little or no waste anesthetic gas is produced when flow rates are low.

In many situations (for example, where continuous monitoring of the patient and the anesthetic machine is not possible) the anesthetist may prefer to use a partial rather than a total rebreathing setup for the safety reasons just enumerated. The anesthetist may choose to err on the side of wasting some gas by using higher gas flow rates rather than risk accumulation of carbon dioxide and depletion of oxygen within the circuit. Conversion from a total rebreathing system to a partial rebreathing system can be easily achieved by keeping the pop-off valve at least partially open (except when bagging the patient) and by maintaining a higher oxygen flow rate.

If a total rebreathing (closed) system is used, the anesthetist should take the following active steps to ensure patient safety:

- Very close monitoring of the patient and anesthetic machine is essential.
- Check the machine for leaks before use. If leaks are present, oxygen may escape from the circuit. This is not normally of critical importance to the patient; however, in a total rebreathing system the oxygen flow rate is low and any loss of oxygen may be detrimental. To prevent oxygen escape, the pop-off valve is normally closed, or almost so.
- Induction is the most challenging period of anesthesia when low oxygen flows are used. The reservoir bag should be emptied and filled with oxygen 2 to 3 times during the first 15 minutes of anesthesia and every 30 minutes thereafter to help prevent patient hypoxia. Alternatively, the anesthetist may provide 5 to 10 minutes of high oxygen flow (200 ml/kg/minute) at the start of anesthesia, until the patient reaches a surgical plane. The pop-off valve should be open when these flow rates are used. This flushes room air out of the system and replaces it with oxygen. Thereafter, much lower flow rates (5 to 15 ml/kg/minute) can be used, and the pop-off valve should be closed. This amount of oxygen will meet the metabolic oxygen requirements of the anesthetized patient.
- Closely monitor the reservoir bag if a total rebreathing system is used. If the bag becomes smaller, either a leak is present in the system, the pop-off valve is open too much, or the flow rate of oxygen is inadequate. On the other hand, if the bag becomes distended, too much air is present in the circuit. In this case, either the oxygen flow rate should be reduced or the pop-off valve should be opened.
- It may be difficult to change the patient's depth quickly. If a rapid change in anesthetic depth is required, convert to a partial rebreathing system by increasing the oxygen flow rate and opening the pop-off valve. If low oxygen flow rates are maintained, changes in the vaporizer setting may not affect the concentration of anesthetic in the circuit for several minutes.
- If a precision vaporizer is used, the setting required during the maintenance period will often be well above the normal setting used to maintain surgical anesthesia with a semi-closed or open system. In a total rebreathing system with an out of circle vaporizer, the vaporizer concentration required may be 1% to 2% higher than that used for a partial rebreathing system. In contrast, if an in-circle vaporizer is used, the required vaporizer setting will usually be lower than that used for a partial rebreathing system. Close patient monitoring and accurate depth assessment are essential to determine if the vaporizer setting is ap-

propriate for the patient. It may be necessary to turn off the vaporizer if the patient's depth seems excessive.

- The low oxygen flow rates used in a total rebreathing system may be inadequate for accurate delivery of anesthetic by some vaporizers. Consult the vaporizer manual for minimum recommended flow rates, and be aware that the anesthetic concentration indicated by the dial may be incorrect at lower flows. Total rebreathing systems should not be used at all with certain vaporizers, including the Fluothane Tek-2, Copper Kettle, and Vernitrol.
- Nonprecision vaporizers are sometimes used to deliver halothane or isoflurane in a closed, total rebreathing system. Ohio No. 8 vaporizers (nonprecision) can be used with halothane or isoflurane, but the wick should be removed and no more than 100 ml of anesthetic should be put into the vaporizer. For the first 2 minutes, a setting of 6 to "fully open" should be used, and thereafter a setting between 2 and 6 is usually adequate.
- If a Stephen's vaporizer (nonprecision) is used to deliver halothane or isoflurane at low oxygen flow rates, the metal sleeve should be fully retracted and the anesthetic should only be filled to the anesthetic level line. A vaporizer setting of 4 to 8 is used for the first 2 minutes, and for the maintenance period a setting between "off" and 4 is usually adequate.
- Low flow rates are unsuitable for Bain or other nonrebreathing systems.

■ CARE AND USE OF ANESTHETIC EQUIPMENT
Setting up Anesthetic Equipment

Before use, the anesthetic machine should be assembled and thoroughly checked for problems. Procedure 4-1 is a checklist to be followed when setting up anesthetic equipment.

Maintenance of Anesthetic Equipment

As with any piece of equipment, the anesthetic machine requires periodic maintenance to ensure proper performance. A routine maintenance checklist includes the items listed below.

Oxygen and nitrous oxide tanks.   After use, the outlet valve of each tank should be closed by turning it clockwise (that is, to the right). Failure to turn off the gas valve will result in excessive pressure on the regulator and, in some cases, leakage of gas from the tank.

Oxygen pressure remaining in the machine after closure of the tank (line pressure) should be removed by using the oxygen flush valve or by turning the flowmeter to a high rate of flow. Failure to evacuate line pressure may damage the pressure gauge and pressure-reducing valve.

Petroleum or petroleum distillate products (for example grease and gasoline) should not be used on oxygen tanks or their connections. An explosion may occur when the tank is opened and these materials contact oxygen released from the tank.

Flowmeter.   The dial of each flowmeter should be returned to the off position (full clockwise) for storage. Failure to do so may result in a sudden rush of air into the flowmeter when the oxygen tank is opened, which may jam the float or ball at the top of the flowmeter tube. Care should be taken not to overtighten the flowmeter knob when turning the flowmeter off.

▼ **PROCEDURE 4-1**
Setting Up Anesthetic Equipment

1. Assemble all needed supplies.
2. Inflate the endotracheal tube cuffs and record the amount of air required.
3. Check the laryngoscope light.
4. Draw up and label the injectable preanesthetic and anesthetic agents.
5. Warm intravenous fluids to be used.
6. Rotate the vaporizer dial to ensure smooth function.
7. Check the amount of anesthetic in the vaporizer and replenish as necessary.
8. Turn on the gas tanks using a cylinder wrench or similar device. Tanks should be opened slowly and turned to full open position for use. The oxygen tank should be changed if the tank pressure gauge indicates a pressure less than 100 psi (680 kPa). A cutoff of 200 psi (1360 kPa) is advisable if a long anesthesia is planned or if high flow rates are to be used. A nitrous oxide tank should be changed if nitrous oxide pressure is less than 500 psi (3400 kPa).
9. With the oxygen tank open, check the flowmeter controls to ensure proper function.
10. Assemble the appropriate circuit (nonrebreathing circuit or hoses and Y piece) and connect to the machine. The gas flow should be mentally traced from the tank to the patient and back to the machine and scavenger to ensure that connections are correctly assembled.
11. Attach the reservoir bag to the machine or nonrebreathing circuit.
12. Change the carbon dioxide absorber canister contents if necessary. This procedure is best done immediately after machine use, when color changes are most evident.
13. Test the machine for leaks. (See Chapter 5.)

Flowmeter accuracy can be assessed easily by setting the flow at, for example, 2 L/minute and ensuring that a 2-liter bag connected to the machine fills in approximately 1 minute.

Vaporizer.   Vaporizers should be turned off when the machine is not in use.

It is not necessary to routinely empty the anesthetic from the vaporizer after each anesthetic procedure. However, precision vaporizers designed for halothane or methoxyflurane should be emptied of anesthetic every 6 to 12 months to help remove the build-up of preservative within the vaporizer. Isoflurane is supplied without a preservative, and periodic flushing is not usually necessary.

Despite periodic emptying, a precision vaporizer may eventually become clogged with preservative and other residue. When this occurs, the anesthetic levels produced by the vaporizer will not correlate with the percentage indicated by the dial. The anesthetist may become aware of the problem when patients can no longer be maintained at a satisfactory anesthetic depth even at high vaporizer settings. To prevent this problem, precision vaporizers should be cleaned and recalibrated by the manufacturer or other qualified personnel every 6 to 12 months. It may be necessary to remove the vaporizer from the anesthetic machine and send it away for servicing. Many companies provide a "loaner" replacement during the servicing period.

Carbon dioxide absorber canister.   Barium hydroxide lime or soda lime granules should be checked after each anesthetic procedure. Granules that change color or that cannot be crushed with finger pressure should be replaced. Because the granules contain corrosive chemicals (NaOH and KOH) they should not be handled with bare hands (use latex gloves for this purpose). Care should be taken to avoid inhalation of dust when the granules are removed or replenished. Use of a ventilation fan or breathing protection (a mask or respirator) may be necessary.

When replacing the granules, it is important to ensure that they are not tightly packed. At least 1 centimeter (one half inch) of air space should be left between the granules and the top of the canister to allow unimpeded airflow out of the canister. Gentle shaking of the canister after filling helps prevent channels from forming in the granules, which could reduce the efficiency of the absorber.

When replenishing soda lime or barium hydroxide lime granules, the technician must ensure that dust does not enter the tubing or hoses of the machine, because it may be inhaled by the patient and is corrosive to mucous membranes.

Water may collect in the trap below the CO_2 canister and should be periodically removed.

Flutter valves.   Flutter valves require periodic removal and cleaning with a disinfectant to prevent a buildup of water vapor, mucus, dust from the soda lime or barium hydroxide lime, and other material. Access to the valves is obtained by unscrewing the plastic caps that lie over the valves. Valves that are not cleaned may become sticky and adhere to the machine housing, impeding airflow through the circuit.

Other machine parts.   After each anesthetic procedure, removable machine parts (such as the hoses, Y piece, Bain circuit or other nonrebreathing system, and the reservoir bag) should be washed in a mild soapy solution and thoroughly rinsed with water. A surgical scrub brush or bottle brush is useful in cleaning equipment surfaces. After cleaning, the equipment should be air dried. Other machine parts (such as the compressed air tanks, pop-off valve, and CO_2 canister) should be wiped with a disinfectant solution on a weekly basis.

In some cases anesthetic equipment will require more effective disinfection. This is particularly true of equipment that contacts the patient's airway or oral cavity, including the endotracheal tube, laryngoscope blade, esophageal stethoscope, and face mask. If the equipment is used on a patient harboring certain viruses or bacteria (including feline upper respiratory viruses, *Bordetella*, and other respiratory pathogens), infection may be transmitted to the next patient. To prevent disease transmission between patients, these items should be soaked in a disinfectant solution such as 2% glutaraldehyde or sterilized in an ethylene oxide system or autoclave (if the material allows this). Gauze, adhesive tape, and the adapter should be removed from an endotracheal tube before disinfection.

Unfortunately, there is no ideal agent for cleaning anesthetic supplies. Agents such as chlorhexidine are relatively harmless to tissues but are not effective against all microorganisms and spores. Glutaraldehyde solutions (2%) are effective against many microorganisms but are stable for only 2 to 4 weeks and must be periodically replaced. Glutaraldehyde solutions also are irritating to the skin, and the technician should wear rubber gloves when working with this substance. All items exposed to any chemical solution should be thoroughly rinsed with water after cleaning. Some chemicals may be absorbed by rubber and, if not completely removed by rinsing, may cause burns when in contact with the patient's airway or skin. Ethylene oxide is particularly well absorbed by materials being sterilized, and endotracheal tubes exposed to this substance have been known to cause tracheal necrosis.

After prolonged use rubber items deteriorate and must be replaced. Autoclaving causes rubber surfaces to become brittle and crack. Prolonged exposure to disinfectants or rubber-soluble anesthetics (such as methoxyflurane) may also cause rubber surfaces to deteriorate. Endotracheal tubes, masks, and reservoir bags should be periodically checked for wear and discarded if necessary. Endotracheal tubes with leaking or nonfunctional cuffs should also be discarded.

✔ KEY POINTS

1. Many different types and sizes of endotracheal tubes are available for use in veterinary patients.
2. The anesthetic machine delivers volatile gas anesthetic and carrier gases (oxygen with or without nitrous oxide) to the patient and moves exhaled gases away from the patient. If gases are reused, the machine removes carbon dioxide from them before returning them to the patient.
3. Anesthetic machines can be used as a source of oxygen in emergencies.
4. Compressed oxygen cylinders contain oxygen gas under high pressure (up to 2200 psi or 15,000 kilopascals). Various sizes of oxygen cylinders are available; these may be freestanding or attach to the anesthesia machine, but are always white or green. Large cylinders contain more liters of oxygen and function for a longer time than small cylinders. For all oxygen cylinders, tank pressure is gradually reduced as the cylinder empties. Cylinders should be changed when the pressure reaches 100 to 200 psi.
5. Nitrous oxide cylinders are blue and contain nitrous oxide gas and liquid at a pressure of up to 770 psi (5170 kilopascals). As the tank empties, tank pressure is maintained until most of the nitrous oxide is gone. Therefore tanks should be changed when the pressure starts to drop below 500 psi.
6. The pressure regulator (pressure-reducing valve) allows a constant flow of gas to enter the machine and provides a safe operating pressure (50 psi) for the machine.
7. For each type of carrier gas, the flow rate is set by its respective flowmeter. Flows are generally expressed in liters per minute. The flow rate indicates to the anesthetist how much gas is being delivered to the patient at any given time. When using nitrous oxide, the anesthetist should set a nitrous oxide/oxygen ratio of 2:1.
8. Liquid anesthetic is evaporated and added to the carrier gas in the vaporizer. The combination of vaporized anesthetic, oxygen, and nitrous oxide (if present) is called fresh gas. Vaporizers may be precision or nonprecision, based on their construction. Precision vaporizers are commonly used for anesthetics with high vapor pressures and provide compensation for variations in temperature, gas

flow rate, and back pressure. Precision vaporizers are found outside of the anesthetic circuit (VOC), whereas nonprecision vaporizers are found inside the anesthetic circuit (VIC).

9. The reservoir bag (rebreathing bag) can be used to monitor the animal's respiration and to deliver oxygen (with or without anesthetic) to the patient by a process called bagging.

10. Inhalation and exhalation flutter valves allow one-way passage of gas through the machine.

11. Waste gas exits the machine at the pop-off valve, which is usually connected to a scavenger.

12. Carbon dioxide is removed from the circuit by an absorber canister containing granules. Most types of granules exhibit a color change when they have become depleted and require replacement.

13. The pressure manometer measures the pressure of gases within the anesthetic circuit.

14. Anesthetic circuits may be classified as rebreathing (either closed or semiclosed) or nonrebreathing. Rebreathing systems use lower oxygen flow rates but must provide for carbon dioxide absorption. Nonrebreathing systems, such as the Bain system, require relatively high flow rates and are commonly used in small patients.

15. Carrier gas flow rates vary with the period of anesthesia and type of anesthetic circuit used (that is, rebreathing or nonrebreathing). High flow rates are used during induction and recovery and also during the maintenance period of anesthesia if a nonrebreathing system is used.

16. Anesthetic equipment requires routine cleaning, care, and maintenance.

 REVIEW QUESTIONS

1. When the oxygen tank is half full, the pressure gauge will read approximately:
   a. 1000 psi
   b. 2000 psi
   c. 500 psi
   d. 2200 psi
   e. None of the above

2. The pressure gauge of a nitrous oxide tank will read _____ psi when the tank is full.
   a. 2200
   b. 1100
   c. 900
   d. 500
   e. 750

3. When the nitrous oxide tank is half full, the pressure gauge will read ____ psi.
   a. 750
   b. 350
   c. 100
   d. 500
4. Nitrous oxide is present in the tank as a _____.
   a. Liquid
   b. Gas
   c. Liquid and a gas
5. The amount of oxygen an animal is receiving is indicated by the:
   a. Oxygen tank pressure gauge
   b. Flowmeter
   c. Pressure manometer
   d. Vaporizer setting
6. Flowmeters that have a ball for reading the gauge should be read from the _____ of the ball.
   a. Top
   b. Bottom
   c. Middle
7. The best flow rate to use with nitrous oxide and oxygen would be a combination of _____.
   a. 50% oxygen and 50% nitrous oxide
   b. 80% oxygen and 20% nitrous oxide
   c. 23% oxygen and 77% nitrous oxide
   d. 77% oxygen and 23% nitrous oxide
   e. 33% oxygen and 67% nitrous oxide
8. The minimum size for the reservoir bag can be calculated as _____.
   a. 20 ml/kg
   b. 60 ml/kg
   c. 80 ml/kg
   d. 100 ml/kg
9. The flutter valves on an anesthetic machine help _____.
   a. Control the direction of movement of gases
   b. Maintain a full reservoir bag
   c. Remove carbon dioxide
   d. Vaporize the liquid anesthetic
10. The pop-off valve is part of the anesthetic machine and helps:
    a. Vaporize the liquid anesthetic
    b. Prevent excess gas pressure from building up within the breathing circuit
    c. Keep the oxygen flowing in one direction only
    d. Prevent waste gases from reentering the vaporizer
11. When the pressure manometer reading exceeds ____ cm of water pressure, it indicates there is a buildup of pressure within the circuit that could be dangerous.
    a. 5
    b. 10
    c. 15
    d. 20

12. Rebreathing systems are best reserved for animals over 7 kg.
    True   False
13. Rebreathing is determined primarily by the:
    a. Fresh gas flow
    b. Design or type of circuit
    c. Presence of a reservoir bag
    d. Open or shut pop-off
14. Nonrebreathing systems should have maintenance flow rates that are:
    a. Very high ($\geq$130 ml/kg/minute)
    b. Very low (10 ml/kg/minute)
    c. Moderate ($\geq$50 ml/kg/minute)
15. The negative pressure relief valve is particularly useful when:
    a. Nitrous oxide is being used
    b. There is no scavenging system
    c. There is insufficient oxygen flow through the system
    d. The carbon dioxide absorber is no longer functioning
16. The tidal volume of an animal is considered to be ____ ml/kg of body weight.
    a. 5-10
    b. 15
    c. 20
    d. 25

For the following questions, more than one answer may be correct.

17. A reservoir bag that is not moving may indicate:
    a. The endotracheal tube is not in the trachea
    b. The animal has a decreased tidal volume
    c. There is a leak around the endotracheal tube
    d. The vaporizer is empty
18. The anesthetist will know when the granules in the carbon dioxide absorber have been depleted because the:
    a. Anesthetist will smell waste carbon dioxide
    b. Granules will be brittle
    c. Granules may change color
    d. Granules may be hard
19. An increase in the depth of anesthesia can be achieved quickly by:
    a. Having high oxygen flow rates
    b. Having high vaporizer settings
    c. Using a closed anesthetic system
    d. Bagging the animal with the vaporizer on
20. The concentration of anesthetic delivered from a nonprecision vaporizer may depend on the:
    a. Temperature of the liquid anesthetic
    b. Flow of the carrier gas through the vaporizer
    c. Back pressure
21. The advantages of a nonprecision vaporizer include:
    a. It is economical to buy
    b. It can be readily used with all anesthetics

  c. It is easy to clean and service
  d. It can be used out of circle
22. Low-flow anesthesia means:
  a. Using oxygen flows of 5 to 50 ml/kg/minute
  b. Using flows that only meet the metabolic requirements of the animal on oxygen
  c. Using flows that allow accurate measurement of halothane or isoflurane output
  d. Using flows that allow you to open the pop-off valve
23. The disadvantages of low-flow anesthesia include:
  a. Production of excess waste anesthetic gas
  b. It may allow carbon dioxide to accumulate in the circuit
  c. It results in the use of more anesthetic in the maintenance period
  d. It cannot be used with nitrous oxide
24. Using special techniques, nonprecision vaporizers can be used for:
  a. Low-flow anesthesia
  b. Delivery of nitrous oxide
  c. Elimination of carbon dioxide from the circuit
  d. Delivery of isoflurane

Answers for Chapter 4

1. a   **2.** e   **3.** a   **4.** c   **5.** b   **6.** c   **7.** e   **8.** b   **9.** a
10. b   **11.** c   **12.** True   **13.** a   **14.** a   **15.** c   **16.** a
17. a, b, c   **18.** b, c, d   **19.** a, b, d   **20.** a, b, c   **21.** a, c   **22.** b
23. b, d   **24.** a, d

Selected Readings

BEDNARSKI RM, GAYNOR JS, MUIR WW III: Vaporizer in circle for delivery of isoflurane to dogs, *J Am Vet Med Assoc* 202(6):943-948, 1993.

BEDNARSKI RM: Use of in-circle vaporizers to deliver isoflurane, *Compendium* 17:1377-1382, 1995.

DYSON DH: Influence of oxygen flows during anesthetic management, *Can Vet J* 32:752-754, 1991.

HASKINS SC: Opinions in small animal anesthesia, *Vet Clin North Am Small Anim Pract* 22(2):326-469, 1992.

LUDDERS JW, STAFFORD KL: Basic equipment for small animal anesthesia: use and maintenance, part II, *Compendium* 12(1):35-40, 1991.

MUIR WW III, HUBBELL JAE: *Handbook of veterinary anesthesia,* St Louis, 1989, Mosby.

PADDLEFORD RR: *Manual of small animal anesthesia,* New York, 1988, Churchill Livingstone.

SHORT CE: *Principles and practice of veterinary anesthesia,* Baltimore, 1987, Williams & Wilkins.

WARREN RG: *Small animal anesthesia,* St Louis, 1983, Mosby.

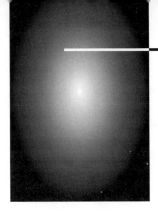

C H A P T E R 5

Workplace Safety

A veterinary technician may participate in the anesthetic management of several thousand animals during the course of his or her career. It is therefore essential that the technician be familiar with the human safety considerations involved in veterinary anesthesia. These can be divided into two categories: (1) hazards of waste anesthetic gas, and (2) safety considerations when handling compressed gas cylinders.

This chapter outlines the precautions that the anesthetist can take to reduce as much as possible the health risks of working with anesthetic equipment and gases.

■ HAZARDS OF WASTE ANESTHETIC GAS

Concerns have been raised regarding the possible adverse effects resulting from exposure of hospital personnel to waste anesthetic gas. The term *waste anesthetic gas* refers to the nitrous oxide, halothane, isoflurane, or methoxyflurane vapors that are breathed out by the patient or that escape from the anesthetic machine. These vapors are inadvertently breathed by all personnel working in areas in which animals are anesthetized or are recovering from inhalation anesthesia. Significant exposure to anesthetic vapors can also occur when emptying or filling anesthetic vaporizers. In addition, short-term exposure to high levels of anesthetic vapors can occur as the result of an accidental spill of liquid anesthetic.

Since the first study of waste anesthetic gas was published in 1967, many investigators have attempted to determine the toxicity of halothane, methoxyflurane, nitrous oxide, and other anesthetic agents to operating room personnel. Although some of the evidence is contradictory, it is generally accepted that exposure to high levels of waste anesthetic gas is associated with a higher than normal incidence of some health problems. The suspected health hazards can be divided into two categories: (1) short-term problems that occur during or immediately after exposure to these agents, and (2) long-term problems that may become evident days, weeks, or years after exposure.

Short-term Problems

The short-term problems associated with breathing waste gas appear to arise from a direct effect of anesthetic molecules on brain neurons. Symptoms such as fatigue, headache, drowsiness, nausea, depression, and irritability have been reported by persons working in environments in which a high level of waste gas is present. Although these symptoms usually resolve spontaneously when the affected person leaves the area, the recurrence of these symptoms may indicate that excessive levels of waste gas are present and that a potential for long-term toxicity exists.

Long-term Effects

Long-term inhalation of air polluted with waste gas may be associated with serious health problems, including reproductive disorders, liver and kidney damage, and chronic nervous system dysfunction. The mechanism of long-term anesthetic gas toxicity is not fully understood, but is thought to be the result of toxic metabolites produced by the breakdown of anesthetic gases within the liver and their subsequent excretion by the kidneys. These metabolites include inorganic fluoride or bromide ions, oxalic acid, and free radicals, all of which are known to have harmful effects on animal tissues.

It is widely accepted that anesthetic agents that are retained by the body and metabolized will have greater long-term toxicity than will those that are quickly eliminated through the lungs. For this reason, isoflurane is believed to be the least toxic inhalation agent in common use (0.2% of the amount inhaled is retained and metabolized). In contrast, 20% to 50% of halothane and 50% to 80% of methoxyflurane administered to a patient are retained within body fat, metabolized, and excreted through the kidneys. Although the patient may appear completely recovered from anesthesia induced by these agents, this indicates only that the level of anesthetic in the brain is very low. Significant amounts of anesthetic may linger in the liver, kidney, and body fat stores. Metabolites of halothane have been recovered from the urine of patients as long as 20 days after anesthesia. Human patients who inhale 50% nitrous oxide for 1 hour may have over 100 parts per million (ppm) nitrous oxide in their expired breath for the next 3 hours. In the same way, the anesthetist who inhales waste anesthetic gas may retain the gas or its metabolites for a considerable period. For example, anesthetists may show traces of halothane in their breath 64 hours after administering this gas to a patient.

Although it is generally accepted that isoflurane is safer for staff than other halogenated anesthetics, safety concerns (including NIOSH recommendations and OSHA* regulations) apply to *all* anesthetics.

---

*OSHA, the United States' Occupational Safety and Health Administration, is the government body that enforces safety and health regulations in the workplace. NIOSH, the National Institute for Occupational Safety and Health, conducts research into the prevention of work-related illness and injury, and publishes recommendations on safety procedures.

Effects on reproduction.   The most convincing evidence of waste anesthetic gas toxicity has emerged from numerous studies into the adverse effects of these agents on reproduction.

A comprehensive survey of nurse and physician anesthetists, undertaken by the American Society of Anesthesiologists, found that the *risk of spontaneous abortion* in this group was 1.3 to 2 times that of the normal population. Another study showed that the frequency of spontaneous abortion among working hospital anesthetists (18.2%) was higher than that observed among nonworking anesthetists (13.7%) and a control group (14.7%). The same study showed that 12% of the working anesthetists interviewed were infertile, compared with 6% of the control group.

Exposure to anesthetic gases also has been linked to an increase in *congenital abnormalities* in the children of pregnant operating room personnel. One study reported a 16% incidence of congenital abnormalities in children of practicing nurse-anesthetists, compared with a 6% incidence in a control group. Other studies have failed to show a statistically significant correlation between waste gas exposure and an increased incidence of congenital abnormalities.

It is difficult to interpret or compare the results obtained by these and other studies because there are wide variations in the types of anesthetics used, the amounts of waste gas exposure, and in control measures (such as the availability of scavengers). In most cases, operating room personnel were exposed to several agents simultaneously, and it is difficult to determine which agent or combination of agents was responsible for the adverse effects. It appears, however, that nitrous oxide may be at least partially responsible for the reproductive hazards associated with waste anesthetic gas. Experimentally, exposure of rats to high levels of nitrous oxide results in abnormalities in sperm morphology, in reduced ovulation, and in retarded fetal development. The adverse reproductive effects associated with exposure to nitrous oxide also were evident in a survey of dentists and dental assistants. Female dental assistants exposed to nitrous oxide for more than 9 hours per week showed a 1.7 to 2.3 times increase in spontaneous abortion rates compared with the normal population. An increase in the rate of spontaneous abortions also was noted in the wives of male dentists who administered nitrous oxide to their patients. Another study found that dental assistants exposed to unscavenged nitrous oxide for more than 5 hours per week were significantly less fertile than women who were exposed to lower levels of nitrous oxide. This reduced fertility may be a reflection of early fetal loss.

Given the weight of this evidence, it is prudent for women to avoid exposure to high levels of waste anesthetic gas (particularly nitrous oxide) during pregnancy.

Oncogenic effects.   Given that waste anesthetic gases may exert their adverse reproductive effects by altering DNA, investigators have attempted to determine whether these agents have the potential to cause other DNA-related changes, such as cancer. Several studies undertaken in the 1970s appeared to suggest that operating room personnel suffer from an increased incidence of some types of cancer. These studies, however, have been criticized for inappropriate data collection and statistical analysis, and it is now generally believed that none of the commonly used anesthetic agents is carcinogenic at the levels found in veterinary hospitals.

Effects on the liver.   Several studies have investigated the incidence of liver disorders in personnel exposed to waste anesthetic gas. Halothane, in particular, is recognized as being potentially hepatotoxic. Metabolism of halothane in certain rare anesthetized individuals produces toxic by-products that may result in massive hepatic necrosis, termed "halothane hepatitis."

The possible adverse effects of waste anesthetic gas on the liver were revealed by a study showing that the risk of liver disease in hospital operating room personnel is 1.5 times that of the general population. However, it is difficult to say with certainty whether the increased incidence of liver disease is associated with exposure to waste anesthetic gas or the result of other occupational hazards.

Effects on the kidney.   It is well established that methoxyflurane has the potential to cause renal toxicity in humans anesthetized with this agent, but the risk to operating room personnel has been more difficult to assess. Studies have indicated that there is a 1.2- to 1.4-fold increase in renal disease in female operating room personnel and a 1.2- to 1.7-fold increase in renal disease in female dental assistants compared with the general population. It has not been determined whether this increase is the result of the effect of methoxyflurane, nitrous oxide, other anesthetic agents, or other occupational factors working alone or in combination.

Neurologic effects.   Because the mechanism of action of anesthetic agents involves their effect on neurons, various studies have investigated the effect of waste anesthetic gas on the central nervous system. It has been suggested that exposure to high levels of anesthetics produces a decline in performance of motor skills and short-term memory. However, the threshold at which they begin to affect performance has not been established.

Some studies have indicated that exposure to even low concentrations of anesthetic gas mixtures (for example, nitrous oxide 500 ppm, halothane 15 ppm) results in decreased cognitive and motor skills. Chronic exposure to nitrous oxide has been associated with increased risk of neurologic disease: a study of female dental assistants exposed to high levels of nitrous oxide showed them to have a 1.7- to 2.8-fold increase in the incidence of neurologic disease compared with the normal population. Dentists and dental assistants exposed to high levels of waste nitrous oxide reported muscle weakness, tingling sensations, and numbness.

Assessment of Risk

Despite the alarming list of potential health hazards, the average veterinary technician working in a veterinary clinic is not necessarily at high risk. It is difficult to determine a clear-cut assessment of risk for several reasons, including the following:

- Caution must be used in interpreting the epidemiologic evidence provided by these studies. The evidence produced by various studies (or within one study) is sometimes contradictory. For example, some studies have failed to show any association between the incidence of spontaneous abortion or congenital abnormalities and a history of exposure to waste gas, whereas other studies suggest the opposite.
- Although many epidemiologic studies indicate an increased incidence of health problems in people working in an environment where exposure to waste gas occurs, it does not necessarily follow that the anesthetic gases themselves are the causative agents. Other chemicals or other factors present in the operating room or dentist's office may contribute to increased incidence of health disorders.
- Many studies of the adverse effects of waste anesthetic gases did not measure the level of waste gas present in the working environment. Epidemiologic stud-

ies do not give information regarding the use of scavengers and procedures that reduce waste gas pollution. Without this information, interpretation of the studies is difficult.

Despite the difficulties noted here, most authorities and regulatory agencies agree that exposure to high levels of waste anesthetic gas should be avoided and that controls should be introduced to reduce exposure. The safe level of anesthetic gas in the working environment has not yet been determined. After reviewing the available literature, the U.S. National Institute for Occupational Safety and Health (NIOSH) recommended that the concentration of halothane, methoxyflurane, or isoflurane not exceed 2 parts per million when used alone and not exceed 0.5 ppm when used with nitrous oxide. (The concentration at which the odor of halothane can be detected by the average person is 50 ppm or more, which is 25 times the maximum recommended level.) It is also suggested the nitrous oxide concentration not exceed 25 ppm. These levels were chosen because they were believed to be the lowest levels realistically achievable given current technology. The NIOSH levels have been adopted by OSHA and most state and provincial regulatory bodies. It is generally accepted that exposure to this level of anesthetic gas is associated with minimal risk to employees, including those who are pregnant.

Surveys of human and veterinary hospitals reveal a wide variation in the levels of waste anesthetic gas present in different locations within the clinic (Tables 5-1 and 5-2). The halothane concentration in the air of unscavenged surgery suites in human hospitals has been reported to be as high as 85 ppm, and concentrations of nitrous oxide have been measured as high as 7000 ppm. As expected, air samples taken from surgery suites, surgical preparation rooms, and anesthetic recovery

TABLE 5-1

Waste Anesthetic Gas (Halothane) Concentrations in Various Locations Within the Veterinary Hospital (Semiclosed Circuit, 1 L/Minute Oxygen Flow)

Sampling Site	Level of Contamination (ppm)
PERSONNEL BREATHING ZONE	
With scavenging	1.45
No scavenging	2.00
NOSE AND MOUTH OF PATIENT JUST REMOVED	
FROM ANESTHETIC CHAMBER	10.00
AIR AROUND UNSCAVENGED ANESTHETIC CHAMBER	10.00
NOSE AND MOUTH OF ANESTHETIZED PATIENT	
Intubated, cuff inflated	3.25
Intubated, cuff not inflated	6.10
AIR OUTSIDE RECOVERY CAGE DOOR	1.07
NOSE OF PATIENT IN RECOVERY CAGE	5.43

Modified from Short CE, Harvey RC: Anesthetic waste gases in veterinary medicine, *Cornell Vet* 73(4):363-374, 1983.

TABLE 5-2

Sources of Anesthetic Gas Contamination

Technique or Situation	Level of Contamination (ppm)
ROOM AIR WHEN FILLING VAPORIZER	10
RESERVOIR BAG EMPTIED INTO ROOM AIR	2.5->10
ROOM AIR AFTER SPILL OF AGENT	10
HANDS OF PERSONNEL FILLING VAPORIZER	2.5->10
HANDS AFTER WASHING	0
CLOTHING OF PERSONNEL FILLING VAPORIZER	5.0-8.75
RESIDUES IN UNWASHED RUBBER COMPONENTS	1.8->10

Modified from Short CE, Harvey RC: Anesthetic waste gases in veterinary medicine, *Cornell Vet* 73(4):363-374, 1983.

rooms are more likely to contain waste gas than samples taken elsewhere in the clinic. During the anesthetic period itself, the level of waste gas is highest immediately adjacent to the anesthetic machine, but the actual level varies with the duration of anesthesia, the flow rate of the carrier gas, the type of anesthetic system used (rebreathing or nonrebreathing), and most importantly, whether an effective scavenging system is used.

Reducing Exposure to Waste Anesthetic Gas

Given the potential health hazards associated with exposure to waste anesthetic gas, it is obviously in the technician's best interest to minimize exposure as much as possible. The American College of Veterinary Anesthesiologists recommends that any veterinary facility using inhalant anesthetics should institute and maintain a control program for waste anesthetic gases, based on the possibility that trace gases may adversely affect human health.

If proper equipment, techniques, and procedures are used, it is possible to reduce waste gas exposure to a level well below the NIOSH standards. This can be achieved through several means, including use of a gas scavenging system, testing equipment for leaks, and practicing techniques and procedures that minimize exposure to waste gas.

Use of a scavenging system.   The installation and use of an effective gas scavenging system is the single most important step in reducing waste gas exposure. A 1982 survey of veterinary hospitals showed that scavenging reduces waste halothane concentrations by 64% to 94%. A scavenger consists of tubing attached to the anesthetic machine pop-off valve (or in the case of a nonrebreathing system, to the outlet port or tail of the reservoir bag). The function of a scavenger is to collect waste gas from the machine and conduct it to a disposal point outside the building.

From the regulatory perspective, OSHA's Hazard Chemical Standard (1910.1200) requires the employer to install adequate engineering controls to ensure that occupational exposure to any chemical never exceeds the permissible exposure limit. This is difficult or impossible to achieve unless a waste anesthetic gas scavenger or activated charcoal canister is used.

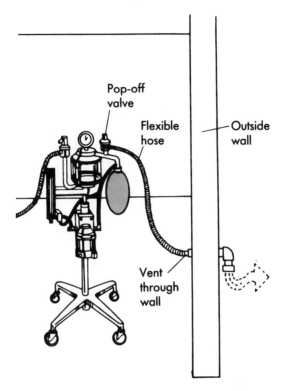

FIG. 5-1   Passive scavenging system.

Scavenging systems may be passive or active (Figs. 5-1 and 5-2). An active system uses suction created by a vacuum pump or fan to draw gas into the scavenger, whereas a passive system uses the positive pressure of the gas in the anesthetic machine to push gas into the scavenger. Both active and passive scavenging systems appear to be effective when correctly assembled and operated. The most efficient system, however, appears to be an active one with a dedicated vacuum pump.

Active scavenging systems are more costly than passive systems and require more maintenance. Activation with a switch is required for active systems. Passive systems are well suited for rooms adjacent to the exterior of the building, but are ineffective for interior rooms where the distance to the outlet is more than 20 feet (4 meters).

Ideally, scavenging systems should be professionally installed when the veterinary clinic is built. However, it is not difficult to assemble and install an effective scavenging system in an established veterinary hospital. Scavenger parts may be purchased or can be readily assembled using simple materials. The hose or tubing of the scavenger may be constructed from plastic tubing, PVC pipe, or other flexible, gas-impermeable material. Most modern anesthetic machines are equipped with adapters to allow connection to a scavenging system. Older machines can be retrofitted with pop-off valves that can be connected to a scavenger hose.

The most commonly used type of passive system discharges waste gas to the outdoors through a hole in the wall. Another type of passive system can be set up

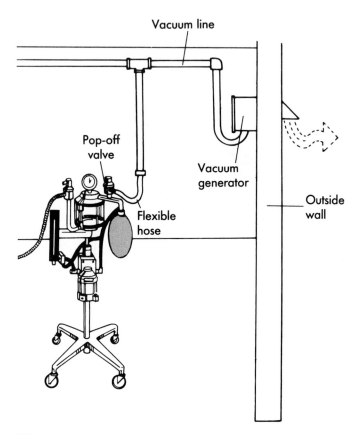

FIG. 5-2   Active scavenging system.

by placing the end of the transfer hose adjacent to the room ventilation exhaust or nonrecirculating air conditioning system. This is acceptable provided the air is not recirculated within the building and the transfer hose is no more than 10 feet in length. Because anesthetic vapors are heavier than room air, the transfer hose should travel a downward course toward the exhaust. The waste gas must be discharged outdoors: passive systems that simply vent gases to the floor level are not effective.

Once the waste gas is collected, it must be expelled outside of the building, away from doors, windows, and air intakes. Waste gas collected in the tubing should be totally confined within the scavenger hose from the pop-off valve to the point of discharge and must not be recirculated into the building air. Scavenger hoses that end on the floor of a room, in an attic or basement, or that conduct the waste gas into a recirculating central vacuum system or recirculating ventilation exhaust merely contaminate all building rooms with the waste gas.

Normally, use of a scavenging system with an anesthetic machine does not alter the operation of the machine. The anesthetist should, however, be aware of two potential difficulties that can occur when a scavenging system is present:

1. When using an active scavenging system, it is important to prevent the negative pressure (vacuum) from the scavenger from entering the breathing circuit. If this is allowed to occur, the reservoir bag will collapse. Many machines are equipped with a negative pressure relief valve, adjacent to the pop-off valve, which opens automatically if negative pressure is detected in the circuit. The open valve admits room air to the circuit, thereby ensuring that a vacuum does not develop. When using a machine that is not equipped with a negative pressure relief valve, it is important to ensure that the reservoir bag is at least partially inflated with air at all times.

2. If either a passive or active scavenging system is in use, the anesthetist must be aware of the potential for a blockage to occur such that waste gas cannot enter the scavenging system. If this happens, gas will accumulate within the anesthetic circuit. This situation is analogous to operation of a machine with a closed pop-off valve and may result in excessive pressure developing within the circuit. To prevent this occurrence, many machines are equipped with a positive pressure relief valve, which opens automatically if excessive pressure starts to build up within the circuit.

Regardless of whether an active or passive system is used, the anesthetist must be able to connect an anesthetic machine or anesthetic chamber to a scavenger in every room in which the machines are used. It is sometimes impractical to use a scavenger (for example, in a specialized room such as the x-ray room, or when a mobile anesthetic machine is used). In this case, either anesthesia can be maintained using an injectable agent or an anesthetic machine with an activated charcoal cartridge can be used (for example, f/air canister, A.M. Bickford, Inc). These cartridges can effectively absorb isoflurane, halothane, and methoxyflurane vapors. To be effective, however, these cartridges must be replaced after 12 hours of use or after a weight gain of 50 grams. An additional drawback of these units is their inability to filter nitrous oxide.

For additional protection, masks with activated charcoal filters can be worn by personnel who are at special risk (such as pregnancy). Like the activated charcoal canister for anesthetic machines, these are not effective in filtering out nitrous oxide vapors.

Equipment leak testing.   Although the installation of a scavenging device is the most important step in reducing anesthetic gas pollution, there are many other procedures and techniques that significantly reduce the anesthetist's risk of exposure. One of these is leak testing of anesthetic machines. Leakage of gas from anesthetic machines is a significant source of operating room pollution, and it is *not* reduced by a scavenging system. Leakage may occur from any part of the machine in which nitrous oxide or gas anesthetic (for example, methoxyflurane, isoflurane, and halothane) is present. The most common problems that can result in waste gas leakage are the following:

- The connections for nitrous oxide gas lines are not tightly secured
- O rings, washers, and other seals joining nitrous oxide gas tanks to the machine hanger yokes are missing, worn, or out of position
- The covering over a unidirectional valve is not tightly closed
- The carbon dioxide absorber canister is not securely sealed. Leaks are often caused by improper positioning of the canister or by the presence of absorber granules on the seals around the canister.
- Holes in the reservoir bag or hoses

- A connection between the pop-off valve and scavenger that is not airtight
- Breathing hoses, reservoir bag, or endotracheal tube not securely connected to the machine
- A vaporizer cap not replaced after the vaporizer is filled

The anesthetist should routinely perform leak tests to determine the presence and location of waste gas leaks. There are two types of tests:

1. High-pressure tests for nitrous oxide or oxygen leakage. High-pressure leaks arise between gas tanks and the flowmeter, where the pressure is 50 pounds per square inch (psi) or greater.
2. Low-pressure tests for the escape of anesthetic gas from the anesthetic machine itself. The pressure of gas within the machine is approximately 15 psi. Low-pressure leaks may arise between the flowmeter and the patient, or within the anesthetic circuit and attachments.

High-pressure system tests.   One test of the high-pressure system is to turn the nitrous oxide tank on and place a 10% detergent solution on all tank connections and joints. Each location is then observed for bubble formation, which indicates a leak.

Another useful high-pressure test is conducted by first turning on the nitrous oxide cylinder, noting the reading on the tank pressure gauge, and then turning the cylinder off. Throughout this procedure the flowmeter is set to zero, maintaining the pressure in the system (that is, line pressure is not evacuated). The tank pressure gauge should be checked again in 1 hour. If the pressure gauge reading is unchanged, the high-pressure system is leak-free. If the pressure is at or near zero, there is a leak somewhere between the cylinder and the flowmeter, and nitrous oxide is escaping into the room air. The most likely location of the leak is at the connection of the cylinder to the machine yoke.

It is also possible to check for high-pressure leaks of oxygen by following the same procedure as that outlined for the nitrous oxide. Although the escape of small amounts of oxygen obviously poses little or no risk of health problems to the anesthetic machine operator, it may lead to premature emptying of the oxygen tank.

Low-pressure system tests.   Low-pressure leaks are best detected by securing all connections, closing the pop-off valve, and placing a hand or stopper over the Y piece, thus closing off all avenues of gas escape from the machine. The oxygen tank is turned on and the flowmeter is adjusted to supply a flow rate of at least 2 L/minute, and the reservoir bag is allowed to gradually fill with oxygen. The anesthetist should be able to squeeze the inflated bag with gentle pressure without causing escape of air from the bag. Because the only exits from the system (the pop-off valve and the Y piece) are closed, any escape of air indicates that a leak is present. Alternatively, the anesthetist can close the pop-off valve, occlude the Y piece, and pressurize the system to 30 cm of water, using the flowmeter. When the oxygen flow meter is turned off, the pressure should be maintained for 10 seconds. When the system is pressured to 30 cm of water, the quantity of leakage can be measured by determining the flow rate of oxygen necessary to maintain a constant pressure in the system. The leak rate should be less than 300 ml/minute.

Nonrebreathing systems such as the Bain apparatus can be checked for leaks by applying pressure to the system (with all ports occluded) using guidelines as for circle systems. For both nonrebreathing and rebreathing systems, the location of leaks may be determined by listening for the hiss of escaping air or by using a detergent solution as previously described.

High-pressure leak testing should be performed at least weekly if nitrous oxide is in use. Low-pressure leak testing should be done every time the machine is assembled. If leaks are detected that cannot be resolved by the technician, the machine should be serviced by a manufacturer's representative or other qualified person.

Anesthetic techniques and procedures.   The anesthetist, by his or her choice of anesthetic techniques, has considerable control over the amount of waste gas released into the room air. One survey of human hospitals found faulty work practices were to account for 94% to 99% of waste anesthetic gas released in scavenged operating rooms.

The steps in Procedure 5-1 are recommended to minimize waste gas release.

 PROCEDURE 5-1
Minimizing Waste Gas Release

1. Use caution when inducing an animal in an anesthetic chamber. Anesthetic chambers were the greatest source of anesthetic pollution noted in a 1983 survey of veterinary facilities. Not only are large amounts of waste gas released when the chamber is opened, but also the fur of the patient is contaminated with anesthetic vapor. If a chamber is used, a scavenging system should be connected to it. Anesthetic chambers should have 2 inlet holes, to which the breathing hoses from the anesthetic machine can be attached after the Y piece is removed. In this way, the waste gases are evacuated through the machine and regular scavenger. Alternatively, the hose from a Bain system can be attached to one inlet and the scavenger system can be directly attached to the other hole. Either way, the chamber should be closed immediately after the patient is removed, and the oxygen flow should be continued for several minutes to purge waste gas, rather than releasing waste gas into the room air. Anesthetic chambers should be tightly sealed to avoid leakage, and used only in a well-ventilated area. Chambers should be washed with soap and water after each use to remove residual anesthetic.

2. Avoid using masks to maintain anesthesia. Significant amounts of anesthetic gas may escape from around the diaphragm of the mask and enter the room air. If the situation dictates the use of a mask, it should be fitted tightly over the animal's face. Face masks are available in a variety of sizes and should be chosen to fit the patient snugly but comfortably. When a mask is used, the sequence of events is the same as for an endotracheal tube: turn the oxygen on, place the mask on the patient, then turn the vaporizer on. This order should be reversed when ending the procedure.

3. Use cuffed endotracheal tubes when possible. Endotracheal tubes significantly reduce the escape of waste gas into room air, as compared with masks. To be effective, however, the tube must be of adequate size and the cuff must be inflated and in good repair. Before use, inflate cuffs with air to check for leaks. After intubation of the patient, check the fit of the endotracheal tube
Continued

▼ **PROCEDURE 5-1**
Minimizing Waste Gas Release—*cont'd*

within the trachea by closing the pop-off valve and gently squeezing the reservoir bag (To prevent overinflation of the patient's lungs, ensure that the circuit pressure displayed on the manometer does not exceed 20 cm of water when applying pressure to the bag to check the cuff). The cuff should be inflated to its "minimum no leak volume," the minimum amount of air that results in no air escape around the cuff when the bag is gently squeezed.

4. When using a rebreathing system, ensure that the reservoir bag inflates and deflates regularly with the patient's respirations. If this does not occur, one should suspect either an air leakage around the endotracheal tube or esophageal intubation. Significant release of waste gas can occur in both cases. (It is also likely that the patient will wake up because a significant amount of room air enters the lungs in either case.)

5. The use of closed rebreathing systems may help minimize waste gas pollution. Anesthesia using open systems and high gas flows (that is, greater than 3 L/minute) is associated with greater release of waste gas, particularly if effective scavenging is not available.

6. Do not turn the vaporizer or flowmeters on until the anesthetic machine is connected to the endotracheal tube and the cuff is inflated. The practice of filling the machine and reservoir bag with anesthetic gas before connecting the machine to the patient should be discouraged. Once the anesthetic procedure is under way, avoid disconnecting the patient from the breathing circuit unnecessarily. If the patient is to be disconnected from the machine, the vaporizer setting and flowmeters should be turned to zero.

7. Do not release the contents of the reservoir bag into the room air. If it is necessary to empty the reservoir bag, leave it attached to the machine and evacuate the contents into the scavenger.

8. Maintain the connection between the animal and the machine, having the animal breathe pure oxygen at 2 to 3 times the maintenance flow rate for several minutes after the vaporizer is turned off. Periodically flush the system with oxygen by emptying the rebreathing bag through the pop-off valve. If possible, leave the patient attached to the machine until extubation occurs. This allows expired anesthetic to enter the scavenging system rather than the room air.

9. Ensure that all rooms in which anesthetic gases are released (for example, surgical prep room, operating room, recovery room, and radiography room) have adequate ventilation that provides at least 15 air changes per hour. A properly designed ventilation system helps eliminate residual waste gases not collected by the scavenging system (for example, those that arise from leaks or improper work practices).

10. One study found that concentrations of halothane and nitrous oxide were higher in recovery areas than in scavenged operating rooms. To reduce waste

PROCEDURE 5-1
Minimizing Waste Gas Release—*cont'd*

gas levels, it is usually necessary to have an exhaust fan or nonrecirculating ventilation system operating in the room where patients are recovering from anesthesia. Whenever possible, avoid being closer than 3 feet from the nose of an animal recovering from anesthesia.

11. Have anesthetic machines serviced at least annually by a qualified service technician to ensure minimal leakage through machine components. A log of evaluation and maintenance procedures and leakage testing should be maintained for each anesthetic machine, ventilator, and vaporizer.

12. Inspect equipment often. The routine maintenance procedures for anesthetic machines are usually explained in the operations manual.

13. Hoses, reservoir bags, and endotracheal tubes that are cracked or worn should be discarded. Endotracheal tubes with nonfunctional or leaking cuffs should not be used.

14. Wash hoses, reservoir bags, masks, endotracheal tubes, and all other rubber components of the anesthetic circuit with soap and water and allow them to air dry after each procedure. These components may absorb considerable amounts of anesthetic during use. Washing not only removes absorbed waste gas, but also reduces transfer of microorganisms between patients.

15. Emptying and filling vaporizers may release significant amounts of anesthetic vapor into the surrounding air. Anesthetics may also be spilled onto the technician's hands and clothing. (See Table 5-2.) Ideally, vaporizers should be filled at the end of the workday, as personnel are leaving the hospital. Use a filling device (a specialized attachment that transfers anesthetic directly into the vaporizer) rather than pouring from a bottle to replenish liquid anesthetic in the machine. Agent-specific keyed filler systems are preferred. If no filling device is available, use a bottle adapter with a spout to prevent spillage. Fill vaporizers in a well-ventilated area (ideally, outside of the building). Use of an approved respirator (a device that fits over the mouth and nose and filters incoming air), vinyl or plastic gloves, a lab coat or plastic apron, and other protective equipment will also minimize exposure to anesthetic liquid or vapors. Hands should be washed immediately after filling a vaporizer because liquid anesthetics are readily absorbed through intact skin.

16. If liquid anesthetic is spilled, high concentrations of anesthetic vapor will be present in the immediate area of the spill. Accidental spillage of even 1 ml of liquid anesthetic will vaporize up to 200 ml of gas with a concentration of 1,000,000 ppm. If a spill occurs, increase ventilation as much as possible during the cleanup by opening windows or using fans. Close doors to the rest of the building and turn off the central vacuum system to avoid spreading the fumes throughout the building. All personnel not involved in the cleanup should leave the area, and the remaining staff should wear approved

Continued

▼ PROCEDURE 5-1
Minimizing Waste Gas Release—*cont'd*

protective clothing, vinyl or plastic (not latex or rubber) gloves, and respirators (for a large spill). Remove all contaminated articles, including lab coats. Pour absorbent material such as kitty litter on the spill so that the liquid is completely absorbed. Dispose of the litter in an airtight container outside the clinic. If the spill is large or if protective equipment is not available, all personnel should leave the building and the local fire department should be notified.

17. Cap empty anesthetic bottles when discarding them because residual anesthetic in the bottle may evaporate into the room air. For the same reason, store vaporizer-filling devices in a sealed plastic bag between uses.

Monitoring Waste Gas Levels

It is advisable to periodically monitor waste anesthetic gas levels to ensure that the NIOSH levels are not exceeded. If professional monitoring is required, an accredited industrial hygiene laboratory can be contacted for assistance. (Industrial hygienists are found in the yellow pages of the telephone directory under "occupational safety.") An occupational hygienist will usually visit the hospital to evaluate ventilation and scavenging techniques and to interview the anesthetist regarding procedures used to minimize waste gas release. Air samples should be collected from all areas in which anesthetics are used, and the level of waste gas in the collected air is determined using an infrared spectrometer. The cost of such a visit ranges from $250 to $700.

Professional monitoring services are not always required. Clinic employees can inexpensively monitor waste gas levels using detector tubes or badges. The badges are worn by personnel in the operating room during a timed period when anesthetic gases are being used. Alternatively, the badge may be placed in a room for area monitoring. Badges may detect only one chemical, such as halothane, isoflurane, or nitrous oxide, or may be sensitive to all halogenated anesthetics. After use, the badge is returned to the supplier (usually an industrial health and safety supply house or a company specializing in OSHA compliance) for analysis. Results are given as a time-weighted average in parts per million. Cost, including analysis, is approximately $40 to $50 per badge.

■ SAFE HANDLING OF COMPRESSED GASES
Fire Safety Precautions

There is a potential for fire in any room where oxygen or nitrous oxide is used. Oxygen and nitrous oxide are not flammable; however, both support combustion and cause fuels to burn more readily. It is recommended that no flames or sources of ignition (for example, matches, lighters, or Bunsen burners) be present in any room in which oxygen or nitrous oxide cylinders are stored or used. For obvious reasons, smoking must be prohibited in all rooms in which oxygen is stored or used. Even static electricity can cause fires in areas in which oxygen and flammable materials are used together. (This is one of the reasons why ether, which is extremely flammable, is no longer used in anesthesia.)

Use and Storage of Compressed Gas Cylinders

Another potential danger of compressed gases is the damage that may result from a sudden release of gas from the cylinder. When the tank is turned on, compressed gas may exit the cylinder nozzle with great force. Persons connecting compressed gas cylinders to an anesthetic machine or gas piping system should wear impact-resistant goggles to protect their eyes from jets of gas. If a cylinder leak occurs, never use your hand to try to stop the leak.

A sudden gas release can have catastrophic consequences if a cylinder is damaged. Gas will be suddenly released if the cylinder is punctured or if it is knocked over and the regulator (the metal attachments at the top of the tank) or cylinder neck is broken off the tank. If this happens, the force of the gas suddenly escaping from the tank may cause the tank to move like a rocket through a wall or roof. To prevent this occurrence, large cylinders should be chained or belted to a wall and should always be stored in an upright position. To protect the regulator from damage, valve caps should be used on all large cylinders that are not connected to gas lines.

Gas cylinders should be stored away from emergency exits or areas with heavy traffic. If a cylinder must be moved to another location, a hand cart should be used, rather than rolling the cylinder.

Full tanks should be kept separate from empty tanks and also should be clearly labeled for quick identification. The use of tear-off labels helps eliminate confusion regarding the empty, in-use, or full status of a given compressed air cylinder. In reading these labels, the current status of the tank is given on the outermost section of the label (Fig. 5-3). Cylinders should be used in the order that they are received (that is, first in, first out).

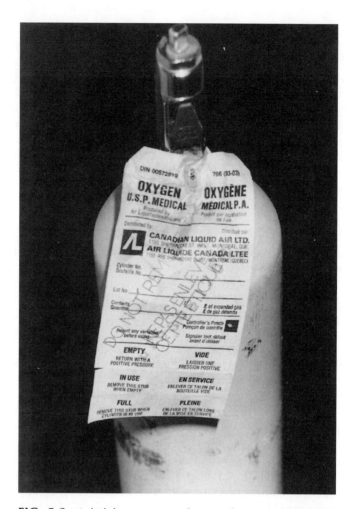

FIG. 5-3 Label for compressed gas tanks. Current status of tank is shown by printing at the bottom of the label. Label shown is from newly purchased tank and reads "FULL." When tank is connected to machine, lower portion of the label is removed so that remaining label reads "IN USE." When tank is empty, "IN USE" stub is removed, leaving the label that reads "EMPTY."

✔ **KEY POINTS**

1. Anesthesia presents several potential health risks to hospital personnel, including exposure to waste anesthetic gas and the handling of compressed gas cylinders.
2. Waste anesthetic gas vapors are breathed by all personnel working in areas in which animals are anesthetized or are recovering from inhalation anesthesia. Filling or emptying vaporizers and the cleanup of accidental spills also may result in significant exposure.

3. Exposure to waste anesthetic gas is associated with short-term problems such as fatigue, headache, drowsiness, nausea, depression, and irritability.

4. Long-term exposure to waste anesthetic gases may be associated with reproductive disorders, liver and kidney damage, and nervous system dysfunction. The evidence of epidemiologic studies is sometimes contradictory and difficult to interpret. Most authorities recommend that exposure to high levels of waste anesthetic gas be avoided, particularly by pregnant women.

5. Anesthetics such as methoxyflurane and halothane, which are eliminated significantly by hepatic metabolism and renal excretion, are considered to be a greater hazard than anesthetics eliminated by respiration.

6. Waste anesthetic gases apparently do not have oncogenic (cancer-causing) effects.

7. The NIOSH recommendations for waste anesthetic gas concentrations limit exposure to 2 parts per million (ppm) or less for halothane, isoflurane, and methoxyflurane (0.5 ppm or less if nitrous oxide is concurrently used). Surveys of veterinary clinics show wide variations in waste gas levels, depending on the sampling site, scavenging system, and anesthetic techniques used.

8. Installation and use of an effective gas scavenging system greatly reduces waste gas exposure. Caution should be used to prevent negative pressure from the scavenger from entering the breathing circuit.

9. Equipment leak testing should be done on a daily basis to detect and allow correction of leakage from the anesthetic machine and compressed air cylinders. Tests should be done on both the high-pressure and low-pressure components of the machine, particularly if nitrous oxide is in use.

10. Certain anesthetic techniques are associated with excessive waste gas release. These include the use of anesthetic chambers, masks, and uncuffed endotracheal tubes. Procedures such as turning off the vaporizer before disconnecting the animal from the machine are helpful in reducing waste gas contamination of hospital air.

11. Vaporizers should be filled and emptied with care, using appropriate equipment and protective clothing.

12. Waste gas levels may be monitored by professional occupational hygienists or by the use of detector tubes or badges.

13. Compressed air cylinders should be transported, used, and stored with care. Special hazards include risk of fire in areas in which cylinders are stored and the risk of sudden release of pressurized gas from cylinders.

 REVIEW QUESTIONS

1. Waste anesthetic gases are a potential hazard to personnel, but problems that arise are really only of a short-term nature.
   True   False

2. Long-term toxicity of inhalation anesthetics is thought to be caused by the release of toxic metabolites during the breakdown of these drugs.
   True   False

3. The anesthetic thought to be the least toxic to hospital personnel is:
   a. Isoflurane
   b. Halothane
   c. Methoxyflurane
   d. Nitrous oxide
4. In the United States, the National Institute for Occupational Safety and Health recommends that the levels of waste anesthetic gases for anesthetics such as isoflurane, halothane, or methoxyflurane should not exceed _____ ppm.
   a. 0.2
   b. 2
   c. 20
   d. 200
5. The odor of halothane may be detected by a person when the levels reach _____ ppm.
   a. 5
   b. 50
   c. 500
   d. 5000
6. Rooms in which animals are recovering from anesthesia may be highly contaminated with waste gas.
   True   False
7. It is recommended that for a passive scavenger system, the hose be no longer than _____ feet if it discharges into the room ventilation exhaust.
   a. 1
   b. 10
   c. 20
   d. 50
8. How often should a test for low-pressure leaks be conducted?
   a. Each time the machine is used
   b. At least once per week
   c. At least once per month
   d. When the anesthetist smells anesthetic gases
9. The safest way to transport a high-pressure tank, such as an oxygen tank, is by:
   a. Carrying it
   b. Rolling it along the floor
   c. A hand cart
   d. Dragging it by the neck
10. Rooms in which waste anesthetic gases are at risk of being released should have a minimum of _____ air changes per hour.
    a. 5
    b. 10
    c. 15
    d. 20

For the following questions, more than one answer may be correct.

11. Long-term hazards that may occur from exposure to anesthetic waste gases include:
    a. Reproductive disorders
    b. Liver damage
    c. Kidney damage
    d. Nervous system dysfunction
12. A technician may reduce the amount of waste gases by:
    a. Using cuffed endotracheal tubes
    b. Ensuring the anesthetic machine has been tested for leaks
    c. Using an induction technique other than mask or chamber
    d. Using high fresh gas flows
13. To conduct a low-pressure test on an anesthetic machine, you must:
    a. Close the pop-off valve and occlude the end of the circuit
    b. Turn off the oxygen tank
    c. Compress the reservoir bag
    d. Pressurize the circuit with a volume of gas

Answers for Chapter 5

1. False   **2.** True   **3.** a   **4.** b   **5.** b   **6.** True   **7.** b   **8.** a
9. c   **10.** c   **11.** a, b, c, d   **12.** a, b, c   **13.** a, c, d

Selected Readings

AD HOC COMMITTEE OF THE AMERICAN SOCIETY OF ANESTHESIOLOGISTS: Occupational disease among operating room personnel: a study, *Anesthesiology* 41(4):321-340, 1974.

AMERICAN COLLEGE OF VETERINARY ANESTHESIOLOGISTS: Commentary and recommendations on control of waste anesthetic gases in the workplace, *J Am Vet Med Assoc* 209(1):75-77, 1996.

BURKHART JE, STOBBE TJ: Real-time measurement and control of waste anesthetic gases during veterinary surgeries, *Am Ind Hyg Assoc J* 51(12):640-645, 1990.

GROSS ME, BRANSON KR: Reducing exposure to waste anesthetic gas, *Vet Tech* 14(3):175-177, 1993.

HARVEY RC: *Anesthetic waste gas management in veterinary medicine*, Knoxville, 1991, University of Tennessee (unpublished).

LIETZEMAYER DW: Current methods for removal of anesthetic gas, *Vet Tech* 11(4):213-220, 1990.

OSHA OFFICE OF SCIENCE AND TECHNOLOGY ASSESSMENT: Anesthetic agents—workplace exposures, *OSHA Instruction TED* 1.15 (H-2), 1996.

PADDLEFORD RR: *Manual of small animal anesthesia*, New York, 1988, Churchill Livingstone.

PURDHAM JT: *Anaesthetic gases and vapours*, Hamilton, Ontario, Canada, 1986, Canadian Centre for Occupational Health and Safety.

SHORT CE: *Principles and practice of veterinary anesthesia*, Baltimore, 1987, Williams & Wilkins.

SHORT CE, HARVEY RC: Anesthetic waste gases in veterinary medicine, *Cornell Vet* 73(4):363-374, 1983.

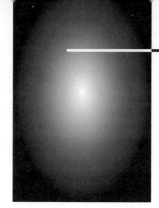

CHAPTER **6**

Anesthetic Problems and Emergencies

PERFORMANCE OBJECTIVES

After completion of this chapter, the reader will be able to:

- List the most common reasons why anesthetic emergencies occur, including problems arising from human error, equipment failure, and the adverse effects of anesthetic agents.
- Explain how anesthesia of geriatric and pediatric patients differs from anesthesia of healthy adult dogs and cats.
- Describe the problems involved in anesthetizing each of the following: brachycephalic dogs; sighthounds; obese animals; and patients suffering from trauma or cardiovascular, respiratory, hepatic, or renal disease.
- Describe the role of the veterinary technician in responding to anesthetic emergencies.
- List the most common causes of the following anesthetic problems: inadequate anesthetic depth, excessive anesthetic depth, pale mucous membranes, prolonged capillary refill, dyspnea, tachypnea, bradycardia, tachycardia, and cardiac arrhythmias.
- Describe the appropriate response to common emergencies, including dyspnea, respiratory arrest, and cardiac arrest.
- List the most common problems that may arise in the recovery period, and the appropriate action that can be taken to prevent or treat these problems.

G eneral anesthesia poses little risk to most patients when performed by capable personnel using an anesthetic protocol appropriate for the animal. Emergencies are uncommon, and the overwhelming majority of patients recover from anesthesia with no lasting ill effects. After successfully anesthetizing hundreds of patients, it is easy for the technician to be lulled into a false sense of security. However, it is vitally important that the anesthetist remembers that every anesthetic procedure has the potential to cause the death of the animal. The anesthetist must remain watchful for problems that may arise in even the most routine anesthetic procedure.

A survey of British veterinary clinics revealed a mortality rate of one death for every 870 anesthetic procedures in healthy dogs and one death for every 552 procedures in healthy cats. The same study found a mortality rate of 1 in 30 patients where systemic disease was present. An American study of 3,239 cases found the incidence of anesthetic complications to be 12% in dogs and 10.5% in cats, with a mortality rate of 0.43% (4.3 per 1000) in both dogs and cats.* A Canadian study of 16,000 anesthetized animals found the incidence of cardiac arrest to be approximately 1 in 900 patients. Of the dogs with anesthetic complications, bulldogs, Pekingese, and other brachycephalic breeds; weimaraners; and Jack Russell terriers were disproportionately represented. Emergency anesthesia was associated with a much greater risk than elective anesthesia.

This chapter describes problems that may arise during anesthesia, ranging from minor (such as maintaining appropriate anesthetic depth) to major (including respiratory arrest and cardiac arrest). Appropriate responses to various anesthetic emergencies are presented, and the reasons the anesthetic problems may arise (and procedures for their prevention) are emphasized. The challenges associated with anesthesia of patients with special problems such as heart disease or brachycephalic conformation are also discussed.

■ REASONS WHY ANESTHETIC PROBLEMS AND EMERGENCIES ARISE

Although an awareness of the correct response to an anesthetic emergency is essential, it is even more important to understand why emergencies arise and how they may be prevented. Most anesthetic emergencies are the result of one or more of the following factors: human error, equipment failure, the adverse effect of anesthetic agents, and patient-related factors.

Human Error

Human error is, unfortunately, a contributing cause in some anesthetic deaths. Common human errors committed by anesthetists in veterinary practice include the following:

1. Failure to obtain an adequate history or physical examination on the patient
2. Inadequate experience with the anesthetic machine or anesthetic agents being used
3. Failure to devote sufficient time or attention to the anesthetized patient
4. Fatigue
5. Failure to recognize and respond to early signs of patient difficulty

Failure to obtain an adequate history or to perform a physical examination. Ideally, every patient scheduled for anesthesia should have a complete physical examination, and a thorough history should be obtained. In practice, this is not always possible. Animals are sometimes dropped off at the veterinary clinic by owners who are in a hurry and reluctant to stop and answer questions about their pet. Animals may be brought in by neighbors or friends of the owner or by other persons unfamiliar with

---

*The death rate related to general anesthesia in human patients has been variously estimated to be as high as 1.5 per 1000 and as low as 1 per 10,000 patients.

the animal's history. The receptionist or other person admitting the animal to the hospital may fail to ask important questions or may not transmit the information to the anesthetist or veterinarian. The physical examination is sometimes cursory or omitted entirely. The net result is that significant information may be overlooked. For example, the anesthetist may be unaware that a patient has not been fasted or that an animal scheduled for surgery is dehydrated as a result of vomiting and diarrhea. An anesthetic protocol that is safe for a healthy patient could be inappropriate for these animals, and an anesthetic problem or even death of the patient could result.

Lack of familiarity with the anesthetic machine or drugs used.   It is the responsibility of the veterinarian to ensure that his or her personnel are sufficiently trained and knowledgeable to perform competently all required procedures. Some simple anesthetic tasks, such as adjusting a vaporizer setting, can be done by unskilled personnel working under a veterinarian's direct supervision. More demanding tasks, such as induction of anesthesia and monitoring of anesthetized patients, are best assigned only to personnel (veterinarians or technicians) who have sufficient training, knowledge, and experience to recognize abnormalities and danger signals and to respond appropriately.

Incorrect administration of drugs.   Many anesthetic agents have a narrow margin of safety between therapeutic and toxic doses. The incorrect administration of drugs may have serious or even fatal consequences, and may arise from any of the following:

- Failure to weigh the patient and calculate an accurate dose
- Mathematical errors (particularly decimal errors, which can result in an error of 10 times or 100 times in the amount of drug given)
- Use of the wrong medication (for example, calculating a dose of atropine and drawing up xylazine instead)
- Use of the wrong concentration of a medication. This is a common problem with drugs that are available in several different concentrations (for example, atropine and acepromazine). Obviously, the concentration used in calculating the dose must be the same as that drawn up into the syringe.
- Administration of anesthetics by the incorrect route (for example, administration of the intramuscular dose of ketamine by the intravenous route)
- Confusion between syringes drawn up for two different patients. This involves either a failure to label the syringes or a failure to read the labels correctly.

Personnel who are preoccupied or in a hurry.   Although efficiency is desirable in any anesthetic procedure, it is not necessary or advisable that the anesthetist feel hurried. A technician who is feeling rushed is more likely to inject barbiturates perivascularly or to insert an endotracheal tube into the esophagus. Unfortunately, it is common for the technician working in a busy practice to feel pressured and distracted. The technician responsible for anesthesia may be simultaneously called on to restrain patients for examination or procedures, answer the phone, perform laboratory tests, take radiographs, discharge animals, clean soiled kennels, and carry out other similar tasks. However, when an animal is anesthetized, the technician's top priority must be monitoring that patient because failure to satisfactorily perform this duty may result in the death of the animal.

The technician usually does not have the luxury of being constantly by the animal's side throughout the procedure. In most work situations, periodic absences are necessary. However, the anesthetist should return to check the patient at least once every 5 minutes, or more frequently if the patient's status requires close monitoring. If necessary, other tasks must be temporarily set aside to allow the anesthetist to return to the patient.

Fatigue.   Fatigue is an ailment common to many veterinarians and technicians, particularly at the end of a busy day. Anesthetic emergencies may arise when personnel are tired and less alert than normal, possibly because minor problems are not detected and corrected at an early stage. If possible, surgeries that are lengthy or difficult should be scheduled early in the day.

Inattentiveness.   One of the most serious human errors in anesthesia is the failure to monitor and recognize danger signals. It is obviously better for the patient—and easier for the anesthetist—to detect and address anesthetic problems early, rather than late. For example, an animal experiencing respiratory depression while under an inhalation anesthetic will show a gradually decreasing respiratory rate, from 12 breaths per minute to 8 breaths per minute (at which point the anesthetist should consider adjusting the vaporizer to a lower setting); then from 8 breaths per minute to 4 (at which point the vaporizer should be turned off and the animal bagged with oxygen); then from 4 breaths per minute to 0 (at which point cardiac arrest is likely to occur).

The anesthetist's attitude toward patient care is a key factor in the safety of anesthesia. The conscientious anesthetist will monitor the animal often to ensure that the patient is not in trouble. A brief check of the parameters listed on page 72 takes less than 1 minute and gives the anesthetist a good assessment of the patient's status. The best attitude is one of low-level anxiety, which is relieved only when a quick examination of the patient reveals that all vital signs and depth indicators are within acceptable limits.

Equipment Failure

Equipment failure is an uncommon cause of anesthetic emergencies, but it does occur. In many cases, failure of the anesthetic machine is, in fact, a failure of the operator to maintain and monitor the machine properly. The importance of a preanesthetic check of the anesthetic machine, as described in Chapter 4, cannot be overemphasized.

The following anesthetic machine problems are occasionally encountered in routine anesthesia.

Carbon dioxide absorber exhaustion.   Patients on a rebreathing system rely on the carbon dioxide absorber to remove expired CO_2 from the circuit, preventing inhalation of excessive levels of this toxic gas. If CO_2 is not removed from the circuit, the patient will experience hypercapnia (elevated blood CO_2). Signs of this disorder include tachypnea (rapid respiration), tachycardia, and cardiac arrhythmias. Examination of the CO_2 absorber crystals will reveal an obvious color change, if exhaustion of the crystals has occurred.

Empty oxygen tank.   Failure to deliver oxygen to the patient is one of the most serious and yet one of the most easily prevented mistakes that an anesthetist can make. Before starting an anesthetic procedure, the anesthetist must ensure that the tank contains sufficient oxygen for the duration of the surgery. (For information on calculating the amount of oxygen present in a tank, refer to page 158.) During the procedure, the oxygen tank pressure and flowmeter should be checked every 5 minutes during anesthesia.

The anesthetist must ensure that either oxygen or room air is continuously provided to the patient. At the end of a procedure, the patient should be disconnected from the machine before the oxygen flowmeter is turned off.

It is important to be able to recognize when the machine is no longer delivering oxygen to the patient. If the oxygen flowmeter reads zero flow, the system is not receiving any oxygen, regardless of the oxygen tank pressure. Occasionally, the situation arises in which the oxygen tank pressure gauge reads zero, but the flowmeter indicates some oxygen flow; in this case the tank is still delivering a small amount of oxygen, but loss of oxygen pressure is imminent and the tank should be changed immediately.

The anesthetist must be aware of the proper response when oxygen delivery to the patient is stopped, whether because of machine malfunction or the tank running out of oxygen. If the oxygen flow stops (that is, the flowmeter reads zero despite the efforts of the anesthetist to establish flow) and the patient is on a nonrebreathing system, the anesthetist should immediately disconnect the hose from the endotracheal tube, allowing the patient to breathe room air until the oxygen delivery is reestablished. (If a circle system with a full reservoir bag is in use, the patient can remain connected for a short period of time.)

Misassembly of the anesthetic machine.   It is essential that the person handling the anesthetic machine be familiar with every connection, hose, dial, and component of the machine. Before using an unfamiliar machine, the anesthetist should take a few minutes to examine it carefully for the location of the controls and to understand the direction and path of gas flow within the machine. Every time a connection, such as a Bain circuit, is added or removed, the anesthetist must trace the flow of gas, ensuring that the correct pattern of flow is maintained and that all connections are secure. Failure to do so can result in the patient not receiving anesthetic gases or rebreathing expired CO_2.

Endotracheal tube problems.   Although the endotracheal tube is, strictly speaking, not a part of the anesthetic machine, it is a critical component of the anesthetic delivery system and is subject to many problems. Endotracheal tubes may become blocked during anesthesia, cutting off the flow of anesthetic gas and oxygen to the patient. Blockages may be the result of twisting or kinking of the tube; accumulation of material such as blood, mucus, or saliva within the tube; or inappropriate positioning of the tube (as may occur when the neck is flexed). The endotracheal tube should be premeasured from the incisor teeth to the midneck, and it should be advanced no further than the position of the carina. If the tube is accidentally advanced into a bronchus, the patient may become hypoxic and hypercapnic. Endotracheal tube blockage (if complete) results in a cessation of oxygen flow to the patient and retention of carbon dioxide. The patient may become dyspneic and may develop cardiac arrhythmias. Eventually, respiratory arrest may occur. The anesthetist usually becomes aware of the problem by observing the patient's exaggerated breathing pattern or by noting that the reservoir bag no longer inflates and deflates with the patient's respirations. If a problem is suspected, the anesthetist should quickly check the endotracheal tube function in two ways:

1. Attempt to bag the patient and observe if the chest rises. If the endotracheal tube is blocked, no chest movement will be seen, and there will be considerable resistance to the passage of air into the patient.

2. Disconnect the animal from the machine. With the endotracheal tube still in place, feel for air coming out of the tube when the patient's chest is compressed. If no air movement is felt, a blockage may be present. In this case, the tube should be removed and another endotracheal tube or mask used to deliver oxygen to the patient.

If blood, mucus, or similar material is causing the obstruction, suction with a 20-cc syringe and a cut-down feeding tube may be helpful.

Vaporizer problems. A potentially disastrous problem can arise if the wrong anesthetic is put into a vaporizer. In particular, the inadvertent use of isoflurane or halothane in a nonprecision vaporizer designed for methoxyflurane may result in delivery of extremely high concentrations of anesthetic gas to the patient. (The use of isoflurane or halothane in this type of vaporizer is safe if special techniques are used, as discussed in Chapter 4 under low-flow anesthesia.)

Vaporizers should not be tipped. Tipping may lead to leakage of anesthetic into the oxygen bypass.

Occasionally, a vaporizer dial may stick or become jammed. If the dial cannot be adjusted, the patient should be transferred to another machine.

Anesthetic machines equipped with two vaporizers in series should be monitored carefully to ensure that both vaporizers are not turned on at the same time.

Vaporizers should not be overfilled. If too much anesthetic is put into the vaporizer, it should be drained until the fluid level is at, or below, the indicator line.

Pop-off valve problems. Occasionally, an anesthetist inadvertently leaves the pop-off valve in a closed position. If the pop-off valve is closed and the oxygen flow rate is greater than the patient's oxygen requirement, pressure within the circuit will rapidly rise. (An example of this situation is a closed system in which the oxygen flow rate is greater than the metabolic oxygen consumption, approximately 10 ml/kg/minute.) As pressure rises in the circuit, the reservoir bag will expand, as will the patient's lungs. This prevents exhalation and also decreases the venous return to the heart. This in turn may decrease cardiac output, cause blood pressure to fall rapidly, and lead to death within a short time.

To detect the problem at an early stage, the anesthetist should frequently monitor the reservoir bag size and attempt to maintain it at no more than two-thirds full of gas during anesthesia. The reservoir bag size is easily adjusted by changing the oxygen flow rate or by opening and closing the pop-off valve.

Anesthetic Agents

Each injectable or inhalation agent has the potential to harm a patient and, in some cases, cause death. Several strategies are used to reduce this potential:

- The anesthetic protocol must be chosen to reflect the special needs of the patient. For example, acepromazine is a poor preanesthetic for patients with low blood pressure because this agent may cause vasodilation, further decreasing the blood pressure. Similarly, halothane is not the preferred inhalation agent for patients suffering from cardiac arrhythmias because it may cause arrhythmias to worsen. Animals that are fearful or excited may undergo cardiac fibrillation if they are induced with halothane by mask, because of the combined arrhythmogenic effect of halothane and epinephrine. In each case, the veterinarian might choose to use an alternative agent.

- The anesthetist must be familiar with the side effects and contraindications associated with each of the preanesthetic and general anesthetic agents used in the hospital. For example, the anesthetist who administers xylazine should be aware of its potential to cause bradycardia, cardiac arrhythmias, vomiting, bloating, abortion, and respiratory depression.
- Multidrug use to achieve balanced anesthesia can be safer than anesthesia using a single drug, provided that the dosages of the individual drugs are appropriately reduced. For example, the concentration of halothane needed to anesthetize an animal is significantly reduced if the animal is premedicated with acepromazine and butorphanol, as compared with an animal given halothane without premedications. If the same halothane concentration was used in both situations, the multidrug regimen could be dangerous for the patient.

A detailed description of the pharmacology and physiologic effects of preanesthetic and general anesthetic agents is given in Chapter 1 (preanesthetic agents) and in Chapter 3 (general anesthetic agents).

Patient Factors

Animals presented for anesthesia may be suffering from systemic abnormalities that considerably increase anesthetic risk. Patients with a preoperative status of class IV or class V are particularly difficult to anesthetize successfully. Challenging patients routinely encountered in veterinary practice include geriatric animals, neonates, brachycephalic animals, sighthounds, and obese animals. Cesarean delivery of puppies or kittens also places unique demands on the anesthetist because the response of both the dam and the offspring to anesthetic agents must be considered. Animals suffering from recent trauma may be presented for emergency surgery, and the anesthetist must be prepared to deal with shock, respiratory difficulties, and cardiac arrhythmias in these patients. Animals with cardiac problems such as heartworm disease or congestive heart failure may require anesthesia for diagnostic or therapeutic procedures. Similarly, animals may require anesthesia despite the presence of renal or hepatic disease. Although a detailed discussion of the anesthetic challenges posed by these and other patients is beyond the scope of this book, it is desirable that the technician be familiar with some of the special problems encountered when anesthetizing these animals. These are summarized in Table 6-1.

Geriatric patients.   A geriatric patient is one who has reached 75% of the average life expectancy for that species and breed. In these patients the functions of critical organs such as the heart, lungs, kidneys, and liver are reduced in comparison with the healthy, young patient. Geriatric animals have less functional reserve than do younger animals, and a relatively poor response to stress. Often they are less able to adequately maintain their state of hydration than younger patients. In addition, geriatric animals are often affected by degenerative disorders such as diabetes mellitus, cancer, mitral valve insufficiency and the resulting congestive heart failure, and chronic renal disease, all of which are of concern to the anesthetist. Because of the high incidence of health problems in these animals, the importance of a thorough history and physical examination cannot be overemphasized. Preoperative tests such as a blood chemistry panel, urinalysis, chest radiographs, and an electrocardiogram may be advisable for these patients.

TABLE 6-1

Patient Factors That Increase Anesthetic Risk

Patient Factor	Anesthetic Problems Encountered	Strategies Used to Decrease Risk
GERIATRIC PATIENTS	Reduced organ function; poor response to stress; degenerative disorders common; increased risk of hypothermia and overhydration	Reduce anesthetic dosages by 30% to 50%; allow longer time for response to drugs; administer fluids at reduced rate; keep patient warm
PEDIATRIC PATIENTS	Increased risk of hypothermia and overhydration; inefficient excretion of drugs; difficult intubation and intravenous catheterization	Avoid heat loss; avoid prolonged fasting; administer 5% dextrose in lactated Ringer's using accurate methods of delivery; weigh accurately; dilute injectable drugs; reduce anesthetic dosages; inhalant agents preferred to injectable agents
BRACHYCEPHALIC DOGS	Conformational tendency toward airway obstruction; abnormally high vagal tone	Include anticholinergic in anesthetic protocol; preoxygenate; rapid induction using intravenous agents; delay extubation; observe closely during recovery period
SIGHTHOUNDS	Increased sensitivity to barbiturates	Use alternative agents
OBESE ANIMALS	Accurate dosing difficult; poor distribution of anesthetics; may have respiratory difficulties	Dose according to ideal weight; preoxygenate; induce rapidly; assist ventilation if necessary; delay extubation; observe closely in recovery period
CESAREAN PATIENTS	Dam: increased workload to heart; respiration may be compromised; increased tendency to vomit or regurgitate; increased risk of hemorrhage	Dam: administer intravenous fluids; clip patient before induction; preoxygenate; use lowest effective dose of general anesthetic; avoid pentobarbital and ketamine/diazepam
	Offspring: anesthetic agents cross placenta and may reduce respiratory and cardiovascular function	Offspring: use reversing agents and doxapram; administer oxygen by face mask; administer atropine for bradycardia
TRAUMA PATIENTS	Respiratory distress common; cardiac arrhythmias seen for 72 hours after incident; shock and hemorrhage common; internal injuries often present	Stabilize before anesthesia; obtain thoracic radiographs and ECG; thorough physical examination necessary to check for concurrent injuries
CARDIOVASCULAR DISEASE	Circulation is compromised; pulmonary edema common; increased tendency to develop arrhythmias and tachycardia	Alleviate pulmonary edema with diuretics; preoxygenate for 5 minutes before induction; avoid agents that depress myocardium or cause arrhythmias; avoid overhydration
RESPIRATORY DISEASE	Poor oxygenation of tissues; patient may be anxious and difficult to restrain; respiratory arrest common	Avoid stress and unnecessary handling; preoxygenate; avoid nitrous oxide; induce with injectable agents; intubate rapidly and control ventilation if necessary; monitor closely during recovery

Continued

217

TABLE 6-1		
Patient Factors That Increase Anesthetic Risk—cont'd		
Patient Factor	**Anesthetic Problems Encountered**	**Strategies Used to Decrease Risk**
HEPATIC DISEASE	Delayed metabolism of anesthetic agents; decreased synthesis of blood clotting factors; may be hypoproteinemic; dehydration common; may be anemic and/or icteric	Preanesthetic blood chemistry tests; may omit preanesthetic medication; inhalation agents preferred over injectable agents; expect prolonged recovery
RENAL DISEASE	Delayed excretion of anesthetic agents; electrolyte imbalances common, including hyperkalemia, hyperphosphatemia, and metabolic acidosis; dehydration usually present	Rehydrate before surgery; obtain renal function tests and electrolyte values; reduce dosages of anesthetic agents; use caution with barbiturates; may require intraoperative intravenous fluids
URINARY OBSTRUCTION	Dehydration, acidosis, uremia and hyperkalemia common; bradycardia may be present	Avoid barbiturates; treat for hyperkalemia if present

Geriatric animals typically have reduced anesthetic requirements, and doses of anesthetic agents are often decreased by one half to one third compared with the healthy, young patient. In the case of barbiturates, dose requirements may be as little as one twentieth of the normal dose. Response to drugs is slower, and the technician should allow more time for intravenous injections to take effect. Recovery from anesthesia also may be prolonged in geriatric animals, partly because of decreased renal and hepatic function (and hence, decreased ability to excrete drugs). Geriatric patients also have a tendency to develop hypothermia because they have a reduced ability to regulate body temperature.

The use of intravenous fluids is generally advocated in geriatrics because they have less tolerance for hypotension and often have reduced kidney function. Geriatric animals are at increased risk for developing overhydration problems such as pulmonary edema, however, and intravenous fluids should be given with care.

Pediatric patients.   A veterinary patient under 3 months of age is generally considered to be at increased risk when anesthetized, compared with a mature animal. When working with these patients, the anesthetist must be aware of special considerations during preanesthesia, the anesthetic period, and recovery.

Preoperative fasting of the pediatric patient may not be advisable because hypoglycemia and dehydration can occur after even a short period of fasting. Oral fluids are usually allowed up to 1 hour before induction. To prevent hypoglycemia during surgery, many veterinarians use 5% dextrose in lactated Ringer's for intravenous fluid therapy of anesthetized pediatric patients. (This can be formulated by adding 100 ml of 50% dextrose to 1 liter of lactated Ringer's solution.) The fluid administration rate should not exceed 5 ml/kg/hr unless shock or dehydration is present, because these animals are prone to overhydration if fluid administration is rapid. The use of a syringe driver or pediatric minidrips (60 drips/ml) and a burette is helpful in preventing inadvertent overinfusion of fluid.

To calculate drug dosages, it is necessary to obtain an accurate weight. For animals weighing under 5 kg, a pediatric or lab animal scale gives more reliable weights than does a conventional scale. Injectable agents may require dilution because otherwise the dose may be too small to measure or administer accurately. The dose of injectable anesthetics given to pediatric animals is often one half to two thirds of the dose given to mature animals because very young animals have less plasma protein binding of drugs and lack an efficient mechanism to metabolize drugs within the liver. Injectable anesthetic agents that require liver metabolism for inactivation (for example, thiopental and pentobarbital) can be expected to have a prolonged effect in puppies or kittens less than 8 weeks of age and should be avoided. Renal function is also inefficient, compared with the adult animal, and excretion of drugs by this route may be slow.

Many veterinarians prefer to anesthetize pediatric patients with inhalant agents (particularly isoflurane) because administration and elimination of these agents is accomplished through the respiratory tract and patient recovery tends to be rapid.

Certain anesthetic procedures such as intubation and intravenous catheterization are difficult in pediatric patients because of their small body size. The larynx is difficult to see, and use of a laryngoscope may be required. It is often necessary to cut endotracheal tubes short to avoid bronchial intubation.

Apart from obvious differences in size, the monitoring of pediatric patients is similar to adults. The anesthetist should be particularly watchful for bradycardia, which is associated with poor cardiac output in the anesthetized animal less than 4 weeks of age. Xylazine may cause significant bradycardia in animals under 4 weeks of age and should be avoided. Premedication with atropine may not be effective because response to atropine is unpredictable in patients less than 14 days old.

Pediatric patients are prone to hypothermia because of their lack of subcutaneous fat, their relatively large surface area, and their inability to shiver. Particular care should be taken to avoid heat loss during surgery. This is accomplished through the use of warmed intravenous fluids and circulating warm water heating pads. It is also essential to make sure that all air is removed from IV lines to avoid the risk of air embolism.

Brachycephalic dogs.   Technicians are often called on to anesthetize brachycephalic dogs such as the English bulldog, pug, Boston terrier, and Pekingese. Because of their conformation, these animals may suffer from one or more anatomic characteristics that impede air exchange. These include very small nasal openings, an elongated soft palate, and a small-diameter trachea. Any anesthetic agent that depresses respiration or reduces muscle tone in the pharyngeal and laryngeal area will cause increased respiratory difficulty in these animals. In some cases this may be fatal, particularly if the animal is not intubated and if an open airway cannot be maintained. These problems are most evident in animals undergoing surgery to correct conformation defects in the pharyngeal region (for example, soft palate resection) because postoperative swelling or hemorrhage may occur, increasing the risk of respiratory difficulty.

In addition to their respiratory problems, many brachycephalic animals also have abnormally high parasympathetic tone, which may cause bradycardia. Use of atropine or glycopyrrolate in these patients is helpful in increasing heart rates before surgery.

The induction period is particularly difficult for brachycephalic dogs. If possible, the anesthetist should preoxygenate brachycephalic patients for 5 minutes before induction. This is done by gently restraining the animal and administering oxygen through a face mask. This procedure helps maintain adequate blood oxygen levels and gives the animal an extra margin of safety during the induction period that follows.

Induction should be rapid, and for this reason intravenous induction agents are generally preferred over mask induction. Agents that are rapidly metabolized (for example, propofol, ketamine/diazepam, and methohexital) are preferred. The dog must be adequately anesthetized to allow rapid and efficient intubation. Difficulties may be encountered because of the large amount of redundant tissue in the pharynx. This reduces visibility of the laryngeal opening, and the use of a laryngoscope is helpful in these patients. The anesthetist may find that the endotracheal tube that fits the trachea is smaller than that expected, considering the size and weight of the dog.

Anesthesia usually can be safely maintained through the use of an inhalation anesthetic. With the help of an endotracheal tube, breathing during anesthesia may, in fact, be superior to that of the normal awake brachycephalic animal. Agents that allow rapid recovery (particularly isoflurane) are preferred because dyspnea is common in these dogs during the early recovery period.

After surgery, the patient should be observed closely until it is extubated and breathing well. Vigilance is necessary well into the recovery period because patients have suffered airway obstructions even after attempting to stand. The endotracheal tube should be left in place as long as possible because the animal will maintain an open airway as long as the tube is in place. Oxygen should be delivered until the patient is extubated. Once the endotracheal tube is removed, the animal's head and neck should be extended, and the animal should be watched closely for dyspnea and cyanosis. If dyspnea is seen, the mouth should be kept open with a mouth gag and the tongue pulled forward. Administration of oxygen by mask or even reinduction (with ketamine/diazepam, propofol, or other IV induction agent) and reintubation may occasionally be necessary. It is advisable to have supplemental oxygen and supplies for reintubation (that is, a laryngoscope, endotracheal tube, and the appropriate dose of an inducing agent) readily available in the recovery area in case dyspnea occurs after extubation.

Excitement and stress should be minimized as much as possible in the recovery period, especially if airway surgery was carried out. Some patients may require mild tranquilization or the use of opioid analgesics to reduce the rapid respirations that can worsen laryngeal swelling. Corticosteroids are also helpful in some patients.

Sighthounds.   Several canine breeds (including the greyhound, saluki, Afghan hound, whippet, and Russian wolfhound) show increased sensitivity to anesthetic agents, particularly tranquilizers and barbiturates such as thiopental. The reason for this increased sensitivity is not entirely understood, but it may involve a lack of body fat for redistribution of the drug and inefficient hepatic metabolism of many drugs. Fortunately, many inducing agents (including diazepam and ketamine, methohexital, propofol, halothane, and isoflurane) can be safely used as alternatives to thiobarbiturates in these animals.

Obese animals.   Some patients presented for anesthesia have a high percentage of body fat. Because the blood supply to fat is relatively poor, anesthetics are not efficiently distributed to fat stores. Obese dogs, therefore, require less anesthetic on a per kilogram basis than do normal dogs. It is advisable to decrease the dose of preanesthetic and anesthetic agents so that the animal is dosed according to a weight halfway between the normal breed weight and the actual weight.

Obese animals also may suffer from some degree of respiratory difficulty, further complicating the anesthetic process. Dogs that show respiratory difficulties should receive oxygen by face mask for 5 minutes before induction. They may also require the use of induction techniques similar to those used in brachycephalic dogs.

Obese dogs and toy breeds often exhibit rapid shallow respirations during anesthesia. This breathing pattern may result in hypercapnia. The anesthetist who observes persistent rapid and shallow respirations should assume control over respiration by bagging the patient with oxygen and anesthetic, once every 5 seconds, until increased anesthetic depth and slower respirations are observed. The anesthetist can also slow down the respiratory rate by administering opioids such as hydromorphone or oxymorphone, especially if the elevated rate is a result of surgical stimulation.

Cesarean sections.   The anesthetist for animals undergoing cesarean surgery must be aware of the special needs not only of the patient undergoing the surgery, but also of the neonates being delivered. Essentially, all anesthetic drugs administered to the pregnant patient (with the exception of neuromuscular blocking agents and local anesthetics) will readily cross the placenta and affect the newborn. Although it is essential that the patient receive adequate anesthetic agent to provide immobilization and analgesia for the surgery, it is advisable to use minimal doses of those agents that depress respiration in the puppies or kittens.

The pregnant female patient is at increased anesthetic risk for several reasons. Advanced pregnancy greatly increases the workload of the heart, particularly when the patient is in dorsal recumbency. Additionally, respiratory function will be compromised by the pressure of the abdominal organs on the diaphragm. Pregnant animals are prone to vomiting because of pressure from the uterus on the stomach. (Studies of human cesarean procedures have shown that inhalation of vomit causes approximately 50% of maternal anesthetic deaths.) Additionally, the patient may be exhausted before the surgery starts, particularly if the owner has delayed bringing the animal in for veterinary attention.

Hemorrhage from the uterus is a common complication of cesarean surgery, and even nonhemorrhaging patients have an increased risk of shock. It is therefore advisable that an intravenous catheter and intraoperative fluid administration be routinely used in cesarean patients.

It is helpful to do as much preoperative preparation of the cesarean patient as possible, thereby reducing the anesthesia time. If possible, clipping and prepping should be initiated in the awake patient. Whether awake or anesthetized, it is advisable that patient clipping and surgical preparation be done as much as possible with the patient gently restrained in left lateral recumbency rather than in dorsal recumbency. The latter position may cause the heavy uterus to compress the vena cava, decreasing venous return to the heart.

Various anesthetic techniques are used for cesarean surgeries, depending on the preference of the veterinarian:

- Epidural analgesia combined with a tranquilizer or neuroleptanalgesic is popular because this technique, once mastered, provides inexpensive but effective anesthesia with minimal depression of the patient or the neonates. IV fluids and oxygen should be administered in conjunction with epidural analgesia.
- General anesthesia using a variety of injectable and inhalant agents is also commonly used, with anesthetics given at the lowest effective dose to maintain

anesthesia without unnecessarily depressing pediatric respiration. Because of the dam's increased sensitivity to medications, the dose of inhalant anesthetic required is often reduced by up to 40%. Propofol or low-dose thiopental are commonly used.

- Preoxygenation is helpful, regardless of the anesthetic protocol.
- Opioid agents are favored by some veterinarians for cesarean anesthesia because they are reversible in both the dam and the neonates through the use of naloxone or other reversing agent.
- The use of nitrous oxide may be helpful to supplement opioids or inhalation agents because it reduces the amount of other agents required and has minimal effects on fetal respiration. The anesthetist should be aware of the possibility of diffusion hypoxia in newborn animals delivered from mothers receiving nitrous oxide, and oxygen should be administered to each puppy or kitten immediately after delivery.
- Pentobarbital is considered to be a high-risk agent and pediatric mortality may approach 100%.
- Use of diazepam should be avoided because this agent is poorly metabolized by pediatric animals.

Puppies or kittens delivered by cesarean section often show signs of reduced respiratory and cardiovascular function when first delivered. If respiration appears inadequate or if cyanosis is present, oxygen should be administered by face mask. If necessary, the newborn animal can be intubated with a 16- or 18-gauge intravenous catheter and gently bagged with oxygen every 5 seconds. Aspiration of fluid from the mouth and nose with an eyedropper or bulb syringe may also be useful. The use of reversing agents and doxapram (0.1 to 0.2 ml injected into the root of the tongue) is common. If bradycardia is present, a drop of dilute atropine (0.25 mg/ml) can be administered under the tongue or injected into the tongue. Gentle cardiac massage and oxygen may also be helpful.

The newborn should be allowed to nurse as soon as the mother appears to be recovered from anesthesia (or, with supervision, during the recovery period). The dam may be disoriented and should be closely watched to ensure the safety of the newborn puppies or kittens. Anesthetic agents excreted in the milk appear to have little effect on nursing ability or neonatal viability. Postoperative analgesics such as butorphanol or buprenorphine assist the mother's recovery.

Trauma patients.   Animals that have recently undergone trauma, such as being hit by a car, may be suffering from numerous ailments that greatly increase anesthetic risk. Respiratory difficulties are common and may be the result of pneumothorax, pulmonary contusions and hemorrhage, or diaphragmatic hernia. Cardiac arrhythmias are common in the 12 to 72 hours after chest trauma. Shock is also common in animals that have undergone significant trauma, particularly if hemorrhage has been severe. Serious internal injuries such as fractures and herniated or ruptured organs may pose further difficulties for the veterinarian and anesthetist.

Very few trauma patients require anesthesia immediately after the accident, and as a general rule it is wise to stabilize these animals before anesthesia. Delaying anesthesia offers two advantages: (1) it allows time for a thorough workup to assess the extent of the injuries, and (2) it provides some time to stabilize the animal's condition (which reduces anesthetic risk). The patient should be closely monitored for signs of dyspnea, cardiac arrhythmias, or decreased mentation. It is advisable to obtain thoracic radiographs before anesthesia for repair of internal injuries (such as fractures) resulting from trauma. This is because studies have shown that one third of patients with traumatic forelimb, hind limb, or pelvic injuries have concurrent thoracic injuries that could jeopardize the safety of anesthesia. It is obviously advisable to identify and treat a disorder such as pneumothorax before anesthetizing an animal for the repair of a fractured femur. The veterinarian may also request an electrocardiogram as part of the preanesthetic workup because cardiac arrhythmias may be seen as long as 3 days after chest trauma. Fortunately, many thoracic injuries improve with cage rest, and if anesthesia can be delayed for 24 to 72 hours after the traumatic incident, the anesthetist usually encounters fewer problems.

Cardiovascular disease.   The most common cardiovascular disorders found in patients scheduled for anesthesia include anemia, shock, cardiomyopathy (primary, or secondary to hyperthyroidism), and congestive heart disease (secondary to mitral valve insufficiency). In some areas, heartworm disease is also common. Many animals with heart disease have concurrent pulmonary disease, particularly pulmonary edema, which further complicates anesthesia. Diuretics such as furosemide (Lasix) may be helpful in alleviating pulmonary edema before anesthesia.

As with patients that have undergone recent trauma, before initiating anesthesia it is generally advisable to stabilize the patient's condition by treating cardiovascular and respiratory disease to alleviate the symptoms as much as possible. Preoxygenation using a face mask or oxygen chamber for 5 minutes immediately before induction is also extremely helpful in reducing anesthetic risk in animals with cardiovascular or respiratory difficulties.

The veterinarian and anesthetist should ensure that anesthetic agents that depress the myocardium or that exacerbate arrhythmias (for example, xylazine and halothane) are avoided as much as possible in these animals. Opioid agents, diazepam, and isoflurane offer the advantage of relative lack of toxicity to the heart.

When anesthetizing animals with cardiovascular problems, the anesthetist should be aware of the increased risk of overhydration through excessive or too rapid administration of intravenous fluids. Even an infusion rate of 10 ml/kg/hr may be dangerous for these animals. It is advisable to frequently monitor the anesthetized patient for signs of pulmonary edema such as ocular or nasal discharge, increased lung sounds, and increased respiratory rate. Central venous pressure monitoring, if available, is useful to detect overhydration.

Respiratory disease.   Of all the animals to undergo anesthesia, those with respiratory problems are perhaps the most challenging for the anesthetist. Examples of these patients include animals with pleural effusion (that is, free fluid present in the chest cavity), diaphragmatic hernia, pneumothorax, pulmonary contusions resulting from trauma, pneumonia, tracheal collapse, and pulmonary edema. Poor oxygenation is often present in these animals, and many show signs of tachypnea, dyspnea, and cyanosis. If possible, anesthesia should be delayed until respiratory function has improved. If surgery is absolutely required (for example, to place a chest tube), local analgesia and gentle manual restraint may be preferable to general anesthesia. Administration of oxygen through a nasal line (described on pages 244-245) is helpful for patients with respiratory compromise.

Nitrous oxide should be avoided in patients with respiratory distress because the administration of 100% oxygen is usually necessary to maintain adequate oxygenation.

Before anesthesia, it is important to thoroughly evaluate the animal and, if possible, to find the cause of the respiratory distress. Radiographs and thoracocentesis are particularly helpful. Thoracocentesis is not only useful in diagnosis, but also may be therapeutic if large volumes of air or fluid can be removed from the chest.

One of the most common procedures requiring anesthesia of an animal in respiratory distress is surgical repair of a diaphragmatic hernia. When preparing to anesthetize these patients, as with all patients showing signs of dyspnea, it is advisable to preoxygenate for 5 to 10 minutes before surgery. Head-down positions should be avoided before and during anesthesia because they may result in further movement of abdominal contents into the thorax. If possible, an induction method that allows rapid intubation (that is, use of an injectable agent) is preferred over mask induction. After induction, some patients may show signs of respiratory depression and even respiratory arrest, and the anesthetist must be prepared to intubate rapidly and assist or control ventilation. Nitrous oxide should not be used; this avoids diffusion of the gas into the displaced stomach and intestines and further distention of these organs. Ventilatory assistance may be provided by periodic or continuous "bagging" of the patient, or a ventilator may be used. The animal should be closely observed for cyanosis. Pulse oximetry, capnography, and arterial blood gas determination are helpful aids for assessing ventilation.

These patients require close observation during the recovery period. Administration of oxygen may be helpful if signs of respiratory distress are seen. Pneumothorax is common after chest surgery, and affected patients may require chest tube placement or removal of air from the pleural space using a syringe and needle.

Hepatic disease.   Animals with liver disease are subject to increased anesthetic risk because of the central role that organ plays in drug metabolism, synthesis of blood clotting factors and other serum proteins, and carbohydrate metabolism. Some animals with liver disease are hypoproteinemic, which may lead to increased potency of barbiturate agents. Patients with chronic liver failure are also commonly dehydrated, thin, and icteric, and may be anemic.

Preanesthetic medication should be given with care or omitted from the protocol because most of these agents require hepatic metabolism before they can be excreted. Xylazine and acepromazine in particular may have long-lasting effects in patients with compromised hepatic function. Use of ketamine and diazepam should also be avoided. Induction and maintenance of anesthesia is best achieved using isoflurane or propofol, which require little or no hepatic function for elimination.

Renal disease.   The kidneys are the organs most involved in maintaining the volume and electrolyte composition of body fluids. This helps explain why animals with renal disease are often dehydrated and may have severe electrolyte imbalances, including metabolic acidosis and hyperkalemia. General anesthesia may be particularly stressful for these patients because renal blood flow is decreased during anesthesia and renal function may be further compromised, particularly if the animal is hypotensive. Use of injectable nonsteroidal antiinflammatory agents such as ketoprofen during anesthesia may reduce renal perfusion even further.

Renal function tests such as urine specific gravity, BUN, and creatinine may be useful in obtaining an accurate picture of renal function. Preoperative water deprivation may not be advisable in some patients with renal disease because dehydration may occur rapidly after withdrawal of oral fluids. Water should be offered up to 1 hour before premedication. The patient with renal disease should be rehydrated as much as possible before surgery, and electrolyte problems should be identified and addressed. Administration of intravenous fluids is often continued throughout the anesthetic and postanesthetic period until the animal is fully hydrated and able to drink unassisted.

Many preanesthetic and anesthetic agents and their metabolites are eliminated from the body by renal excretion. For this reason, animals with compromised renal function may show prolonged recovery after anesthesia if conventional dosages are used. It is prudent to reduce dosages of anesthetic drugs (including acepromazine, xylazine, diazepam, ketamine, and barbiturates) in these patients. Barbiturates, in particular, have increased potency in acidotic and uremic animals and should be used with great caution in patients with renal disease. Inhalation agents (particularly isoflurane) have some advantages over injectable agents, although halothane and methoxyflurane can produce fluoride ions, which are damaging to the kidneys.

Animals with urinary blockages (including male cats with urethral obstructions caused by struvite crystals) pose similar problems to the anesthetist. Many of these cats are depressed, dehydrated, uremic, acidotic, and hyperkalemic. Hyperkalemic animals are at particular risk of cardiac arrest. Hyperkalemic patients may sometimes be identified by auscultation because bradycardia is often seen if plasma potassium levels exceed 6 mEq/L. Treatment of hyperkalemia may require the use of sodium bicarbonate, 10% calcium gluconate, and/or dextrose, and should be done only with close supervision and guidance from the veterinarian. Conditions stressful to the animal should be avoided as much as possible because the release of epinephrine from the adrenal glands may potentiate cardiac arrhythmias.

The administration of inhalation agents (particularly isoflurane) to cats with urinary blockages may be less hazardous than the use of injectable drugs because renal excretion is not required for patient recovery. Propofol or ketamine/diazepam may be used intravenously with caution and at reduced dosages, provided normal kidney function is present. Obstructed cats showing extreme depression may not require general anesthesia, particularly if a local anesthetic such as lidocaine gel is administered as part of the urethral catheterization procedure.

■ RESPONSE TO ANESTHETIC PROBLEMS AND EMERGENCIES

Despite every precaution, the veterinary technician is likely to encounter anesthetic emergencies several times during the course of a career. The nature of the technician's response may mean the difference between life and death for the anesthetized patient.

Role of the Veterinary Technician in Emergency Care

Ideally, emergency response is a team effort involving the veterinarian, technician, and other hospital staff. Normally the veterinarian acts as the team leader, directing the staff in emergency procedures. However, the veterinarian may be performing surgery on the patient when an anesthetic emergency arises and therefore may have other pressing concerns besides anesthesia. The technician must be prepared to take an active role in resuscitating the patient and not rely solely on the already-busy veterinarian. Constant communication between the veterinarian and the technician is obviously important under these circumstances.

It is a good idea to conduct periodic "dress rehearsals" or mock resuscitations in which all staff members participate. Everyone in the hospital should be familiar with the location of the crash kit and IV fluids. Procedures such as warming towels in a clothes dryer, making up hot water bottles, and drawing up drugs into a syringe can be readily taught to hospital staff and, once mastered by them, will free the veterinarian and technician to perform more demanding tasks.

Occasionally an emergency arises when the veterinarian is absent from the hospital or unavailable to assist. For example, seizures may occur in the postoperative recovery period. Most provincial and state regulations allow the technician to undertake emergency care if the veterinarian is absent. To protect the veterinarian and technician from liability, however, it is advisable to discuss in advance the procedures that the veterinarian will authorize the technician to do in an emergency. It is helpful to have written instructions available in the form of an emergency protocol authorized by the veterinarian.

General Approach to Emergencies

It cannot be assumed that every anesthetic emergency should be treated in the same way. For example, the veterinarian and animal owner may elect not to resuscitate a severely ill or debilitated animal that undergoes cardiac arrest during anesthesia. Cost considerations may influence the treatment given in some cases. Emergency care is labor-intensive, and treatment costs may be considerable. Most veterinarians, however, will not stop to consider cost if the emergency arises during a routine surgery, such as a spay, and will do everything possible to revive the animal.

When responding to an emergency, the technician should bear in mind the principles of emergency care listed in Procedure 6-1.

Emergency Situations That May Arise During Anesthesia

Although anesthetic emergencies are by their nature unpredictable, certain problems occur with some frequency. The following situations will be addressed in detail:

Animals that will not stay anesthetized
Animals that are too deeply anesthetized
Pale mucous membranes
Prolonged capillary refill
Cyanosis and dyspnea
Tachypnea
Abnormalities in cardiac rate and rhythm
Respiratory arrest
Cardiac arrest

Animals that will not stay anesthetized.   Occasionally, the anesthetist will have difficulty in maintaining a patient at sufficient anesthetic depth. Often the veterinarian becomes aware of the problem when the patient shows signs of movement in response to surgical stimulation. If depth appears inadequate, the anesthetist should check the following:

PROCEDURE 6-1
Responding to an Emergency

1. The technician should take a few seconds to think before doing anything. After consulting with the veterinarian, the technician should mentally list the most important things to be done and undertake them in order of priority.
2. Every veterinary practice should have a well-stocked crash kit for use in emergency situations within the hospital. A list of supplies that may be useful in a crash kit is given in Appendix C.
3. Useful emergency drugs are listed in Tables 6-2 and 6-3. Doses for emergency drugs should be posted or listed on a paper kept in the crash kit. Emergency drugs kept in the crash kit should be periodically checked to ensure that they have not expired. In particular, epinephrine has a short shelf life and should not be used if a brown discoloration is present.
4. Above all, the technician should do no harm. In an emergency it is easy to panic and do things that are not only unnecessary but also potentially harmful to the animal, including performing cardiac compressions on an animal whose heart is still beating. Sometimes the best course of action is to watch, monitor, and wait.
5. After an anesthetic emergency, the technician, veterinarian, and hospital staff should discuss the reasons why the emergency arose and determine what could be done to prevent the same thing from happening again. The adequacy of the resuscitation efforts should be analyzed, and if a problem exists, it should be addressed.

- Has the vaporizer been turned off, or is the setting too low to maintain an adequate depth of anesthesia?
- Does the vaporizer contain anesthetic?
- Is the endotracheal tube in the esophagus? This can be easily determined by checking to see if the reservoir bag expands and contracts as the animal breathes. If so, the endotracheal tube is in the trachea. Movement of the reservoir bag also tells the anesthetist that the endotracheal tube is connected to the Y piece and that the tube is not blocked. Other procedures used to determine the location and patency of the endotracheal tube include palpation of the neck, and compression of the reservoir bag to see if the chest expands.
- Is air leaking around the endotracheal tube? If so, the patient is probably breathing room air, which dilutes the anesthetic gas entering the lungs. Air leakage can be detected by closing the pop-off valve, inflating the reservoir bag, and gently pressing on the bag while listening for the sound of air escaping from the animal's mouth. A soft hiss of escaping air is acceptable, but a large gush of exiting air should alert the anesthetist that either the endotracheal tube is too small or the cuff is not sufficiently inflated. If this is the case, the cuff can be further inflated, or the pharyngeal area can be packed with damp gauze.
- Is the animal holding its breath? This is most commonly seen immediately after the intubated animal is connected to the machine, particularly if propofol or

ketamine/diazepam was used for induction. Prolonged breath-holding may lead to arousal from anesthesia because vaporized anesthetic is not entering the lungs or the bloodstream. If arousal appears imminent, it may be necessary to periodically bag the animal with a mixture of oxygen and anesthetic until adequate depth of anesthesia is achieved.

- Are the patient's respirations too shallow to draw sufficient anesthetic into the lungs? Rapid, shallow respiration, commonly seen in toy dogs and obese animals, may be associated with insufficient anesthetic depth. The anesthetist should assist ventilation by bagging these patients (with vaporizer on) every 5 seconds.
- Is the anesthetic machine assembled correctly and are all connections tight? Occasionally, hoses become detached from the machine or the endotracheal tube, in which case the patient obviously does not receive any anesthetic from the machine.
- Is the oxygen flow rate adequate to vaporize anesthetic? For most precision vaporizers, a minimum flow rate of 500 ml/minute is necessary for accurate delivery of anesthetic. Very high oxygen flow rates or excessive use of the oxygen flush valve may also result in unpredictable vaporization of anesthetic.
- Is the anesthetic machine functioning correctly? Repeated episodes of awakening during anesthesia may indicate poor vaporizer function. If a halothane or isoflurane vaporizer setting of 3% to 4% seems necessary to maintain anesthesia in many patients, cleaning and recalibration of the vaporizer is probably necessary.
- Is the exaggerated respiratory movement actually an agonal (near death) phenomenon, indicating dangerous anesthetic depth rather than a light plane?

If none of the reasons listed above can explain the patient's arousal, the anesthetist should consult with the veterinarian. It may be necessary to increase the vaporizer setting, administer an analgesic, or switch to a different anesthetic in order to achieve the desired anesthetic depth.

Animals that are too deeply anesthetized.   An animal that is too deeply anesthetized will usually show the following signs:

- Respiration rate is 8 breaths per minute or less; respirations may be very shallow or the patient may be breathing with difficulty.
- Mucous membranes are pale and may be cyanotic.
- Capillary refill is greater than 2 seconds.
- Bradycardia is present (less than 60 to 70 bpm in a dog or 100 bpm in a cat).
- Pulse is weak; systolic blood pressure is less than 80 mm Hg (indirect measurement).
- Cardiac arrhythmias may be present; QRS complexes (ventricular contractions) are irregular on the ECG, or abnormal complexes such as ventricular premature contractions (VPCs) may be present.
- The animal's extremities and ears are cold; body temperature is often less than 35° C.
- Reflexes are completely absent, including palpebral and corneal reflexes.
- Muscle tone is flaccid.
- Pupils may be dilated and pupillary light reflex is absent.

The anesthetist should use judgment in interpreting the signs listed above. The presence of one or two signs may not indicate excessive depth, provided the other

PROCEDURE 6-2
Treating Excessive Anesthetic Depth

1. After concluding that the anesthetic depth is excessive, the anesthetist should immediately decrease the vaporizer setting (to zero, if necessary) and inform the veterinarian.

2. If the veterinarian decides that the animal's condition has deteriorated so that resuscitation efforts are warranted, the anesthetist should begin to bag the animal with pure oxygen. (This assumes that the patient is intubated and is undergoing gas anesthesia. If an injectable agent has been used, intubation and oxygen delivery by means of an anesthetic machine should be initiated immediately.)

3. To bag the animal, the pop-off valve is closed part way, the reservoir bag is filled with oxygen, and the bag is gently squeezed until the animal's chest rises slightly.

4. This procedure should be repeated every 5 seconds until the animal shows signs of recovery (such as increased heart rate, stronger pulse, and improved mucous membrane color and refill).

5. The use of intravenous fluids, external heat, and drugs such as doxapram and specific reversing agents (yohimbine, naloxone) may also expedite recovery.

6. Occasionally the anesthetist may be unsure of whether a patient's anesthetic depth is excessive. If the veterinarian is not immediately available to advise on the patient's condition, it is safest to assume that the animal is too deep and to decrease the vaporizer setting, while observing the animal carefully for signs of arousal.

---

signs are absent. Vital signs also vary depending on the preanesthetic and general anesthetics used (for example, atropine may affect heart rate and pupil dilation). The more parameters that the anesthetist considers, the more accurate the depth assessment is likely to be.

There are several reasons why anesthetic depth may be excessive. In most cases, the vaporizer setting is too high for the patient being anesthetized, or in the case of injectable agents, too high a dose has been given. Occasionally, the animal may have a preexisting problem such as shock or anemia that increases susceptibility to anesthetic overdose (Procedure 6-2).

Pale mucous membranes.   Pale mucous membranes may arise from several causes. Some patients have preexisting anemia secondary to diseases such as feline leukemia, hemolytic anemia, bleeding disorders, neoplasia, or chronic renal disease. In other cases blood loss may have occurred during surgery. Some anesthetic agents (particularly inhalation agents, xylazine, and acepromazine) cause vasodilation and decrease blood pressure, resulting in poor perfusion of capillary beds and pale mucous membranes in some animals. Hypothermia or pain can also reduce blood supply to the tissues and cause pale mucous membranes.

▼ PROCEDURE 6-3
Treating Pale Mucous Membranes

1. The anesthetist should ascertain the animal's anesthetic depth and monitor vital signs including heart rate, respiration, pulse strength, and capillary refill time.
2. The veterinarian should be consulted because it may be necessary to initiate intravenous fluid therapy or a blood transfusion to stabilize the patient's condition.

If pale mucous membranes are observed during surgery, follow Procedure 6-3.

Prolonged capillary refill.   The observation of a prolonged capillary refill (that is, greater than 2 seconds) suggests that blood pressure is inadequate to perfuse superficial tissues. The presence of hypotension should be suspected in any animal with a slow capillary refill time. Hypotension was the most common anesthetic complication found in a recent study of dogs and cats (Gayner et al, 1999). Hypotension may be present before the induction of anesthesia, as in the case of animals undergoing emergency surgery after trauma. Hypotension or shock also may arise secondary to blood loss during surgery, or may occur in patients that are at a very deep plane of anesthesia. Acepromazine and the inhalation agents may also cause hypotension in susceptible patients. Follow Procedure 6-4 if a prolonged capillary refill time is observed.

The treatment for shock in the anesthetized patient is similar to that in the conscious patient and should be done under the supervision of a veterinarian (Procedure 6-5).

Dyspnea and/or cyanosis.   Any patient showing dyspnea or cyanosis during the administration of an anesthetic should be immediately brought to the veterinarian's attention. The presence of dyspnea (respiratory difficulty) indicates that the animal is unable to obtain sufficient oxygen or remove adequate CO_2 using normal respiratory movements. Cyanosis (a bluish coloration of the mucous membranes) indicates that tissue oxygenation is inadequate. Dyspnea and cyanosis often are seen together and may be followed by respiratory arrest, in which respiratory efforts cease and the amount of oxygen available to the tissues rapidly declines.

The most common sources of respiratory distress during anesthesia are:
- The animal is unable to obtain oxygen from the anesthetic machine because the oxygen supply has run out, the flowmeter has been turned off, or the anesthetic circuit or endotracheal tube is blocked.
- The animal is unable to breathe normally because of airway obstruction or respiratory pathology. Causes of airway obstruction include endotracheal tube blockage, excessive flexion of the head and neck, laryngospasm, bronchoconstriction, aspiration of stomach contents after vomiting or regurgitation, and brachycephalic conformation. Common causes of respiratory pathology include pneumothorax, pulmonary edema, diaphragmatic hernia, and pleural effusion. Use of heavy surgical drapings or constricting bandages also may impair normal respiration.

PROCEDURE 6-4
Treating Prolonged Capillary Refill Time

1. The anesthetist who observes a prolonged capillary refill time should immediately check the animal's pulse and blood pressure reading (if available). In a dog or cat, a systolic blood pressure under 80 mm Hg indicates hypotension and poor perfusion.
2. If blood pressure readings are not available, the anesthetist can roughly estimate the systolic pressure by palpating a peripheral pulse. As a general rule, the absence of a palpable pulse at the metatarsal artery indicates a systolic pressure under 60 mm Hg, and the absence of a palpable pulse at the femoral artery indicates a systolic pressure under 40 mm Hg.
3. If pulse pressure is reduced, the anesthetist should closely observe the animal for other signs of shock, including hypothermia and tachycardia (or bradycardia in later stages of shock). As circulation to the extremities deteriorates, the surface temperature of the ears and paws is reduced. The heart may respond to the fall in blood pressure by increased rate and force of contraction, although this effect may not be present in deep anesthesia.

PROCEDURE 6-5
Treatment of Shock

1. Intravenous fluids should be administered at a rapid rate. Over the first 15 minutes, 20 ml/kg should be given, and the animal should be observed closely for a response. The maximum fluid administration rate is 90 ml/kg for the first hour in the dog (or 65 ml/kg in the cat). The use of colloid therapy or blood transfusions may be appropriate in some situations.
2. Anesthetic depth should be reduced, if possible, and 100% oxygen should be administered.
3. The patient must be kept warm through the use of supplemental heat in the form of warm towels, circulating warm water heating pads, hot water bottles, or similar devices.
4. Various drugs are recommended for the treatment of shock, including corticosteroids (prednisone sodium succinate, dexamethasone), sodium bicarbonate, and cardiac inotropes such as dopamine, ephedrine, or dobutamine.

■ The animal is too deeply anesthetized, to the point that respiration and other vital functions are adversely affected.

Respiratory problems are lifethreatening and should be addressed as discussed in Procedure 6-6.

Tachypnea.   Tachypnea, or rapid respirations, must be differentiated from dyspnea, in which respiratory distress is present. Tachypnea may arise at any time during

▼ PROCEDURE 6-6
Treating Respiration Problems

1. The anesthetist must first ensure that oxygen is being delivered to the patient. If the oxygen tank has run out, the patient must be disconnected from the machine until another oxygen source can be secured. If the endotracheal tube is blocked, it must be removed and replaced. Suspected endotracheal tube blockage can be confirmed by disconnecting the endotracheal tube from the Y piece and feeling for air passage through the tube when the patient breathes or the chest is gently compressed. Capnography, if available, will confirm if blockage has occurred.
2. Once oxygen flow has been established, the vaporizer should be turned off and the animal should be bagged with 100% oxygen. If the anesthetic machine is unavailable, an Ambu bag (Fig. 6-1) can be used to deliver room air to the patient. While initiating bagging, the anesthetist should observe the chest for movement. If the chest does not rise when the animal is bagged, the endotracheal tube or airway may be blocked, and the blockage must be relieved. If the chest does rise when the reservoir bag is squeezed, oxygen is

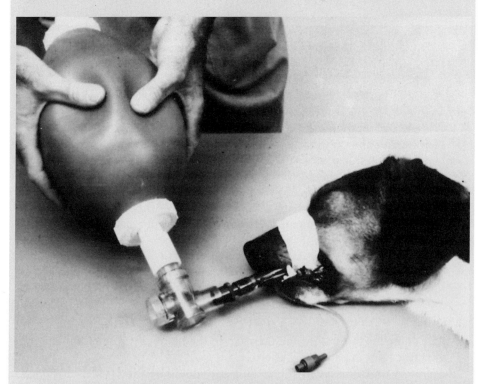

FIG. 6-1 Use of an Ambu bag to deliver room air to an intubated patient. (From Muir WW III, Hubbell JAE: *Handbook of veterinary anesthesia*, St Louis, 1989, Mosby.)

▼ **PROCEDURE 6-6**
Treating Respiration Problems—*cont'd*

being delivered to the lungs and bagging should be continued until the mucous membrane color improves or pulse oximeter readings rise to 90% to 95%. It is best to watch the anterior thorax for chest rise movement in the area of the heart, so as not to be misled by passive movement of the chest because of distention of the stomach by a misplaced endotracheal tube.

3. On rare occasions, dyspnea and cyanosis may be secondary to complete airway obstruction. If intubation is not possible under these circumstances, the veterinarian may elect to perform an emergency tracheostomy, a surgical opening of the trachea to allow the insertion of a breathing tube. Alternatively, a 14-gauge intravenous catheter can be placed through the cricothyroid membrane and into the trachea. The catheter is connected to the barrel of a 3-cc syringe, which is in turn attached to the Y piece of an anesthetic machine for oxygen delivery.

4. Administration of intravenous fluids or emergency drugs such as doxapram may be helpful in reviving patients suffering from respiratory depression or arrest.

5. It is important that the anesthetist closely observes the patient during resuscitative efforts to ensure that cardiac arrest does not occur. If a pulse or heartbeat cannot be detected, cardiac compressions should be initiated in conjunction with continued bagging.

6. If necessary, supplemental oxygen should be continued into the recovery period, using a mask, oxygen cage, or intranasal insufflation.

anesthesia and may be disconcerting to the anesthetist. It is particularly common during procedures utilizing opioids such as oxymorphone. Tachypnea also may be seen if anesthetic depth is inadequate, in which case it is often accompanied by tachycardia and spontaneous movement. Paradoxically, tachypnea also may occur in deep anesthesia as a response to low blood oxygen and high blood carbon dioxide levels. Tachypnea is also seen in hyperthermic patients, including animals with malignant hyperthermia.

If tachypnea is seen, follow Procedure 6-7.

Abnormalities in cardiac rate and rhythm. Abnormalities in cardiac rate and rhythm include tachycardia, bradycardia, and cardiac arrhythmias, all of which may be seen in anesthetized patients.

Tachycardia is present if the heart rate during stage III anesthesia is greater than 160 bpm for a large dog or greater than 180 bpm for a small dog or cat. It may result from the administration of drugs such as atropine, ketamine, or epinephrine. Tachycardia may also be a preexisting condition in animals suffering from hyperthyroidism, shock, congestive heart failure, and other conditions. An elevation in heart rate is also a common response to surgical stimulation, although it does not necessarily indicate insufficient anesthetic depth unless accompanied by rapid respiration, spontaneous movement, or active reflexes.

▼ PROCEDURE 6-7
Treating Tachypnea

1. The anesthetist should assess the anesthetic depth and check the CO_2 absorber crystals to ensure that hypercapnia is not present.
2. If anesthetic depth, body temperature, and vital signs appear to be within acceptable limits, the anesthetist should refrain from changing the vaporizer setting because the condition will usually correct itself within 1 to 2 minutes.
3. If tachypnea arises as a result of surgical stimulation and the perception of pain, intravenous injection of an analgesic such as oxymorphone, hydromorphone, or butorphanol may be helpful.
4. Obese patients are prone to tachypnea, which may result in inefficient ventilation. It may be necessary to assist or control ventilation in these patients.

Not all cases of tachycardia require treatment (for example, those in patients with otherwise normal cardiac function), but the anesthetist should notify the veterinarian before assuming that tachycardia is not significant. It is also important to check the vaporizer setting and anesthetic depth and adjust them if necessary.

Bradycardia can be defined as a heart rate less than 60 bpm in a medium-sized or large dog, a heart rate less than 70 bpm in a small dog, and a heart rate less than 100 bpm in a cat. Bradycardia may be secondary to the administration of xylazine or opioid agents, particularly if preanesthesia with an anticholinergic has been omitted from the anesthetic protocol. Bradycardia also may result from increased activity of the vagus nerve in response to endotracheal intubation, ocular surgery, or handling of the viscera by the surgeon. Bradycardia may also occur if the animal is very deeply anesthetized, and when seen in this context it is a warning that respiratory and cardiac arrest may be imminent. Other causes of bradycardia include hyperkalemia, hypothermia, and hypoxia.

Not all cases of bradycardia require treatment. If capillary refill, pulse oximeter readings, and pulse strength appear normal, tissue perfusion may be adequate and treatment may be unnecessary. The veterinarian should be consulted and should direct treatment. If anesthetic depth is excessive, the vaporizer setting should be adjusted and bagging with 100% oxygen may be helpful. Bradycardia as a result of the administration of drugs or because of excessive vagal stimulation is best treated with intravenous administration of atropine or glycopyrrolate.

The term *cardiac arrhythmia* (or cardiac dysrhythmia) refers to any one of a number of abnormalities, including "dropped beats," premature ventricular contractions (PVCs) arising spontaneously from individual heart muscle cells, and sustained episodes of tachycardia. These abnormalities are most easily detected through the use of an ECG. The alert technician also may note that a pulse deficit is present in animals with some types of arrhythmias.

Cardiac arrhythmias commonly arise in animals given arrhythmogenic drugs such as barbiturates, xylazine, and halothane. Such arrhythmias may be of short duration and well tolerated in young, healthy patients, but may be a significant problem in animals with preexisting heart disease and in geriatric patients. Arrhythmias

▼ PROCEDURE 6-8
Treatment of Cardiac Arrhythmias

1. The anesthetist should rule out inadequate oxygen flow or carbon dioxide accumulation within the circuit.
2. Ventilation should be increased by periodic bagging or use of a ventilator.
3. In some cases, antiarrhythmic drugs such as atropine or lidocaine (without epinephrine) may be administered on the veterinarian's orders.

are particularly common during induction and light anesthesia, and in some cases may be the result of respiratory depression and subsequent hypoxia. Other causes of cardiac arrhythmias include preexisting heart disease, gastric volvulus, thoracic surgery, and endotracheal intubation. Electrolyte imbalances and hypercapnia also may cause arrhythmias. Hypercapnia may arise from poor anesthetic technique, including exhaustion of the CO_2 absorber crystals or inadequate oxygen flow rates.

Treatment of cardiac arrhythmias should be done in consultation with the veterinarian (Procedure 6-8).

Respiratory arrest. Respiratory arrest is the cessation of respiratory efforts by the patient. It may lead to cardiac arrest and is therefore a potentially fatal condition.

Not all cases of respiratory cessation require immediate action by the anesthetist. Respiratory efforts may temporarily cease after the intravenous injection of ketamine, barbiturates, propofol, and other respiratory depressants. Minimal respiratory efforts may also be seen after a period of prolonged bagging with oxygen and, in this case, reflect low blood carbon dioxide and high blood oxygen levels. In both types of ventilatory arrest (whether the result of drug administration or bagging with oxygen) the anesthetist must be sure that other vital signs, particularly heart rate and mucous membrane color, are normal. If the heartbeat is regular, the heart rate is greater than 80 bpm, the pulse is strong, and mucous membranes are pink, the patient does not usually require immediate treatment for respiratory arrest. Pulse oximeter readings are helpful in indicating if the patient's oxygenation status is adequate (that is, a reading greater than 90% usually indicates that bagging is not necessary). To be safe, occasional "breaths" of oxygen (one every 30 seconds) can be delivered to the patient during this period to prevent hypoxia. However, premature bagging with oxygen may extend the period of apnea by removing carbon dioxide from the blood, which is a stimulus for the patient to resume breathing. The anesthetist who suspects that respiratory efforts have temporarily ceased because of administration of drugs or ventilation with oxygen should closely monitor the patient's heart rate and mucous membrane color for 1 to 2 minutes before assuming that a serious condition exists. If spontaneous respiration does not resume within this time, the veterinarian should be consulted, and it may be advisable to begin bagging the patient with oxygen.

True respiratory arrest is much more serious and requires immediate attention. This condition may arise because of anesthetic overdose, cessation of oxygen flow, or preexisting respiratory disease such as pneumothorax or diaphragmatic hernia. Affected animals may show warning signs such as dyspnea and/or cyanosis before respiratory arrest occurs. Other vital signs, such as heart rate, capillary refill, pulse strength, and pupil dilation, are often abnormal. Pulse oximetry values rapidly fall below 90%.

The treatment of respiratory arrest involves the steps shown in Procedure 6-9.

Bagging should continue until the heart rate, mucous membrane color, and pulse oximeter values have been restored to normal. Once this is achieved, the anesthetist should discontinue bagging for 15 to 30 seconds and closely observe the patient for respiratory efforts. If none are seen, bagging should resume.

On occasion, the anesthetist may be faced with a patient in respiratory arrest in the absence of an anesthetic machine. It is possible to substitute an Ambu bag or even institute mouth-to-endotracheal tube or mouth-to-muzzle resuscitation in these cases. (See Fig. 6-1).

Cardiac arrest.   Cardiac arrest may occur at any time during anesthesia. In most cases the anesthetist receives some warning that arrest is imminent, in the form of a short period in which cyanosis, dyspnea or respiratory arrest, and prolonged capillary refill are evident. If cardiac arrest appears imminent, the anesthetist should immediately alert the veterinarian and the hospital staff while continuing to monitor the heart by auscultation, by palpation of the chest, or through the use of an ECG. A patient suffering from cardiac arrest rapidly develops the following signs:

- No heartbeat can be auscultated or palpated, and normal QRS complexes are absent from the ECG tracing.
- There is no palpable arterial pulse, and blood pressure readings (if available) are 25 mm Hg or less.

 PROCEDURE 6-9
Treatment of Respiratory Arrest

1. Inform the veterinarian.
2. If the patient is not intubated, an endotracheal tube should be immediately inserted and the patient connected to an anesthetic machine delivering 100% oxygen.
3. Check the heart rate to ensure that cardiac arrest has not occurred.
4. Turn off the anesthetic vaporizer and nitrous oxide flow.
5. Ensure oxygen flow is adequate by checking the tank pressure gauge and flowmeter.
6. Ensure the airway is not obstructed by bagging the patient and observing that the chest rises on "inspiration."
7. Bag with oxygen at a rate of once every 3 to 5 seconds. Continue bagging until vital signs improve (particularly mucous membrane color, heart rate, and pulse oximeter readings).
8. If an intravenous catheter is present, administer IV fluids at a rate suitable for treatment of shock.
9. The veterinarian may advise that doxapram, reversing agents, or other drugs be given.
10. Ensure that the patient is kept warm.

- Mucous membranes are gray or cyanotic, and capillary refill may be prolonged.
- Pupils are widely dilated with no response to light.
- Respiration is absent except for intermittent, abrupt gasps.

Coordinated action by all hospital staff members is essential to reverse cardiac arrest. Once arrest occurs, permanent brain damage may result if oxygen delivery to the brain is not reestablished within 4 minutes, either by cardiopulmonary resuscitation or restoration of cardiac function. Ideally, at least five staff members should participate in the resuscitative efforts as follows: (1) performs chest compressions, (2) bags the animal, (3) assesses pulse during compressions and checks the pulse or ECG when compressions are temporarily suspended, (4) draws up and administers drugs on the veterinarian's orders, and (5) maintains a record of patient status and resuscitative treatments.

The essential steps in responding to a cardiac arrest may be summarized with the mnemonic ABCD (Airway, Breathing, Circulation, Drugs):

1. **Airway and Breathing**: If the animal is intubated and connected to an anesthetic machine, one staff member should note the time of arrest and immediately initiate respiratory support by turning off the vaporizer and nitrous oxide flow and bagging the animal with 100% oxygen at the rate of one breath every 3 to 5 seconds. Mask administration of oxygen is inadequate: if an endotracheal tube is not present, it is essential that the animal be intubated immediately. Additionally, the anesthetist must ensure that the patient's chest rises slightly during bagging, indicating that the airway is not blocked.

2. **Circulation**: Cardiac compressions should be initiated. The animal should be turned on its right side with its feet toward the person doing compressions and the head tilted down, if possible.

   - *Cardiac compressions for a large dog:* A firm object such as a book, sandbag, or rolled-up towel should be placed under the dog's chest just behind the elbow. The heel of the compressor's hand should compress the chest against this object, with the pressure applied at the point where the chest is widest. Both hands should be used to compress the chest. The chest wall should be allowed to bounce back rapidly after each compression.
   - *Cardiac compressions for a medium-sized dog:* One hand should be placed under the chest and the other hand placed at the 5th intercostal space, just over the heart itself (Fig. 6-2). The chest is then compressed between the two hands.
   - *Cardiac compressions for a cat or small dog:* Compression may be done by using the thumb to compress the chest against the fingers of the same hand.

   The rate of compressions should be 1 to 2 times per second (for example, 80 times per minute for a large dog and up to 120 times per minute for a small dog or cat). The chest should be compressed by approximately one third the diameter of the chest wall. The aim of the compressions is to manually force blood through the heart and, ultimately, to the tissues. It is believed that compressions also may assist circulation by increasing pressure in the chest, indirectly inducing blood flow. Each compression should result in a palpable femoral pulse, which should be periodically monitored by another staff member, if possible. If a pulse is not detected and the mucous membrane color does not improve, the method of compression should be adjusted by changing the rate or intensity, by repositioning the patient, or by assigning the compression task to another staff member.

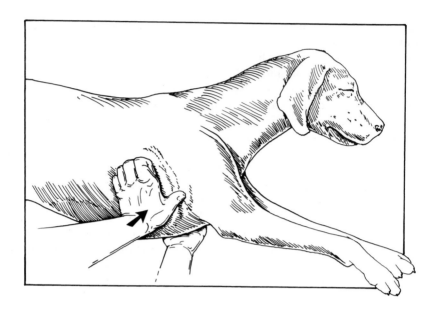

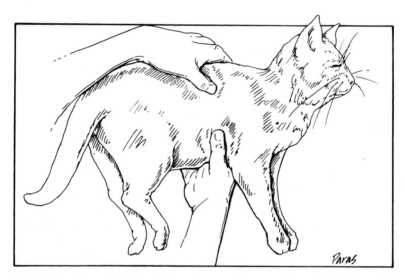

FIG. 6-2   Correct location for cardiac compressions for a medium-sized dog or a cat. (From Muir WW III, Hubbell JAE: *Handbook of veterinary anesthesia,* St Louis, 1989, Mosby.)

If two people are administering CPR, one person should bag every 3 to 5 seconds while the other compresses the chest. Bagging and compressions should be delivered simultaneously. In the case of a technician working alone, 10 compressions should be given alternately with two breaths. Once CPR is initiated, it should not be discontinued for longer than 20 to 30 seconds at a time.

If external cardiac compressions are not effective, as shown by failure to achieve a palpable pulse or pink mucous membranes within 2 minutes, internal compressions may be attempted. In the case of dogs weighing over 20 kg, some authorities suggest that internal compressions should be initiated immediately after cardiac arrest is identified. Investigators have shown that external chest compression in dogs weighing more than 20 kg results in less than 30% of normal cardiac output, whereas internal massage results in outputs of up to 70% of normal. There is understandable reluctance on the part of many veterinarians and technicians to enter the chest to perform internal massage; however, controlled studies have demonstrated that the success rate for resuscitation of large dogs is much greater if internal cardiac massage is performed.

To perform internal compressions, the lateral thorax is quickly shaved and rinsed with alcohol, a self-adhering sterile drape is applied to the prepared area, and a skin incision is made between the seventh and eighth ribs, using a scalpel.* The incision is extended through the muscle until the chest cavity is encountered. Care should be taken to avoid incising lung tissue, which lies immediately below the pleura. The operator's hand is inserted between the ribs (the use of a retractor may be necessary to separate the ribs adequately). The heart is grasped, and gentle but firm pressure is applied to the ventricles at a rate of 80 times per minute. If resuscitation efforts are successful, a palpable heartbeat may return within seconds or minutes. Surgical closure and antibiotic therapy are essential after reestablishment of cardiac function by internal compression.

When doing compressions, it is necessary to stop periodically to determine whether the heart has resumed spontaneous contractions. This is easy to ascertain by palpation when doing internal compressions, but more difficult with external compression methods. Spontaneous contractions can be detected by discontinuing external compression and either palpating for a spontaneous pulse or observing an ECG for QRS complexes. Auscultation may also be useful.

If spontaneous contractions are not observed, external or internal compressions can be resumed, although after 15 minutes they are unlikely to be successful in establishing a heartbeat. Use of a defibrillator is helpful in some situations, but should be authorized and directly supervised by a veterinarian.

If spontaneous contractions are observed, cardiac compressions should be discontinued, although bagging must be maintained until spontaneous breathing is established, which may require up to several hours. The anesthetist should periodically check the capillary refill, mucous membrane color, and heart rate and should discontinue bagging only if these vital signs appear normal. If mucous membrane color deteriorates or if spontaneous respiration does not occur within 1 minute after bagging is discontinued, bagging should be resumed.

3. **Drugs:** Drugs are commonly administered to aid recovery. In all cases, the veterinarian, if present, should authorize the dosage, route, and nature of drugs to be administered.

   If an intravenous catheter is present, the drugs are normally given through it, followed by intravenous fluids at a dosage of 20 ml/kg (cats) or 40 ml/kg (dogs)

---

*In the case of dogs undergoing a laparotomy at the time of arrest, the surgeon may immediately initiate internal compressions by opening the diaphragm, entering the thorax, and compressing the heart.

as rapidly as possible. Caution should be used when administering fluids to patients in cardiac arrest because overhydration and pulmonary edema are common sequelae. If intravenous access is difficult, drugs may be given by injection into the base of the tongue or by intratracheal administration. Intratracheal administration may involve injection of the drug directly into the tracheal lumen, or the drug may be administered by means of a urinary catheter passed through the endotracheal tube. For intratracheal administration, the dose of emergency drug given should be twice the recommended intravenous dose.

Intracardiac injections should be avoided if possible because injections by this route require the interruption of cardiac compressions and have some potential to damage the myocardium.

Commonly administered agents include epinephrine, prednisolone sodium succinate (Solu-Delta Cortef), dopamine, dobutamine, doxapram, atropine, lidocaine, and sodium bicarbonate. The current recommended dosage of emergency drugs is given in Tables 6-2 and 6-3.

Epinephrine is the drug most commonly used for initial treatment of cardiac arrest. The currently recommended dose is 0.5 ml for cats, 1 ml for small dogs, 2 ml for medium-sized dogs, and 3 ml for large dogs, all drawn up from a 1:1000 solution.

TABLE 6-2

Drugs Used in Treating Anesthetic Emergencies in Cats and Dogs

Drug	Dosage for IV Use	Indications for Use
Atropine	0.025 mg/kg, can give 2× dose intratracheal	Treatment for bradycardia
Dexamethasone (Azium)	4-8 mg/kg	Corticosteroid used in treatment of shock
Diazepam (Valium)	0.2-1 mg/kg	Treatment of seizures
Dobutamine (Dobutrex)	5-10 μg/kg/min infusion in 5% dextrose	Increases force of myocardial contractions
Dopamine (Intropin)	2-10 μg/kg/min infusion in lactated Ringer's	Increases force of myocardial contractions, increases heart rate
Doxapram (Dopram)	1-4 mg/kg	Respiratory and CNS stimulant
Epinephrine	0.1-0.2 mg/kg, can give 2× dose intratracheal	Increases rate and force of cardiac contractions, increases systemic vascular resistance
Lidocaine without epinephrine	2 mg/kg, can give 2× dose intratracheal	Antiarrhythmic agent
Naloxone (Narcan)	0.01-0.02 mg/kg	Narcotic antagonist
Prednisolone sodium succinate (Solu-Delta-Cortef)	10-30 mg/kg	Corticosteroid used in treatment of shock
Sodium bicarbonate	1-2 mEq/kg	Treatment of metabolic acidosis
Yohimbine (Yobine)	0.1 mg/kg	Reversing agent for xylazine

TABLE 6-3

Doses of Emergency Drugs Used in Cardiopulmonary Resuscitation of Cats and Dogs

Emergency Drug	Dose	3 kg 6.6 lb	5 kg 11 lb	10 kg 22 lb	15 kg 33 lb	20 kg 44 lb	25 kg 55 lb	30 kg 66 lb	40 kg 88 lb	50 kg 110 lb
Epinephrine 1:1000 1 mg/ml	0.1 mg/kg	0.3 ml	0.5 ml	1 ml	1.5 ml	2 ml	2.5 ml	3 ml	4 ml	5 ml
Atropine 0.54 mg/ml	0.025 mg/kg	0.1 ml	0.2 ml	0.5 ml	0.7 ml	0.9 ml	1.2 ml	1.4 ml	1.8 ml	2.3 ml
Lidocaine 20 mg/ml	2 mg/kg	0.3 ml	0.5 ml	1 ml	1.5 ml	2 ml	2.5 ml	3 ml	4 ml	5 ml
Sodium bicarbonate 1 mEq/ml	1 mEq/kg	3 ml	5 ml	10 ml	15 ml	20 ml	25 ml	30 ml	40 ml	50 ml
Prednisolone Sodium Succinate (Solu-Delta Cortef)	30 mg/kg	90 mg	150 mg	300 mg	450 mg	600 mg	750 mg	900 mg	1200 mg	1500 mg

From Robello CD, Crowe DT: Cardiopulmonary resuscitation: current recommendations, *Vet Clin North Am*, 19(6):1129, 1989.

Dopamine or dobutamine infusions are also advised by many authorities because these drugs increase the force and rate of cardiac contractions. Bicarbonate administration is no longer recommended unless the animal is hyperkalemic or if cardiac arrest has been present for more than 10 minutes. Calcium injections are also no longer advocated, except in hyperkalemic animals.

4. **Aftercare:** Successful cardiac resuscitation often depends on the quality of nursing care given to the patient. As with many recovering patients, restoration of body temperature is important. Other procedures, such as the installation of ophthalmic lubricant and regular repositioning of the patient, are similar to those outlined in Chapter 2 under anesthetic recovery.

Unfortunately, many patients suffering from cardiac arrest cannot be revived. In the case of those patients in which cardiac function is reestablished, conditions such as pulmonary edema and cerebral edema may occur. Cerebral edema is manifested by seizures, failure to return to consciousness, and temporary or permanent neurologic damage.

Repeated cardiac arrests are also common. The type and severity of complications partially depends on the length of time required to reestablish cardiac function.

Problems That May Arise in the Recovery Period

Regurgitation during anesthesia and postanesthesia vomiting.   Regurgitation is a passive phenomenon that may occur even during deep anesthesia. In a regurgitating animal, stomach contents exit through the cardiac sphincter, move up the esophagus, and enter the pharynx, nasopharynx, and oral cavity. Once in the pharynx, stomach contents may be aspirated into the respiratory tract. Regurgitation is most common in animals placed in a head-down position during surgery because this causes increased pressure on the stomach. Unlike vomiting, regurgitation is not accompanied by retching or other outward signs, and in fact, the only sign apparent to the anesthetist may be a small amount of fluid draining from the animal's mouth or nose. Treatment of regurgitation involves immediate intubation (if a cuffed endotracheal tube is not already present) and removal of as much regurgitated material as possible through suction.

Vomiting during or after anesthesia is a relatively common phenomenon, particularly in brachycephalic dogs. Unlike regurgitation, vomiting is an active phenomenon, often accompanied by retching. Vomiting usually occurs as the animal is losing consciousness during induction or as it is returning to consciousness during anesthetic recovery. Vomiting is potentially most dangerous if the animal is unconscious and the airway is not protected with an endotracheal tube. In this situation, the vomitus may be easily aspirated into the trachea. Aspiration of vomitus may cause immediate signs of dyspnea and cyanosis as a result of airway obstruction and bronchospasm. If the patient survives this episode, signs of aspiration pneumonia (including fever, increased respiratory rate, and increased lung sounds) may appear over the next 24 to 48 hours. It is imperative, therefore, that the anesthetist prevents the accumulation of vomitus within the oral cavity of the unconscious patient and the subsequent aspiration of the material into the air passages. To do this, an endotracheal tube should be immediately inserted if time allows. If this cannot be achieved, the animal's head should be placed at a lower level than the rest of its body (for example, over the edge of the surgery table). This helps prevent passive flow of liquid material into the trachea. When the vomiting stops, it may be necessary to manually clean the oral cavity, using suction if available. If respiratory arrest occurs because of airway blockage, the animal should be intubated and bagged with oxygen.

Unconscious animals have a low risk of aspiration if a cuffed endotracheal tube is already in place during the vomiting episode. It is for this reason that the endotracheal tube is customarily left in place until the patient regains the swallowing reflex and is close to consciousness. If vomiting is seen in an unconscious animal that has a cuffed endotracheal tube in place, the anesthetist should ensure that the cuff of the tube is inflated and position the animal's head lower than the rest of its body to prevent accumulation of vomitus within the oral cavity.

Occasionally, an animal may regurgitate after esophageal intubation. If this occurs, the tube should be left in place to direct the contents away from the pharynx. An endotracheal tube should be placed in the trachea, if possible, while the first tube is still in place.

Fortunately, most vomiting episodes occur after the animal has regained consciousness and the ability to swallow. It is not usually necessary to intubate conscious animals during a vomiting episode; however, the anesthetist should ensure that the head is kept extended and as low as possible.

Occasionally the technician may be called on to anesthetize an animal that has not been fasted before induction. These patients may be at risk of vomiting and/or regurgitation during induction, maintenance, and recovery. The anesthetist can help avoid problems by ensuring that rapid induction and intubation techniques are used. For this reason, an injectable agent is preferred over masking in these patients. A cuffed endotracheal tube with adequate diameter is essential. If possible, head-down positions should be avoided during surgery to prevent excessive pressure on the stomach. The anesthetist should also ensure that suction is readily available in case of regurgitation or vomiting. Use of antiemetic drugs such as metoclopramide may be helpful in some cases.

Postanesthesia seizures and excitement.   Seizures are occasionally seen in animals recovering from anesthesia. Seizures may be caused by the administration of ketamine, by diagnostic procedures such as myelography, or by patient disorders such as epilepsy or hypoglycemia.

It is important that the anesthetist differentiate between seizures and excitement during recovery. Excitement usually occurs after barbiturate anesthesia (particularly after the use of pentobarbital) and most often appears as spontaneous paddling of the limbs and occasionally as vocalization. Geriatric animals may also vocalize and appear confused after anesthesia. Usually, treatment is unnecessary other than the calm reassurance of the patient. Sedatives can be helpful, especially if the patient did not receive a sedative in the preanesthetic period.

Occasionally, excitement may be seen after the administration of high doses of opioids to animals that have not been tranquilized (particularly cats). Treatment with naloxone or another opioid-reversing agent may be helpful in these animals. Excitement is rarely observed in animals that receive opioids for moderate or severe pain.

In contrast, seizures appear as spontaneous twitching or uncontrolled movements of the head, neck, and limbs and are often triggered by a stimulus such as sound or touch. Animals given ketamine may show stiff forelimbs, opisthotonus, and exaggerated responses to touch or noise.

Animals undergoing postoperative excitement or seizures should be brought to the veterinarian's attention. Elimination of stimuli such as light, sound, and touch may be adequate to resolve the episode. Adequate postoperative analgesia should be provided. If seizures are present, many animals respond well to administration of intravenous or rectal diazepam at a dosage rate of 0.2 to 0.4 mg/kg. If diazepam is not effective or is unavailable, the animal may be anesthetized with pento-barbital in sufficient quantity to induce sedation and eliminate seizures (5 to 10 mg/kg).

Animals undergoing seizures or excitement during recovery require surveillance and nursing care to prevent self-injury. In the case of cats recovering from ketamine anesthesia, it may be necessary to trim the front claws or to bandage the paws to prevent the animal from scratching its face.

All animals undergoing seizures should be monitored for hyperthermia and cyanosis. Hyperthermia can be treated by the application of cool wet towels. Cyanosis should be treated by the administration of oxygen by face mask or by endotracheal tube (if unconscious).

Dyspnea during the recovery period.   Dyspnea resulting from upper airway obstruction is the most common cause of death in the postanesthetic period. Dyspnea in cats is usually caused by laryngospasm, whereas dyspnea in dogs is most commonly associated with breed-related (for example, brachycephalic) obstruction of the entrance to the trachea.

Laryngospasm is a condition in which the cartilages in the laryngeal area become so tightly closed that air is unable to enter the trachea. This condition commonly arises in cats because of this species' extremely active laryngeal reflex. In some recovering cats, the removal of the endotracheal tube initiates reflex closure of the airway. This reflex is normally useful to the cat in that it prevents the aspiration of food or water into the larynx in the conscious animal; however, in the unconscious animal it may well result in complete airway blockage.

Laryngeal edema may result from repeated attempts to intubate during light anesthesia. Clinically, this resembles laryngospasm.

Cats undergoing laryngospasm or laryngeal edema may breathe with an audible stertor or wheeze. They typically show exaggerated thoracic movements, gasping, and upward movement of the head during inspiration. If conscious, the animal usually appears anxious or excited. Laryngospasm must be differentiated from growling, which is common in cats recovering from anesthesia. In the case of growling, the noises are particularly evident on *expiration*, whereas in laryngospasm the respiration is labored and the noise is most evident during *inspiration*.

If a cat shows signs of laryngospasm during recovery from anesthesia, the anesthetist should check the mucous membrane color and pulse oximeter readings (if available). If the cat's mucous membranes appear pink and the SaO_2 is greater than 90%, the obstruction is likely partial rather than complete. In this case, the situation may resolve without treatment, although administration of oxygen by face mask may be helpful provided it does not stress the cat. It may be helpful to extend the neck and hold the tongue rostrally. If cyanosis is present or SaO_2 readings are less than 90%, and the cat is losing consciousness—and these signs are not alleviated by the administration of oxygen by face mask—the animal must be intubated. If intubation is impossible, the veterinarian may elect to perform a tracheotomy to reestablish airflow. The animal should be kept anesthetized for 2 hours and given furosemide and corticosteroids to reduce swelling. The cat can be extubated once the cords appear less rounded and swollen. Nasal oxygen is useful during extubation.

Laryngospasm is easier to prevent than to treat. When anesthetizing cats, gentle intubation technique is essential to avoid unnecessary laryngeal trauma. Use of lidocaine spray and/or gel is also helpful during intubation. Early extubation is recommended in cats so that the tube is removed before the laryngeal reflex returns.

Dyspnea in brachycephalic breeds of dogs usually occurs because the airway is obstructed by the soft palate or by other redundant tissue in the pharynx. However, there are many other potential causes of obstruction, including foreign objects such as blood clots, gauze sponges, or even extracted teeth. Animals that have undergone surgery of the pharynx or larynx often undergo postoperative tissue swelling that may lead to airway obstruction.

However it arises, airway obstruction will usually not become evident until after the endotracheal tube is removed. Strategies to prevent and treat postoperative dyspnea in brachycephalic dogs are outlined on pages 219-220.

A patient that requires supplemental oxygen during the recovery period can have it administered by one of three routes: face mask, nasal cannula, or oxygen cage/tent. Oxygen can be delivered by means of a nasal cannula (using a 5 French feeding tube for cats and small dogs, and up to a 10 French feeding tube for large dogs), which is inserted into the nostril and secured to the face by a suture. Alternatively, the patient can be enclosed in a temporary "oxygen tent" using an Elizabethan collar that extends beyond the head and is three-fourths covered with plastic wrap. An oxygen line is inserted into the edge of the collar, adjacent to the patient's face.

The flow rate used to deliver supplementary oxygen will depend on the patient's size and the method of administration. As a general rule, the flow rate should be at least 100 ml/kg. If possible, oxygen being delivered to an awake animal should be humidified (for example, by directing the flow of oxygen through a bottle of distilled water before delivery to the patient).

Prolonged recovery from anesthesia.   Animals experiencing prolonged recovery from anesthesia should be examined by the veterinarian. There are many possible reasons why a patient may be slow to recover, including impaired renal or hepatic function, hypothermia, individual susceptibility to a particular anesthetic, breed variation (particularly sighthounds), or the presence of a disorder such as shock or hemorrhage. Excessive anesthetic depth or prolonged anesthesia may also result in delayed recovery. Use of certain agents (including methoxyflurane, intramuscular ketamine, or repeated injections of barbiturates) may be associated with prolonged recovery even in healthy animals.

Recovery may be hastened in several ways (Procedure 6-10).

▼ PROCEDURE 6-10
Expediting Recovery From Anesthesia

1. The patient should be placed in a location where frequent observation is possible. If possible, emergency and monitoring equipment and oxygen should be available in the immediate area.
2. It is often helpful to administer intravenous fluids, which hasten renal and hepatic elimination of anesthetics and support circulation. The recommended rate of fluid administration for most intensive care patients is 3 to 5 ml/kg/hr.
3. Good nursing care is important. The patient should be turned frequently and kept warm. If the patient's temperature is less than 37 °C, active warming procedures should be instituted, including the use of fan heaters, reflective blankets, circulating warm water pads, heat-producing "oat bags," chemical warmers, or towels warmed in a dryer. Expired 1 liter fluid bags can be microwaved for 5 minutes and used as hot water bottles.
4. The animal must be periodically monitored for vital signs, reflexes, and urine production (which should be at least 2 ml/kg/hr).
5. Reversing agents and analeptics are used occasionally to hasten anesthetic recovery. However, the anesthetist whose patients consistently demonstrate slow recoveries should not rely on pharmacologic solutions to solve what may be a problem of technique. The anesthetist should reexamine the anesthetic protocol and consult with the veterinarian to determine whether more appropriate agents or means of administration should be used. It is important to ensure that animals are not maintained at excessively deep levels of anesthesia for routine procedures.

✔ KEY POINTS

1. Although anesthetic complications are uncommon, the technician must be able to anticipate and respond to emergencies in an efficient and knowledgeable fashion.
2. Human error may result in anesthetic problems. Such errors may include the failure to obtain an adequate history or physical examination, a lack of familiarity with the anesthetic machine or drugs used, the incorrect administration of drugs, and fatigue, inattentiveness, or distraction.
3. Examples of equipment failure or operator carelessness include carbon dioxide absorber exhaustion, failure to deliver sufficient oxygen to the patient, misassembly of the anesthetic machine, failure of the vaporizer or pop-off valve, or endotracheal tube problems.
4. Anesthetic agents may cause problems during anesthesia, and the anesthetic protocol must be chosen to reflect the special needs of each patient. The anes-

thetist must be familiar with the adverse side effects associated with the use of each agent in the anesthetic protocol.

5. Some patients are at increased risk of anesthetic complications because of pre-existing factors such as old age, organ failure, recent trauma, or breed-related conformation.

6. Geriatric patients have less reserve than younger patients and have reduced anesthetic requirements. Pediatric patients also require reduced dosages of injectable agents and are prone to hypothermia and hypoglycemia.

7. Brachycephalic dogs have anatomic characteristics that make respiration difficult, particularly during the recovery period. Preoxygenation before induction, rapid induction and intubation, and close monitoring during recovery are essential.

8. Thiobarbiturates should be used with extreme care in sighthounds. Alternative agents are preferable in most situations.

9. Obese animals should receive anesthetic dosages according to their ideal body weight.

10. Pregnant animals presented for cesarean section are at increased anesthetic risk. Various anesthetic techniques (including epidural anesthesia, balanced anesthesia, and neuroleptanalgesia) are sometimes used as alternatives to inhalation anesthesia in these patients. Almost all anesthetic agents may cause depression of fetal respiration and/or circulation, and the use of reversing agents may be advisable.

11. If possible, patients that have undergone recent trauma should be stabilized and thoroughly evaluated before anesthesia.

12. Animals suffering from cardiovascular or respiratory disease may require special anesthetic techniques such as preoxygenation and manual control of ventilation.

13. Hepatic or renal disease may delay excretion of injectable agents, and prolonged recovery times may be seen.

14. Emergency care is ideally a team effort involving all hospital personnel. It is helpful to have preauthorized emergency protocols and periodic "dress rehearsals."

15. It may be difficult to maintain adequate anesthetic depth in some patients. Incorrect placement of the endotracheal tube, incorrect vaporizer setting, inadequate endotracheal tube size, and many other factors may contribute to this problem.

16. Excessive anesthetic depth may result from excessive administration of anesthetic agents or from preexisting patient problems. It may be necessary to bag the patient with 100% oxygen to achieve a lighter plane of anesthesia.

17. Pale mucous membranes may be the result of anemia, hemorrhage, or poor perfusion. Prolonged capillary refill suggests that hypotension (or, if severe, shock) is present.

18. Cyanosis is a critical emergency and arises because of insufficient delivery of oxygen to the tissues. It may result from a machine problem, airway or endotracheal tube blockage, or respiratory difficulties resulting from excessive

Continued

depth, pneumothorax, or respiratory disease. Oxygen delivery to the patient must be reestablished through masking, intubation, or tracheostomy.

19. Abnormalities in cardiac rate and rhythm may result from the administration of anesthetic agents, electrolyte abnormalities, hypercapnia, hypoxia, and many other factors.

20. Respiratory arrest that is accompanied by cyanosis and/or bradycardia is an emergency and must be treated by ventilation with 100% oxygen.

21. Cardiac arrest should be treated according to the principles of ABCD: establish a patent *airway*, *bag* the patient with 100% oxygen, initiate internal or external *cardiac massage*, and administer epinephrine and other *drugs*.

22. Regurgitation and/or vomiting may be dangerous in the anesthetized animal because of the danger of airway obstruction and aspiration pneumonia.

23. Postanesthesia seizures may be treated by eliminating external stimuli and administering diazepam.

24. Dyspnea caused by laryngospasm or brachycephalic airway obstruction may be treated by administration of oxygen by mask, reintubation of the patient, or tracheostomy.

25. Animals experiencing prolonged recovery from anesthesia require close observation and nursing care. An effort should be made to determine the reason for delayed arousal of each patient.

REVIEW QUESTIONS

1. When an animal scheduled for a surgical procedure is brought in by a neighbor who is in a hurry, the best thing to do is:
   a. Instruct the receptionist to have the neighbor sign the consent form
   b. Ask the neighbor to take the animal back home
   c. Ask the neighbor some quick questions about the animal
   d. Have the neighbor sign the consent form and ensure that the owner is called before the procedure is initiated

2. In preparation for an anesthetic procedure, you have drawn up a syringe of barbiturate and an identical syringe of saline. You are then called to the examination room to assist the veterinarian. About 10 minutes later you return to prepare the animal for induction. With the IV catheter in place, you are just about to inject some saline into the animal when you realize that you are not sure if the syringe contains saline. The best thing to do would be to:
   a. Inject a small amount of the solution and see what effect it has
   b. Discard both syringes and start over
   c. Ask the person who was holding the animal which syringe had saline in it
   d. Discard both syringes, label some new syringes, and start over

3. You are about to use the anesthetic machine and notice that although the flowmeter is working, the pressure gauge on the oxygen tank reads close to zero. The best thing to do would be to:

    a. Assume that the pressure gauge may be faulty and wait and see if the flowmeter stops working

    b. Change the oxygen tank

    c. Call the repair person to have the pressure gauge checked

    d. Use low-flow anesthesia techniques and ignore the pressure gauge reading

4. While monitoring a patient on an anesthetic machine, you realize that the oxygen tank has become empty. The best thing to do would be to:

    a. Disconnect the patient from the circuit, put on a new oxygen tank, and then reconnect the patient to the circuit

    b. Remove the circuit from the patient to allow him to breathe room air for the remainder of the procedure

    c. Resuscitate the patient with an Ambu bag

    d. Switch to an injectable anesthetic

5. If the pop-off valve is inadvertently left shut, it will:

    a. Stop the oxygen flow from entering the circuit

    b. Convert the circuit to low-flow anesthesia

    c. Cause a significant rise of pressure within the circuit

    d. Cause the flutter valves to malfunction

6. You look at the oxygen tank and note that 1000 psi of pressure is left in the tank, but the flowmeter now reads 0 and you cannot obtain a flow by twisting the knobs. The best thing to do would be to assume:

    a. The oxygen tank pressure gauge is malfunctioning and you need to recheck the flowmeter

    b. The oxygen pressure is adequate and the flowmeter just is not registering the flow

    c. The animal is not getting oxygen, and you need to remove the animal from the circuit until a new machine is found or the problem is corrected

7. A geriatric patient is considered to be one that:

    a. Is greater than 10 years old

    b. Is greater than 15 years old

    c. Has reached 50% of its life expectancy

    d. Has reached 75% of its life expectancy

8. Brain damage may occur when there is inadequate oxygenation of the tissues for longer than ___ minutes.

    a. 2

    b. 4

    c. 6

    d. 8

    e. 10

9. When a technician is performing CPR alone, the ratio of cardiac compressions to ventilation should be:

    a. 5:1

    b. 10:1

    c. 5:2

    d. 10:2

10. To ensure that the benefit an animal obtains from CPR is not lost, one should not discontinue the CPR for longer than:

    a. 30 seconds
    b. 60 seconds
    c. 90 seconds
    d. 120 seconds
11. Respiratory arrest is always fatal.
    True   False

For the following questions, more than one answer may be correct.

12. One may suspect that the endotracheal tube is malfunctioning even if it is in the trachea because:
    a. Compression of the reservoir bag does not result in the raising of the chest
    b. The animal is dyspneic
    c. The animal cannot be kept at an adequate plane of anesthesia
    d. The reservoir bag is not moving or is moving very little
13. One may suspect that the pop-off valve has been closed or that it is malfunctioning if the:
    a. Reservoir bag is distended with air
    b. Patient has difficulty exhaling
    c. Patient wakes up
    d. Flow rate starts to drop
14. Administration of the normal rate of fluids (10 ml/kg/hr) during an anesthetic procedure may result in overhydration in the:
    a. Patient with cardiac disease
    b. Obese patient
    c. Pediatric patient
    d. Brachycephalic patient
15. Brachycephalic dogs may be an increased anesthetic risk because of their:
    a. Physical size
    b. Excess tissue around the oropharynx
    c. Increased vagal tone
    d. Small trachea in comparison with their physical body size
    e. Increased susceptibility to barbiturates
16. To decrease the anesthetic risk associated with a brachycephalic dog, the anesthetist may elect to:
    a. Use atropine as part of the anesthetic protocol
    b. Preoxygenate the animal before giving any anesthetic
    c. Use an injectable anesthetic to hasten induction rather than masking
    d. Ensure intubation is done quickly after induction
17. Animals that undergo cesarean section are at increased risk during anesthesia because of:
    a. Decreased respiratory function
    b. Increased chance of aspiration vomitus
    c. Increased chance of hemorrhage
    d. Increased workload of the heart
18. Anesthetic agents or drugs that one may want to avoid in the animal with cardiovascular disease include:

 a. Halothane
 b. Isoflurane
 c. Xylazine
 d. Opioids

19. An animal that has liver dysfunction may be hypoproteinemic and therefore requires ____ for induction compared with that needed for a normal dog.
 a. More barbiturate
 b. Less barbiturate
 c. The same amount of barbiturate

20. Too light a plane of anesthesia may be the result of:
 a. A flow rate that is too low
 b. Incorrect vaporizer setting
 c. Incorrect placement of the endotracheal tube
 d. Use of an anesthetic with a low MAC

21. Tachypnea may result from:
 a. Increased levels of arterial oxygen
 b. Increased levels of arterial CO_2
 c. The use of ketamine
 d. Too light a plane of anesthesia

Answers for Chapter 6

1. d **2.** d **3.** b **4.** a **5.** c **6.** c **7.** d **8.** b **9.** d
10. a **11.** False **12.** a, b, c, d **13.** a, b **14.** a, c **15.** b, c, d
16. a, b, c, d **17.** a, b, c, d **18.** a, c **19.** b **20.** a, b, c **21.** b, d

Selected Readings

CLARKE KW, HALL LW: A survey of anaesthesia in small animal practice: AVA/BSAVA report, *J Assoc Vet Anaesth* 17:4-10, 1990.

DODMAN NH, LAMB LA: Survey of small animal anesthetic practice in Vermont. *J Am Anim Hosp Assoc* 28:439-445, 1992.

DYSON DH, MATHEWS K: Recommendations for intensive care management in small animals following anaesthesia, *VCOT* 5:66-70, 1992.

DYSON DH, MAXIE MG: Morbidity and mortality associated with anesthetic management in small animal veterinary practice in Ontario, *J Am Anim Hosp Assoc* 34(4):325-335, 1998.

GAYNOR JS, DUNLOP CI, WAGNER AE, WERTZ EM, GOLDEN AE, DEMME WC: Complications and mortality associated with anesthesia in dogs and cats. *J Am Anim Hosp Assoc* 35(1):13-17, 1999.

HARVEY RC, PADDLEFORD RR: Management of anesthetic emergencies and complications, *Vet Tech* 12(3):237-242, 1991.

HASKINS SC: Opinions in small animal anesthesia, *Vet Clin North Am (Small Anim Pract)* 22(2), Philadelphia, 1992, WB Saunders.

HOLLAND M: Anesthesia for feline cesarean section, *Vet Tech* 12(5):397-402, 1991.

MATHEWS K: *Veterinary emergency and critical care manual*, New York, 1996, Lifelearn, Inc.

PADDLEFORD RR: *Manual of small animal anesthesia*, New York, 1988, Churchill Livingstone.

SAWYER DC: Anesthesia for problem and high-risk patients, *Vet Tech* 15(2):61-69, 1994.

WITTNICH C, BELANGER MP, SALERNO TA, SLUTSKY AS, TRUDEL JL: Canine cardiopulmonary resuscitation: external versus internal cardiac massage, *Compendium* 13(1):50-56, 1991.

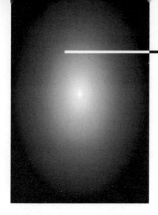

CHAPTER 7

Special Techniques

The anesthetic agents and techniques used for routine procedures on most patients have been described in previous chapters. Occasionally, however, a specialized technique such as local analgesia, mechanical ventilation, and/or the use of neuromuscular blocking agents may be indicated for a patient. This chapter describes these techniques and indicates the circumstances in which they may be useful.

252

■ LOCAL ANALGESIA

The term *local analgesia* refers to the use of a chemical agent on sensory and motor neurons to produce a temporary loss of pain sensation and movement. Although less commonly used than general anesthetics, local analgesics are an effective and practical alternative in many situations involving canine and feline patients. The choice between local analgesia and general anesthesia is made by the veterinarian based on such factors as the temperament, age, and physical status of the patient; cost; time available; the nature of the surgery to be performed; and the anesthetist's skill in performing the local analgesia procedure.

Local analgesia offers the advantages of low patient toxicity, low cost, and minimal patient recovery time. There are several disadvantages, however, including the following:

- There is some risk of overdose, particularly in smaller patients. (See p. 263.)
- Local analgesics may not provide sufficient patient restraint when used alone.
- Effective use of local analgesics often requires precise placement of the drug immediately adjacent to the target nerve. The veterinarian and/or technician performing the procedure must be familiar with the technique involved for each type of nerve block. For example, it is possible to block the sensory nerve of a tooth in a dog to perform a dental procedure; however, accurate and detailed knowledge of the neuroanatomy of the oral cavity is required.
- Local analgesics are relatively ineffective in areas composed of fat, bone, cartilage, fascia, tendon, and other connective tissues.

Agents Used in Veterinary Anesthesia

Many local analgesic agents are available. These agents vary in strength, duration of effect, and method of use (Table 7-1). Lidocaine (Xylocaine), bupivacaine (Marcaine), mepivacaine (Carbocaine), and procaine (Novocaine) are the agents most commonly used for skin infiltration and application to mucous membranes. Tetracaine (Pontocaine) and proparacaine (Ophthaine) are reserved chiefly for ophthalmic use.

Characteristics of Local Analgesia

Local analgesia differs from general anesthesia in several important respects:

- Local analgesics are not anesthetics. The term *anesthetic* is reserved for those drugs such as barbiturates, ketamine, propofol, or inhalation anesthetics that primarily affect neurons in the brain. *Local analgesics* also exert their effect on neurons, but only on those neurons in the peripheral nervous system and spinal cord.
- Because local analgesics normally do not affect the brain, they have little sedating effect. The patient remains fully conscious unless other agents such as tranquilizers or neuroleptanalgesics are used. This is in contrast to general anesthetics, which produce complete unconsciousness.
- When properly used, local analgesics have relatively few effects on the cardiovascular or respiratory systems. In contrast, general anesthetics may cause significant cardiovascular and respiratory depression. For this reason, local analgesia may be preferable to general anesthesia for use in certain high-risk patients.

TABLE 7-1				
Local Analgesics				
Agent (Generic Name)	Agent (Trade Name)	Potency (Procaine = 1)	Dosage	Onset and Duration of Action
Lidocaine	Xylocaine	2	0.5%-2% for injection 2%-4% for topical use Do not exceed 10 mg/kg SC or 2 mg/kg IV in dogs. Cats may be more susceptible to toxic side effects	Immediate onset, 2-hour duration with epinephrine
Mepivacaine	Carbocaine	2.5	1%-2% for injection	Immediate onset, duration 90-180 minutes
Tetracaine	Pontocaine	12	0.1% for injection 0.2% for topical use	Onset 5-10 minutes, duration 2 hours
Bupivacaine	Marcaine	8	0.25%-0.5% for injection 0.75% for epidural, do not exceed 0.5-1mg/kg in cats or 2 mg/kg in dogs.	Delayed onset, duration 4-6 hours

From Skarda RT: Local and Regional Analgesia. In Short CE, *Principles and practices of veterinary anesthesia,* Baltimore, 1987, Williams and Wilkins.

■ Whereas general anesthetics are widely distributed throughout the body, local analgesics primarily exert their effects in the area closest to the site of injection. Unlike general anesthetics, local analgesics are not normally transferred across the placenta to the fetus. For this reason, local analgesia is sometimes used for cesarean sections and obstetric manipulations.

Mechanism of Action

The peripheral nervous system and spinal cord are composed of many types of neurons. From the standpoint of the anesthetist, the most important of these are the neurons that convey sensations (that is, pain, heat, cold, and pressure) from the skin, muscles, and other peripheral tissues to the brain. These neurons are termed sensory neurons and are affected by even small amounts of local analgesics, provided the drug is deposited in close proximity to the neuron. Another type of neuron, called motor neurons, conveys impulses from the brain to muscle fibers and is responsible for initiating and controlling voluntary movements. Motor neurons are also sensitive to the effect of local analgesics, and administration of a local analgesic will cause temporary paresis (weakness) or paralysis (loss of movement) in the area served by the affected motor neurons.

Loss of sensation and loss of motor ability are seen concurrently. For example, use of a local analgesic near the terminal end of the spinal cord (called an epidural block) will result in loss of sensation and voluntary movement to all areas innervated by the affected sensory and motor neurons. The patient sensations that are lost include (in order of loss) pain, cold, warmth, touch, joint sensation, and deep pressure in the caudal abdomen and pelvic limbs. The patient also will be unable to move the pelvic limbs, and the muscles will appear relaxed.

Local analgesics also affect the neurons of the autonomic nervous system. These neurons convey impulses between the brain and the blood vessels and internal organs (including the heart). If these neurons are exposed to local analgesics, their function is lost. This is most important in the sympathetic nervous system, and the loss of function of these neurons is called a *sympathetic blockade*. The main effect in the peripheral tissues is vasodilation, resulting in flushing and increased skin temperature of the affected area. Vasodilation may cause blood pressure to fall in some patients, leading to hypotension. A sympathetic blockade may be seen after epidural blocks with lidocaine and other local analgesics, because sympathetic ganglia adjacent to the vertebrae are affected by the local analgesic. If a sympathetic blockade occurs within the proximal spinal cord (as may occur if local analgesic is allowed to infuse into the thoracic spinal canal), sympathetic innervation to the heart may be blocked, resulting in bradycardia and decreased ventricular contractions.

The mechanism of action of local analgesics is not fully understood, but appears to involve a loss of transmission of electrical impulses along the nerve fiber. The local analgesic appears to block the membrane channels through which sodium flows into the neuron. A local analgesic drug therefore acts as a membrane stabilizer, stopping the process of nerve depolarization. The result is a loss of nerve conduction. Reversal of this effect occurs when the drug is absorbed into the local circulation. Local analgesics are then redistributed to the liver, where they are inactivated.

Route of Administration

Topical use.   Local analgesics are usually ineffective when applied directly to intact skin. This is because the drug molecules are unable to penetrate the epidermis and reach the dermis, where the peripheral nerves are located. A cream formulation containing a mixture of 2.5% lidocaine and 2.5% prilocaine (EMLA cream) can be used to desensitize intact skin. A thick layer of cream is applied to the area to be anesthetized, and covered with an occlusive dressing for 1 hour.

Local analgesics can be absorbed by mucous membranes, including the conjunctiva, larynx, and lining of the urethra. Therefore these drugs can be used in the form of topical sprays, drops, or ointment applied to these areas. For example, lidocaine spray is used to desensitize the larynx and prevent laryngospasm in cats. Another example of topical use of local analgesics is the application of proparacaine or tetracaine to the surface of the eye. This procedure desensitizes the cornea and conjunctiva, allowing procedures such as conjunctival scraping or tonometry. Local analgesics also may be used in the form of a gel and can, for example, be applied to a urinary catheter to ease the catheterization process. In each case, analgesia of the mucous membrane results within 60 to 90 seconds, allowing procedures to be performed with less discomfort to the patient.

Infiltration.   Local analgesics may be infiltrated (injected) into tissues, preferably in close proximity to the nerve that is to be affected. The local analgesic can be given intradermally, subcutaneously, or between muscles, depending on the area to be treated. Infiltration techniques most commonly are used to provide analgesia for surgery involving superficial tissues, including skin biopsies, removal of small skin tumors, and repair of minor lacerations.

The procedure used for local analgesia infusion is relatively simple. Before infiltration of local analgesic, the area must be clipped and a skin antiseptic applied in a manner similar to that used for a surgical prep. This prevents inadvertent contamination of the tissues with skin bacteria when the local analgesic is injected. A small needle (23- or 25-gauge) is often used because these needles create little tissue damage and allow for more precise placement of the drug. The amount of the drug to be injected varies with the location and procedure used, but is typically between 0.5 and 1 ml per site.

The two types of procedures used for local analgesia infusion are nerve blocks and line blocks.

Nerve blocks.   A nerve block is achieved by injecting local analgesic in close proximity to a nerve to desensitize a particular anatomical site. One familiar example is the use of novocaine in human dentistry. Nerve blocks commonly are used in large animal anesthesia, and also may be employed in small animals provided the location of the nerve is known exactly. Reference texts contain illustrations that indicate the exact location of nerve blocks for different species and particular areas of the body. Before placing a nerve block, it is helpful to palpate the nerve to determine its location, although this may not always be possible.

A small amount of local analgesic is injected immediately adjacent to the nerve. The drug diffuses through the tissues to reach the target nerve. Caution should be used to avoid injecting directly into a nerve because temporary or permanent loss of nerve function can occur. It is also important to avoid intravenous injection of the local analgesic, which not only is ineffective in producing analgesia, but also may cause unwanted central nervous system and cardiovascular effects. For this reason, it is advisable to aspirate before injecting a local analgesic. If blood appears in the syringe, the location of the injection should be changed.

Line blocks.   Often the veterinarian will do surgery on an area of tissue that is served by numerous small neurons. In this situation, a line block consisting of a continuous line of local analgesic can be placed in the subcutaneous or subcuticular tissues immediately proximal to the target area (Fig. 7-1). Line blocks should be positioned between the target area and the spinal cord, because this will block the sensory neurons most effectively. Placement of a line block can be easily accomplished by inserting the needle along the proposed line of infiltration and gradually withdrawing the needle while simultaneously injecting a small amount of local analgesic.

Regardless of whether the veterinarian prefers to use a nerve block or a line block, the onset of analgesia is usually 3 to 5 minutes after the injection of lidocaine. Before surgery commences it is advisable to test the effectiveness of the block by gently pricking the skin with a 22-gauge needle. If sensation appears to be present, the anesthetist should wait several minutes longer and consider repeating the infusion or using another anesthetic protocol if the block does not take effect.

The infusion of local analgesics is not universally effective. Deep tissues such as muscles are unlikely to be affected when only superficial neurons are blocked. Additionally, diffusion of local analgesic is impeded by obstacles such as scar tissue or fibrous tissue, fat, edema, and hemorrhage, and the procedure is often ineffective in areas where these occur. Local analgesics are also relatively ineffective when injected into inflamed areas. In areas of active inflammation, tissue pH is acidic, which results in rapid inactivation of the drug.

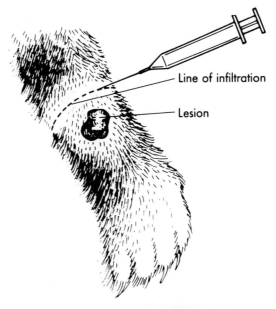

Line of infiltration

Lesion

FIG. 7-1 Procedure for performing a line block.

Once the local analgesic reaches the neuron, the duration of effect depends on the type of drug being used and the rate of absorption by local blood vessels. (See Table 7-1.) This, in turn, depends on whether epinephrine is used with the local analgesic. Lidocaine, the drug most commonly used for local infusion, may be purchased with or without epinephrine. The concentration of epinephrine used is 5 μg/ml (1:200,000 solution).

Epinephrine is added to local analgesics for two reasons:

1. Epinephrine causes blood vessels in the area of the injection to constrict. This decreases the rate of drug absorption and thereby prolongs the effect of the local analgesic.
2. By causing vasoconstriction, epinephrine reduces the concentration of local analgesic that enters the circulation at any given time, thereby reducing toxicity of the drug.

Lidocaine without epinephrine may be preferred to lidocaine with epinephrine in some situations. A solution containing epinephrine should not be used at an incision site because it may impair tissue perfusion and healing. Epinephrine also increases the risk of ventricular arrhythmias and should be used with caution in animals with known cardiac disease. Lidocaine without epinephrine should also be used for intravenous techniques. (See page 262.)

Regional analgesia. Regional analgesia is a technique whereby a local analgesic is injected into a major nerve plexus or in close proximity to the spinal cord. This results in the blockage of nervous impulses to and from a relatively large area, such as an entire limb or the entire caudal portion of the body. Examples of regional analgesia in veterinary practice include epidural, spinal (intrathecal), and brachial plexus blocks. Regional analgesia can be used to provide analgesia during surgery (for example, a cesarean section can be performed using an epidural block).

Regional analgesia techniques are also used to provide effective pain control in the postoperative period (for example, epidural use of lidocaine or morphine after repair of a fractured femur). The provision of analgesia through the use of epidural, intraarticular, and other regional techniques is further discussed in Chapter 8.

Local analgesic techniques are often used in conjunction with neuroleptanalgesics or other injectable medications. This helps to ensure adequate restraint, allowing accurate and safe injection of the local analgesic and preventing patient movement during the surgical procedure.

Epidural analgesia.   Epidural analgesia is a regional analgesia technique that is commonly used in large animal anesthesia and, to a lesser extent, in small animal anesthesia. The procedure is not difficult (Procedure 7-1) and, once mastered, allows the anesthetist to reliably block sensation and motor control of the rear abdomen, pelvis, tail, pelvic limbs, and perineum. The technique therefore can be used for tail amputation, anal sac removal, perianal surgery, urethrostomies, obstetric manipulations, cesarean sections, and some rear limb surgeries.

PROCEDURE 7-1
Epidural Analgesia in the Dog and Cat

1. Gather the necessary equipment. This includes a short-beveled spinal needle with a stylet (18- to 22-gauge, 1.5 inches for small or thin dogs, and 2 to 3 inches for large, overweight dogs) and several sterile 3- or 5-ml syringes. If a catheter is to be placed, a thin-walled, 18-gauge, 3-inch needle is required.
2. Sedate the patient to achieve adequate restraint, and place in sternal or lateral recumbency. The head is positioned higher than the spinal cord for at least the first 10 minutes of analgesia.
3. Identify the right and left cranial dorsal wings of the ilium, the spinous process of L7, and the sacral crest. Shave and surgically prepare the area surrounding the injection site (between L7 and the sacral crest). Wear surgical gloves for the procedure.
4. Palpate the lumbosacral space (between L7 and the sacrum), which is almost exactly midway between the dorsal iliac wings. (See Fig. 7-3.) The lumbosacral space is the depression just caudal to the L7 process and immediately cranial to the sacral crest, which feels like a series of small bumps under the skin. Place the spinal needle in the area of greatest depression, perpendicular to the skin surface and exactly on the midline. The bevel should be directed cranially, and the stylet should be left in the needle. The needle is gently advanced perpendicular to the skin, passing through the skin, subcutaneous fat, supraspinous ligament, interspinous ligament, and ligamentum flavum (Fig. 7-2). Resistance may be encountered, and a distinct pop often can be felt as the needle is advanced through the ligamentum flavum. Immediately after penetrating the ligamentum flavum, the needle enters the epidural space. This usually occurs at a needle depth of 1 to 3 cm,

PROCEDURE 7-1
Epidural Analgesia in the Dog and Cat—*cont'd*

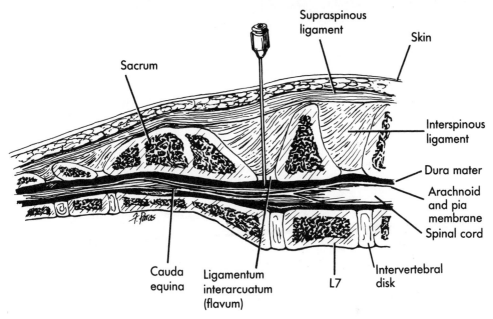

FIG. 7-2 Anatomy of the distal spinal canal, showing the placement of a needle for lumbosacral epidural analgesia. (From Muir WW III, Hubbell JAE: *Handbook of veterinary anesthesia,* St Louis, 1989, Mosby.)

depending on the size of the animal. Occasionally, there is some difficulty in finding the intervertebral space, in which case the needle should be withdrawn, angled slightly caudally or cranially, and reinserted.

5. Remove the stylet and examine the needle hub for blood or cerebrospinal fluid. If cerebrospinal fluid is encountered, the needle is in the subarachnoid space. (If this is the case, the procedure may be abandoned or the anesthetist may choose to administer 50% of the original dose, inducing spinal analgesia, provided the agent used has minimal spinal toxicity). If blood is encountered, the needle has entered the venous sinus and the procedure should be abandoned. If blood and cerebrospinal fluid are not observed, the needle should be aspirated to ensure that neither is present. To further check for proper needle placement, 1 to 2 ml of air can be injected: no resistance to air passage should be felt. For large dogs, it may be easier to remove the stylet as it enters the skin. The hub can be filled with saline, and as the needle penetrates the ligamentum flavum, the liquid will be drawn into the epidural space.

Continued

▼ **PROCEDURE 7-1**
Epidural Analgesia in the Dog and Cat—*cont'd*

Surgery: If the epidural is performed for surgical analgesia and immobilization, lidocaine or bupivacaine is used. The dosage of 2% lidocaine (without epinephrine) or 0.75% bupivacaine will vary with the extent of analgesia required. The anesthetist often will elect to produce anesthesia as far cranial as L2 (which is sufficient for most caudal abdominal procedures and all pelvic and rear limb procedures). The dose used in this case is 1 ml of lidocaine or bupivacaine for each 5 kg of body weight. Inject the calculated dose of lidocaine or bupivacaine over 1 minute. More rapid injection may result in local analgesic infiltrating too far forward along the spinal canal. (See p. 263.) Injection will be resistance-free if the needle is positioned correctly. If continuous epidural analgesia is required, a polyethylene catheter may be advanced through the needle and the needle subsequently withdrawn, leaving the catheter in place. Advance the catheter only 1 cm into the epidural space.

Onset of analgesia is approximately 5 minutes after lidocaine infusion or 20 minutes after bupivacaine infusion. The block normally affects the most distal body parts (toes and tail) first. If a bilateral effect is desired, position the patient in dorsal recumbency for 20 minutes after the injection. If unilateral analgesia is required, place the patient in lateral recumbency, with the desired side positioned ventrally, allowing for gravitation of the local analgesic within the epidural space to the targeted side of the spinal canal.

It has been reported that 12% of correctly performed epidural blocks are ineffective, perhaps because of individual variations in anatomy. Failure of the block may be determined by testing with a needle prick or may become evident during patient preparation or application of towel clamps.

Duration of analgesia is 4 to 6 hours for bupivacaine with epinephrine and 1.5 hours for lidocaine with epinephrine.

Postoperative Pain Control: If the epidural is performed to provide postoperative analgesia, morphine or another opioid agent is used. The procedure used is the same as described above. It is advisable that single-use vials of preservative-free morphine (Duramorph) be used. See Chapter 8 for more information on the use of morphine epidurals for pain control.

Epidural anesthesia is particularly valuable in two classes of patients: (1) debilitated patients that are at high risk for general anesthesia but that may tolerate a lidocaine or bupivacaine epidural block, and (2) patients requiring profound pain control following surgical procedures involving the hind limbs, pelvis, or caudal abdomen. This is provided by an epidural injection of morphine or other opioid drug.

Anatomic considerations for epidural analgesia.   To understand the technique used for epidural analgesia, the anesthetist must be familiar with the anatomy of the terminal spinal cord region. (See Fig. 7-2.) The spinal cord contains sensory, motor, and autonomic neurons and is surrounded by three membrane layers: the

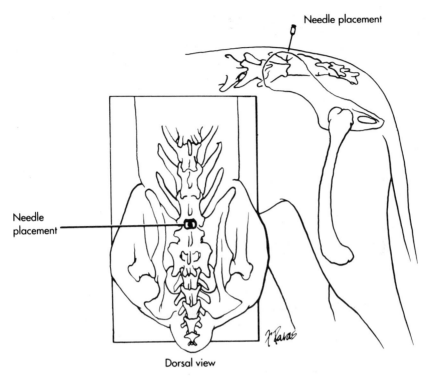

Needle placement

Needle
placement

Dorsal view

FIG. 7-3   Needle placement for lumbosacral epidural anesthesia in the dog.

pia, arachnoid, and dura mater. The subarachnoid space, which is the area between the arachnoid and the pia, is filled with cerebrospinal fluid. This fluid surrounds the entire spinal cord and communicates with the cerebrospinal fluid in the ventricles of the brain. The spinal cord and its membrane layers are encased within the spinal canal. This canal consists of bony vertebrae (cervical, thoracic, lumbar, sacral, and coccygeal) that protect the spinal cord from injury. The vertebral canal is also protected by several ligaments, including the supraspinous ligament (which lies directly under the skin), the ligamentum flavum (also called the ligamentum interarcuatum), and the interspinous ligament. (See Fig. 7-2.) Neurons that supply the tissues exit from the spinal cord at regular intervals, emerging between the vertebrae and ultimately ending in the skin and other tissues. The spinal cord itself terminates in a group of neurons collectively called the cauda equina.

In performing epidural analgesia, local analgesic is deposited in the epidural space, between the dura and the vertebrae. In dogs the location of the block is between the last lumbar vertebra (L7) and the sacrum (Fig. 7-3). When properly performed, injection of local analgesic into this area is unlikely to damage the spinal cord because the cord normally ends at the sixth or seventh lumbar vertebra (L6 or L7). In cats the spinal cord extends further caudally (as far as S1), and there is a slightly increased risk of spinal cord damage when performing an epidural. Inadvertent injection of local analgesic into the subarachnoid space also is more common in the cat than in the dog.

Epidural analgesia must be differentiated from spinal analgesia, which is commonly performed in human patients. In spinal analgesia, the local analgesic is infiltrated into the subarachnoid space, where it mixes with the cerebrospinal fluid.

Intravenous infusion.   Intravenous infusion of local analgesics is not performed routinely in dogs or cats, but may be useful in some situations. In this procedure, a tourniquet is applied just proximal to the area requiring anesthesia (for example, immediately above the elbow if the foreleg is to be anesthetized). A calculated amount of local analgesic is injected into a superficial vein using a 22-gauge, 1.5-inch needle. The usual dose used is 2 to 3 ml of 1% lidocaine without epinephrine, not to exceed 4 mg/kg. Within 3 to 5 minutes, there is total desensitization of the limb distal to the tourniquet, allowing 25 to 30 minutes of analgesia. An additional advantage of this technique is the relatively blood-free surgery site that it affords. As with other local analgesic procedures, however, patient restraint may be a problem unless concurrent sedation or neuroleptanalgesia is provided.

Sensation returns to the affected area within a few minutes of release of the tourniquet. It is important to remove the tourniquet soon after the procedure is completed. If the tourniquet is in place more than 2 hours, prolonged hypoxia of the tissues of the limb may result, leading to tissue necrosis. In all patients, removal of the tourniquet should be gradual (that is, over a 5-minute period) because this helps prevent excessive amounts of local analgesic from reaching the heart and brain.

Toxicity

The use of local analgesics is not without risk, and several adverse side effects have been reported, including the following:

1. If local analgesic is injected into a nerve fiber, temporary or permanent loss of function may result.
2. Tissue irritation may occur with the use of some local analgesics. Mepivacaine (Carbocaine) is preferred over other local analgesics by some veterinarians because it appears to have little local toxicity.
3. Paresthesia, an abnormal sensation of tingling, pain, or irritation, may be present in an anesthetized area during recovery from local analgesia. (Humans also experience this "tingling" sensation during recovery from "freezing" of the oral cavity with Novocaine.) Animals should be monitored during recovery because they may chew or otherwise traumatize affected areas.
4. Humans and animals may exhibit allergic reactions to local analgesics, usually in the form of a skin rash or hives. Anaphylaxis is also occasionally seen. Local analgesics should not be used in patients in which a previous allergic reaction to these drugs has been observed.
5. Systemic toxicity may occur, particularly if a local analgesic is inadvertently given intravenously without the use of a tourniquet. Systemic toxicity may be seen even if the drug is placed in the subcutaneous tissues, particularly if a large amount of local analgesic is injected.

   The most common signs of systemic toxicity originate in the central nervous system and include muscle twitching, sedation or hyperexcitability, convulsions, and respiratory depression. Treatment of CNS signs may include injection of diazepam and administration of oxygen through an endotracheal tube.

Cardiovascular effects may be observed because of the direct effect of local analgesics on the heart. In particular, intravenous injection of lidocaine has a profound effect on conduction of electrical impulses within the heart muscle. This characteristic is undesirable when performing local analgesia, but makes this drug of use in treating certain types of ventricular arrhythmias.

6. Epidural or spinal injection may be hazardous if incorrectly performed. It is possible to traumatize the spinal cord or cauda equina, particularly if the animal is struggling during placement of the needle. Inflammation and fibrosis have been reported after epidural infiltration of local analgesics containing preservatives. Additionally, myelitis (spinal cord inflammation) and meningitis (inflammation of the pia, arachnoid, or dura mater) may occur if asepsis is not maintained.

7. If local analgesics are permitted to infiltrate into the cranial portion of the spinal cord, serious toxicity and even death may occur. If the local analgesic reaches the midthoracic vertebrae, innervation of the intercostal muscles may be blocked, interfering with normal respiration. If local analgesic diffuses as far forward as the cervical spinal cord, the phrenic nerve may be blocked. This nerve innervates the diaphragm, and loss of function may result in respiratory paralysis. Diffusion of local analgesic into the cervical and thoracic spinal cord also may affect sympathetic nerves supplying the heart and blood vessels, resulting in a sympathetic blockade and symptoms of bradycardia, decreased cardiac output, and hypotension.

8. Hypotension resulting from blockade of sympathetic neurons may occur after epidural infusion and other local analgesia techniques. Careful monitoring of the capillary refill time and pulse rate will alert the anesthetist to a fall in blood pressure. Treatment consists of intravenous fluid administration at a rate of 20 ml/kg over a 15- to 20-minute period.

In general, local analgesic toxicity can be minimized by following a few simple rules:

1. The dose of lidocaine given subcutaneously to any patient should not exceed 10 mg/kg. The smallest possible dose should be used. If given intravenously, the dose of lidocaine should not exceed 2 mg/kg. The dose of bupivacaine given subcutaneously should not exceed 2 mg/kg in dogs and 0.5 to 1 mg/kg in cats.

2. Small, undamaged needles must be used for injection.

3. The injection site should be surgically prepared, and the injection should be given in an aseptic manner.

4. The anesthetist should always aspirate before injecting local analgesic, to ensure that inadvertent intravenous administration does not occur.

5. When performing epidural analgesia, care should be taken to keep the head elevated to avoid gravitational flow of the analgesic into the anterior spinal canal around the thoracic and cervical spinal cord. The anesthetist should be prepared to intubate and artificially ventilate any patient undergoing epidural analgesia, because this may be necessary if intercostal and phrenic nerve function is impaired.

■ CONTROLLED VENTILATION

The anesthetist commonly is called on to assist or control patient ventilation during anesthesia. In assisted ventilation, the anesthetist ensures that an increased volume of air is delivered to the patient, although the patient initiates each inspiration. In controlled ventilation, the anesthetist delivers all of the air that is required by the patient, and the patient does not make any spontaneous respiratory efforts. The anesthetist controls the volume of air, rate of respiration, and the pressure of air introduced into the animal.

Types of Assisted or Controlled Ventilation

Ventilation assistance or control may take several forms, including the following:
- Squeezing the reservoir bag once every 5 to 10 minutes. The anesthetist thereby assists the patient's breathing on an intermittent basis.
- Continuous ventilation of the patient by bagging every 5 seconds. Usually, the anesthetist controls patient ventilation in this case.
- Continuous ventilation of the patient by means of a mechanical ventilator. The anesthetist adjusts the ventilator to completely control patient ventilation. Alternatively, mechanical ventilators can be used to assist, rather than control, patient ventilation.

Any procedure by which the anesthetist forcefully delivers oxygen and anesthetic gas to the patient's lungs may be termed positive pressure ventilation (PPV). In positive pressure ventilation, the lungs are filled with oxygen by the pressure of gas entering the airways, either from the reservoir bag or a mechanical ventilator. This differs from normal patient breathing, in which air is drawn into the lungs by the movement of the animal's diaphragm, intercostal, and abdominal muscles. Whether achieved by bagging the patient or by mechanical ventilation, PPV is intended to ensure that the animal receives adequate oxygen and is able to exhale adequate amounts of carbon dioxide. This is a concern in veterinary anesthesia because the patient's own ventilation efforts may be inadequate to achieve these objectives.

Ventilation in the Awake Animal

To understand the use of positive pressure ventilation in anesthesia, it is necessary to first review the mechanics of normal breathing and the reasons why they may be ineffective in the anesthetized animal. Ventilation is the physical movement of air and anesthetic gases into and out of the lungs and upper respiratory passageways. Ventilation has two parts: an active phase (inhalation) and a passive phase (exhalation). Inhalation is initiated by the respiratory center in the brain, which is triggered by an increased level of carbon dioxide in the arterial blood ($PaCO_2$). As $PaCO_2$ rises above a threshold level, the respiratory center initiates the active inspiratory phase by stimulating the intercostal muscles and diaphragm to move, expanding the thorax. This creates a negative pressure (partial vacuum) within the chest, which causes the lungs to expand. As the lungs expand, air moves through the air passages and into the alveoli. When the lungs reach an adequate volume, nerve impulses feed back to the respiratory center, signaling the brain to stop the active phase of respiration. The intercostal muscles and diaphragm then relax, and exhalation takes place as the lungs deflate. Exhalation is passive, which means that no active muscle movement occurs. During exhalation, the carbon dioxide level in the blood begins to rise again, and after a short pause the respiratory center responds by initiating another inspiration.

Normally, inspiration lasts approximately twice as long as exhalation. For example, in an animal breathing 20 times per minute, each inspiration will last approximately 2 seconds and each exhalation will last approximately 1 second.

The amount of air that passes in or out of the lungs in a single breath is the *tidal volume*. Animals that are breathing deeply have a relatively large tidal volume, whereas animals that have shallow breathing or that are panting have a relatively small tidal volume.

The *respiratory rate* is the number of tidal volumes that occurs in 1 minute. The respiratory minute volume is the total amount of air that moves in and out of the lungs in 1 minute. This value can be found by multiplying the average tidal volume by the respiratory rate.

Ventilation in the Anesthetized Animal

Ventilation in the anesthetized animal differs significantly from normal ventilation described above. These differences include the following:

1. Tranquilizers and general anesthetics may decrease the responsiveness of the respiratory center in the brain to carbon dioxide. This means that inspiration does not occur as often in the anesthetized animal as in the normal awake animal, despite the fact that carbon dioxide may be significantly elevated. The respiratory rate of an anesthetized animal is therefore reduced compared with that of a normal awake animal. This explains the observation that a respiratory rate of 12 to 20 breaths per minute is normal in cats and dogs under inhalation anesthesia, whereas the same animal would be expected to have a respiratory rate between 20 and 30 breaths per minute when awake.

2. Tranquilizers and general anesthetics relax the intercostal muscles and diaphragm, causing them to expand less than normal during the inspiratory phase. Because the chest does not expand fully, the tidal volume is reduced. Tidal volume in the normal animal at rest is approximately 10 to 15 ml/kg; in the anesthetized animal, tidal volume may be less than 8 ml/kg. The anesthetist may become aware of the reduced tidal volume by noting that the reservoir bag does not expand appreciably during expiration (that is, the volume of gas exhaled is relatively small).

Because tidal volume and respiratory rate are decreased, respiratory minute volume is also decreased. The amount of air entering and leaving the lungs in the anesthetized animal is therefore considerably reduced compared with the normal awake animal. This has several consequences, including the following:

1. Pa_{CO_2} rises in the anesthetized animal (that is, carbon dioxide produced by the body is not eliminated as rapidly as normal). As blood CO_2 rises, it joins with water molecules in the bloodstream to form bicarbonate ions (HCO_3^-) and hydrogen ions (H^+). The accumulation of hydrogen ions causes the pH of circulating blood to fall, potentially leading to respiratory acidosis. Blood pH in the normal awake animal is between 7.38 and 7.42, whereas in the anesthetized animal, blood pH may be as low as 7.20.

2. If the anesthetized animal is breathing room air, Pa_{O_2} will fall below normal values as a result of the decreased respiratory minute volume. This occurs

because less oxygen is entering the lungs, and therefore less is available to be absorbed into the blood.

3. Because tidal volume is reduced, the alveoli do not expand as fully as normal on inspiration. In fact, some sections of the lung may partially collapse, and the alveoli may not expand at all. This condition is called atelectasis.

The anesthetist has several ways of compensating for these effects. The PaO_2 can be elevated to normal levels (and, in fact, often above normal levels) if the patient is supplied with adequate oxygen. This is easily achieved because animals connected to anesthetic machines normally receive close to 100% oxygen (or a mixture of oxygen and nitrous oxide). The anesthetized patient connected to an anesthetic machine is unlikely to have a reduced PaO_2 unless a problem exists (for example, if the machine runs out of oxygen, if oxygen flow rate is too low, or if insufficient oxygen is provided with nitrous oxide).

It is more difficult to prevent atelectasis or an increase in $PaCO_2$ and resulting respiratory acidosis. In animals anesthetized for prolonged periods or in patients with depressed respiration (such as those undergoing thoracic surgery)* these problems may become significant. The anesthetist should take active steps to counter these changes in the anesthetized patient by assisting ventilation. This can be done in one of two ways:

1. Intermittent or continuous bagging of the patient using the reservoir bag (also called manual ventilation). For most patients, intermittent bagging (once every 5 minutes) is adequate.
2. Mechanical ventilation using a ventilator.

Whatever method is chosen, the patient must be intubated and connected to an anesthetic machine before ventilation can be assisted. (Temporary ventilation assistance also can be given in the absence of an endotracheal tube, using an Ambu bag.) Air enters the respiratory passages under pressure and causes the alveoli to expand. Exhalation is passive and occurs when the positive pressure is discontinued, allowing the lungs to empty. This type of ventilation can be contrasted with normal ventilation, in which active expansion of the chest cavity causes a partial vacuum to form within the alveoli, which draws air into the lungs.

Manual Ventilation

Manual ventilation can be used to assist or totally control the ventilation cycle, by means of pressure placed on the reservoir bag by the anesthetist's hand. The procedure is similar to that used to treat respiratory arrest, described in Chapter 6. The pop-off valve is closed and the reservoir bag is compressed until the lungs are inflated. When pressure is released on the reservoir bag, exhalation can occur. The anesthetist must use caution to ensure that the pressure used is not excessive: the patient's chest should only rise to the same extent as with normal awake respiration, and the pressure manometer reading should not exceed 20 cm H_2O (14 mm Hg).

---

*Animals undergoing thoracic surgery often have preexisting cardiovascular and/or pulmonary disease and are at significant risk of cardiovascular collapse and/or respiratory arrest if conventional anesthesia with unassisted ventilation is pursued. In addition to manual or mechanical ventilation, these patients benefit from preoxygenation and intravenous induction techniques (rather than mask or chamber induction). In these and other patients, mechanical ventilation may be combined with the use of neuromuscular blocking agents. (See following section.)

Manual ventilation can be performed on an occasional basis (once every 5 minutes) on any anesthetized patient. These periodic "sighs" help expand collapsed alveoli and reverse atelectasis.

It is advisable to turn the vaporizer setting to zero before bagging the patient, if an in-circle, nonprecision vaporizer is in use. This helps prevent sudden vaporization of large amounts of anesthetic as a result of the increased flow of carrier gas through the vaporizer. If a precision vaporizer is in use, it is not necessary to turn the concentration setting to zero because back flow compensation is usually present. If continuous manual ventilation is used, however, it may be advisable to reduce the precision vaporizer setting, or the patient's level of anesthesia may become too deep because of increased delivery of anesthetic to the lungs. The anesthetist should closely monitor the patient and adjust the vaporizer setting based on the patient's depth.

For some patients, respiratory depression is so severe that hypercapnia and respiratory acidosis develop despite intermittent bagging. The anesthetist may be able to identify these patients by their shallow breaths (small tidal volume) and infrequent respirations (respiratory rate of 8 breaths per minute or less). These patients require more aggressive ventilation, in the form of continuous manual or mechanical ventilation. In this procedure, ventilation is assisted starting immediately after induction, at which point the anesthetist should use the reservoir bag to superimpose positive pressure on the animal's own spontaneous breathing efforts. The assisted ventilation rate should be 12 to 16 respirations per minute, at a manometer pressure of 15 to 20 cm H_2O (11 to 14 mm Hg). After 3 to 5 minutes, the patient's spontaneous breathing efforts usually disappear, and the anesthetist has gained control over ventilation. If the patient resists the anesthetist's efforts to control ventilation, it may be necessary to use a neuromuscular blocking agent, which paralyzes the muscles of respiration.*

Once control is established, a ventilation rate of 8 to 12 "breaths" per minute is usually adequate. A pressure of 15 to 20 cm H_2O is recommended, unless the chest is open, in which case a pressure of 20 to 30 cm H_2O may be required. When squeezing the reservoir bag, the inspiratory time should be 1 to 1.5 seconds. Expiratory time should be twice as long as inspiratory time. The pop-off valve must be closed when the reservoir bag is squeezed; however, it should be opened briefly between every 2 to 3 breaths to allow gas to escape from the circuit. The anesthetist should not hold on to the reservoir bag between breaths because this causes increased pressure in the lungs, which may in turn cause alveolar rupture or increased intrathoracic pressure.

Continuous manual bagging can be performed using either a rebreathing or a nonrebreathing system. Nonrebreathing systems usually lack a manometer, and the anesthetist must use sight and touch to determine the optimal tidal volume.

When the surgical procedure is nearing completion, it is necessary for the anesthetist to "wean the animal" off the controlled ventilation procedure. This is done by turning off the anesthetic and nitrous oxide while continuing to ventilate the patient with oxygen. If a neuromuscular blocking agent has been used, it should be reversed,

---

*Not all patients require this amount of effort to gain control over ventilation. For many patients it is adequate to give a few large tidal volumes manually, then connect the patient to a ventilator. The initial large tidal volumes depress the animal's urge to breathe by lowering the blood carbon dioxide levels. Once connected to a ventilator or undergoing continuous manual ventilation, the patient usually stops spontaneous breathing efforts within 1 minute.

if possible. The anesthetist should gradually reduce the rate of inspirations to approximately 5 per minute, while observing the animal for evidence of spontaneous breathing. When this is seen, the patient's ventilation can continue to be assisted by squeezing a small amount of air from the reservoir bag with each inspiration. Eventually, the animal regains the ability to maintain a normal rate and tidal volume, and ventilation assistance can be discontinued. This may take several minutes to reestablish, particularly in older and debilitated patients and patients in which ventilation has been controlled for a long time. Stimulation of the patient by pinching the toe pads or gently rubbing the thorax and abdomen may help the patient regain spontaneous respiratory movements.

Continuously assisted ventilation, as described above, offers many advantages. It prevents hypoxia, efficiently eliminates carbon dioxide, and prevents respiratory acidosis. It is particularly useful in animals with compromised respiration, including obese patients, debilitated patients, animals undergoing thoracic surgery, and animals with diaphragmatic hernia, pneumonia, or head trauma. It is also useful in animals showing hypoventilation from any other cause, including prolonged anesthesia.

When assisting or controlling ventilation, it is often difficult for the anesthetist to evaluate the adequacy of the ventilation efforts. Pulse oximetry or end tidal capnography are invaluable aids in monitoring these patients. If, for example, the pulse oximeter reading is 90% or less in a patient undergoing manual ventilation, the patient may need more frequent ventilation, or ventilation at a greater pressure.

Mechanical Ventilation

Mechanical ventilation is similar to continuous manual ventilation in many respects. In mechanical ventilation, however, the patient's breathing is controlled by a ventilator, which replaces continual compression of the reservoir bag. When a ventilator is connected to the breathing circuit, it functionally replaces the reservoir bag and becomes a part of the breathing circuit. The ventilator automatically compresses a bellows, which forces oxygen and anesthetic gas into the patient's air passageways via an endotracheal tube.

There are many types of ventilators that can be used with a veterinary anesthesia machine; they vary in the number and complexity of the controls (Fig. 7-4). Ventilators can be attached to a circle system by removing the reservoir bag and attaching the outlet of the ventilator to the anesthetic machine. The scavenger should be attached to the exhaust port of the ventilator.

Depending on the type of ventilator used, the anesthetist may choose to deliver gases on inspiration according to a pressure cycle, volume cycle, or time cycle. The pressure-cycled ventilator (such as the Bird Mark 7 Respirator) will supply air until the pressure reaches a preset level. A time cycle ventilator (such as the Small Animal Ventilator and Drager) supplies air according to a set inspiratory time. A volume cycle type (such as the Ohio Metomatic) delivers a preset tidal volume regardless of the pressure required. In volume-cycled ventilators, the anesthetist must adjust the volume of gas to be delivered on inspiration (usually 15 to 20 ml/kg; less if respiration is to be assisted rather than controlled). The animal's chest should be observed to rise with each inspiration. Respiratory rate is usually 8 to 12 breaths per minute. Duration of inspiration is set at 1 to 2 seconds, and duration of expiration should be 2 to 4 seconds with an inspiratory/expiratory ratio of 1:2 to 1:3.

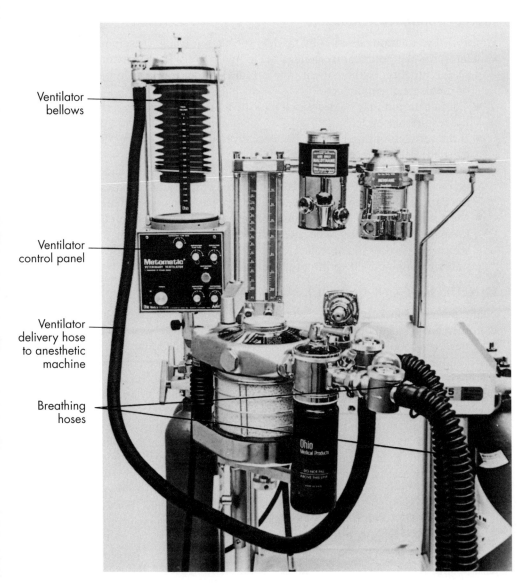

Ventilator bellows

Ventilator control panel

Ventilator delivery hose to anesthetic machine

Breathing hoses

FIG. 7-4   Ventilator for use in small animal anesthesia.

Like manual ventilation, mechanical ventilation is particularly indicated for patients with compromised respiration. It is not normally necessary in healthy anesthetized patients, in which intermittent manual bagging (once every 5 minutes) is usually sufficient. Mechanical ventilation is used most commonly in animals undergoing a thoracotomy or other lengthy surgery, in which continuous manual ventilation would be difficult for the anesthetist.

Risks of Controlled Ventilation

Controlled ventilation, whether by manual ventilation using a reservoir bag or by a ventilator, has the potential to damage the animal's lungs if done incorrectly.

- Overventilation of the patient may rupture alveoli, resulting in pneumothorax or mediastinal emphysema.
- Cardiac output may be decreased if positive pressure is maintained throughout the respiratory cycle.
- If the ventilation rate is excessive, excessive amounts of carbon dioxide can be exhaled, leading to respiratory alkalosis.
- Controlled ventilation using an in-circle vaporizer is difficult and may be dangerous. Because of the lack of back pressure compensation in these vaporizers, the patient may receive excessive amounts of vaporized anesthetic.
- Mechanical ventilation is not intended to relieve the anesthetist of the necessity for patient monitoring. The anesthetist must closely monitor all animals in which ventilation is controlled or assisted to ensure that patient depth and safety are maintained within acceptable limits.

■ NEUROMUSCULAR BLOCKING AGENTS

Neuromuscular blocking agents (also called muscle-paralyzing agents) are often used in human anesthesia, but have found only limited use in veterinary practice. They are used most commonly in conjunction with mechanical ventilation to paralyze the muscles of respiration. The use of neuromuscular blocking agents prevents spontaneous inspiratory efforts by the patient and allows more rapid and complete control of ventilation. These agents also are sometimes used in orthopedic surgery and other surgeries in which profound muscle relaxation is desired. They are used occasionally in conjunction with cesarean surgeries because they produce abdominal muscle relaxation but are not transferred across the placenta to the fetus. Neuromuscular blocking agents also may be useful in facilitating difficult intubation, including animals with laryngospasm. Occasionally muscle-paralyzing agents are used in conjunction with opioids, nitrous oxide, and other general anesthetic agents in "balanced anesthesia" techniques.

Neuromuscular blocking agents should be administered only after the patient has been anesthetized and respiration has been controlled by means of continuous manual or mechanical ventilation. These agents should be considered to be an adjunct to, rather than a replacement for, anesthesia with other agents. Use of neuromuscular blocking agents in a conscious animal is inhumane because these agents have no tranquilizing or analgesic properties. The patient given these drugs as the sole anesthetic agent will have normal sensitivity to pain, but will be unable to move or otherwise resist the surgeon's efforts. Control of respiration is also essential after the administration of these drugs because the respiratory muscles will be paralyzed, making it difficult or impossible for the patient to breathe on its own.

Neuromuscular blocking agents act by interrupting normal transmission of impulses from the motor nerve to the muscle synapse. The site of action is the nerve-muscle junction where chemical transmitters such as acetylcholine are released by the nerve in close proximity to the muscle end plate. There are two ways in which muscle-paralyzing agents may disrupt nervous transmission, and the agents used are classified as depolarizing or nondepolarizing according to which of the two mechanisms applies.

Depolarizing agents, such as succinylcholine, act by causing a single surge of activity at the neuromuscular junction, which is followed by a period in which the muscle end plate is refractory to further stimulation. Animals given these agents may show spontaneous muscle movement, followed by paralysis. *Nondepolarizing agents,* such as gallamine, pancuronium, and atracurium besylate, act by blocking the receptors at the end plates. As their classification suggests, they do not cause an initial surge of activity at the neuromuscular junction.

Muscle-paralyzing agents are normally given by slow intravenous injection. The dose required varies between patients and with the anesthetic protocol used. Most agents take effect within 2 minutes, and the duration of paralysis is approximately 10 to 30 minutes (although this varies considerably, depending on the agent used). If more prolonged paralysis is required, repeated doses can be given. Alternatively, some agents may be given by constant intravenous infusion.

Regardless of the agent used, only voluntary (skeletal) muscles are affected. Involuntary muscles, including cardiac muscle and the smooth muscle of the intestine and bladder, are unaffected by these agents. Skeletal muscles are affected in a predictable order: facial and neck paralysis is seen first, followed by paralysis of the tail, limbs, and abdominal muscles. The intercostal muscles and diaphragm are affected last.

Nondepolarizing agents may be reversed with an anticholinesterase agent, such as edrophonium or neostigmine. Reversing agents have no effect on depolarizing agents. Reversing agents may have undesirable side effects such as bradycardia and increased bronchial and salivary secretions, and should be given only after pretreatment with atropine. Neostigmine should not be given more than two or three times during the course of a single anesthesia because cumulative effects may be seen.

The use of neuromuscular blocking agents carries some risks, including the following:

- Hypothermia is a common side effect resulting from the decreased muscle tone seen in patients given these agents.
- Anesthetic depth may be difficult to assess because of the inhibition or absence of normal reflex responses and the absence of jaw tone.
- Muscle-paralyzing agents should not be used in animals with liver or kidney disease or in animals with glaucoma.
- Concurrent use of isoflurane or halothane increases the potency of neuromuscular blocking agents. Animals that have undergone recent treatments with organophosphate insecticides also show an increased susceptibility to neuromuscular blocking agents. Other drugs, such as corticosteroids, furosemide and other diuretics, anticancer drugs, aminoglycoside antibiotics such as gentamicin, and epinephrine, have been shown to affect the potency of neuromuscular blocking agents.

✔ **KEY POINTS**

1. Local analgesia is the use of a chemical agent on sensory and motor neurons to produce a temporary loss of pain sensation and movement. Because of low patient toxicity, low cost, and minimal recovery time, local analgesia may be preferred to general anesthesia in some patients. Disadvantages include lack of patient restraint, risk of overdose in smaller patients, and technical difficulties.

Continued

2. If sufficient quantities of local analgesics reach the sympathetic ganglia, a sympathetic blockade may result. This causes flushing, increased skin temperature, and, occasionally, hypotension and bradycardia.

3. Local analgesics have many topical uses, including application to the conjunctiva or the epithelium of the respiratory or urogenital tracts.

4. Local analgesics may be injected in close proximity to a peripheral nerve, blocking sensation from the tissues served by the nerve. Surgical preparation of the area is necessary before local analgesia infusion. Epinephrine is commonly added to the local analgesic used for this procedure to delay absorption of the local analgesic agent from the site.

5. Epidural analgesia is achieved by injecting local analgesic in the epidural space, between the dura and the vertebrae. In dogs and cats, the injection is performed between the last lumbar vertebra and the sacrum. This technique is useful for surgical procedures in debilitated patients and in patients requiring profound analgesia of the caudal abdomen, limbs, or pelvis.

6. Intravenous infusion of local analgesics may be useful for distal limb surgery, including amputation.

7. Local analgesics may be harmful if injected into a nerve fiber. They may also cause temporary paresthesia, which may result in self-mutilation.

8. Adverse systemic side effects of local analgesia include hyperexcitability, respiratory depression, and sympathetic blockade. Toxicity may be avoided by limiting the amount of lidocaine administered to the patient (a maximum 10 mg/kg when given subcutaneously).

9. Controlled or assisted ventilation may be used to deliver oxygen and anesthetic to the patient. Either a mechanical ventilator or manual bagging may be used. These procedures are particularly useful in patients with poor respiratory function caused by the use of anesthetic agents or respiratory disease. Controlled or assisted ventilation helps prevent the development of respiratory acidosis and pulmonary atelectasis.

10. Manual ventilation can be achieved by gently squeezing the reservoir bag at a rate of 8 to 12 breaths per minute and a pressure of 15 to 20 cm H_2O. Inspiration time should be 1 to 1.5 seconds, and expiratory time should be 2 to 3 seconds. Manual ventilation is difficult if a nonprecision vaporizer is used.

11. Mechanical ventilators may be incorporated into either a rebreathing or nonrebreathing system. Depending on the type of ventilator used, the anesthetist may control the pressure or volume of gas to be delivered, the respiratory rate, and the length of inspiration and expiration.

12. If controlled ventilation is used, the anesthetist must use caution to avoid excessive expansion of the alveoli, continuous positive pressure, and excessive ventilation rates.

13. Neuromuscular blocking agents may be useful in some anesthetic procedures to allow relaxation of voluntary muscles. They should never be used as the sole anesthetic agent.

14. Neuromuscular blocking agents may be depolarizing or nondepolarizing in their action. Nondepolarizing agents may be reversed by the administration of neostigmine.

15. Neuromuscular blocking agents may cause systemic effects such as hypothermia and respiratory failure. Mechanical or manual ventilation should be available when these agents are used.

16. Many drugs, including isoflurane, halothane, aminoglycoside antibiotics, organophosphates, and diuretics, may alter the effectiveness of neuromuscular blocking agents.

REVIEW QUESTIONS

1. In the normal awake animal, the main stimulus to breathe is the result of:
   a. Excess oxygen concentration in the blood
   b. Excess carbon dioxide concentration in the blood
   c. Insufficient oxygen in the blood
   d. Insufficient carbon dioxide in the blood

2. In the normal awake animal, inhalation lasts _____ times as long as exhalation.
   a. 1/2
   b. 2
   c. 3
   d. 4

3. The normal tidal volume in an awake animal is _____ ml/kg.
   a. 5-10
   b. 10-15
   c. 16-20
   d. 20-25

4. In the anesthetized animal that is breathing room air, the anesthetist may expect to see:
   a. An increase in the $PaCO_2$ and a decrease in the PaO_2
   b. A decrease in the $PaCO_2$ and an increase in the PaO_2
   c. A decrease in the $PaCO_2$ and a decrease in the PaO_2
   d. An increase in the $PaCO_2$ and an increase in the PaO_2

5. When used in a line block, a local analgesic agent will have a direct effect on the:
   a. Peripheral nervous system
   b. Central nervous system
   c. Peripheral and central nervous systems

6. Local analgesic agents may affect:
   a. Sensory neurons
   b. Motor neurons
   c. Autonomic neurons
   d. Sensory, motor, and autonomic neurons

7. Local analgesic agents work because:
   a. They mechanically block nerve impulse transmission
   b. They interfere with the movement of sodium ions
   c. They block the impulses at the spinal cord level

8. When an analgesic agent is infused around a major nerve, the procedure is referred to as a (an):
   a. Line block
   b. Epidural block
   c. Local nerve block
   d. Intravenous analgesia
9. Epinephrine may be mixed with a local analgesic agent to prolong the effects of the drug.
   True   False
10. When performing an epidural, one must be aware that the spinal cord in a cat may extend as far caudally as:
    a. T13
    b. L6
    c. L7
    d. S1
    e. The coccygeal vertebrae
11. The maximum subcutaneous dose of lidocaine for a patient is _____ mg/kg.
    a. 1
    b. 5
    c. 10
    d. 15
12. When performing intravenous analgesia one should use lidocaine
    a. With epinephrine
    b. Without epinephrine
13. The term atelectasis refers to:
    a. Excess fluid in the respiratory system
    b. A lack of breathing
    c. Collapsing of the alveoli
    d. Constriction of the bronchi
14. What is the most common acid-base abnormality in anesthetized patients?
    a. Respiratory alkalosis
    b. Metabolic alkalosis
    c. Respiratory acidosis
    d. Metabolic acidosis
15. When manually ventilating a patient that is connected to a circle system with a precision vaporizer, it is customary to:
    a. Increase the vaporizer setting
    b. Decrease the vaporizer setting
    c. Change the carbon dioxide absorber granules every hour
16. While a patient's breathing is being assisted manually, the exhalation phase should be:
    a. The same length of time as the inhalation phase
    b. Half as long as the inhalation phase
    c. Twice as long as the inhalation phase
    d. Three times as long as the inhalation phase

17. A neuromuscular blocking agent will not only paralyze skeletal muscle, but it will also give some analgesia.
    True   False
18. When an animal is given a _____ drug, an initial surge of muscle activity may be seen before there is paralysis of the muscles.
    a. Depolarizing
    b. Nondepolarizing
19. The muscle type that is most dramatically affected by muscle relaxant drugs is:
    a. Cardiac
    b. Smooth muscle
    c. Skeletal muscle
    d. All types are equally affected
20. Both depolarizing and nondepolarizing drugs can be reversed.
    True   False

For the following questions, more than one answer may be correct.

21. Problems that may result from excessive controlled ventilation may include:
    a. A decreased cardiac output
    b. Muscle twitching
    c. A state of respiratory alkalosis
    d. Ruptured alveoli
22. Local analgesic agents work well when applied:
    a. Topically on the epidermis
    b. Topically on mucous membranes
    c. Topically on the cornea
    d. Only by injection
23. Factors that may interfere with the action of local analgesic agents include:
    a. Fat
    b. Scar tissue
    c. Rapid heart rate
    d. Hemorrhage
    e. Large muscle mass
24. Clinical signs of systemic toxicity from a local analgesic agent may include:
    a. Sedation
    b. Convulsions
    c. Muscle twitching
    d. Respiratory depression
25. The effects that could result from an epidural if the drug reached the cervical spinal cord include:
    a. Sympathetic blockade
    b. Paralysis of intercostal muscles
    c. Paralysis of diaphragm
    d. Hypertension

Answers for Chapter 7

1. b   **2.** b   **3.** b   **4.** a   **5.** a   **6.** d   **7.** b   **8.** c   **9.** True
10. d   **11.** c   **12.** b   **13.** c   **14.** c   **15.** b   **16.** c   **17.** False
18. a   **19.** c   **20.** False   **21.** a, c, d   **22.** b, c   **23.** a, b, d, e
24. a, b, c, d   **25.** a, b, c

Selected Readings

HEATH RB: Lumbosacral epidural management, *Vet Clin North Am Small Anim Pract* 22(2):417-419, 1992.

HUBBELL JA: Disadvantages of neuromuscular blocking agents, *Vet Clin North Am Small Anim Pract* 22(2):351-352, 1992.

ILKIW JE: Advantages of and guidelines for using neuromuscular blocking agents, *Vet Clin North Am Small Anim Pract* 22(2):347-350, 1992.

KO JCH, PABLO LS, HEATON-JONES TG: Epidural injection of anesthetics in dogs and cats, *Vet Tech* 17(3):143-154, 1996.

MUIR WW III, HUBBELL JAE, SKARDA RT, BEDNARSKI RM: *Handbook of veterinary anesthesia,* ed 2, St. Louis, 1995, Mosby.

PASCOE PJ: Advantages and guidelines for using epidural drugs for analgesia, *Vet Clin North Am Small Anim Pract* 22(2):421-423, 1992.

SHORT CE: *Principles and practice of veterinary anesthesia,* Baltimore, 1987, Williams & Wilkins.

VALVERDE A, DYSON DH, McDONELL WN, PASCOE PJ: Use of epidural morphine in the dog for pain relief, *Vet Comp Orthop Trauma* 2:55-58, 1989.

WARREN RG: *Small animal anesthesia,* St Louis, 1983, Mosby.

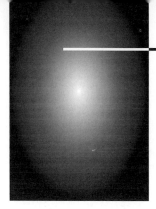

CHAPTER **8**

Analgesia

■ INTRODUCTION

What is Analgesia?

The International Association for the Study of Pain has defined pain as an unpleasant sensory or emotional experience associated with actual or potential tissue damage. Analgesia is the absence of pain, achieved through the use of drugs or other modes of therapy. For both ethical and medical reasons, the veterinarian and veterinary technician must ensure that analgesia is provided for every patient that requires it. The technician must strive to prevent pain whenever possible, and to recognize and bring it to the attention of the veterinarian when it occurs.

277

Why Treat Pain?

In the past, pain control was reserved for animals undergoing extensive orthopedic or thoracic surgery and was seldom provided for painful medical conditions (such as pancreatitis) or for elective surgeries such as castration and ovariohysterectomy. However, this attitude has changed and it is now generally accepted in veterinary medicine, as in human medicine, that most patients benefit significantly if analgesia is routinely provided whenever pain is present. This includes the postoperative period after any major surgery.

The current emphasis on analgesia in veterinary patients has arisen for several reasons:

- Veterinarians and veterinary technicians are becoming more aware of animals' need for analgesia. Although veterinary patients cannot verbally communicate their perceptions of pain, all the available evidence indicates that pain perception in humans and animals is similar. A good rule of thumb is that if a procedure is known to be painful in humans, it should be regarded as such in animal patients. Fortunately, most veterinary technicians are sensitive to their patients' needs for analgesia. A recent survey revealed that veterinary practices that have a veterinary technician on staff are more likely to use postoperative analgesics, compared with practices in which there is no technician.
- Animal owners are increasingly concerned that their pet does not experience unnecessary postoperative pain.
- General anesthetics currently used in small animal practice do not provide significant postoperative pain control. Anesthetics that lack analgesic effect include halothane, isoflurane, propofol, and barbiturates. In addition, recent information has indicated that some of the agents that have traditionally been considered to be good analgesics (for example, meperidine, ketamine, butorphanol, and xylazine) are not effective enough or long-lasting enough to benefit animals with severe postoperative pain, such as that experienced after orthopedic surgery.
- An animal that experiences postoperative pain is more likely to have a poor anesthetic recovery. General anesthetic agents that were in common use before the 1980s (including methoxyflurane and pentobarbital) were characterized by slow recoveries and prolonged sleep after anesthesia. These have been largely replaced by agents that allow arousal within minutes after completion of a surgery (for example, propofol and isoflurane). If no analgesia is provided, these recoveries are not only rapid, but may also be painful!
- It is no longer accepted that animals benefit from pain. In the past, many veterinarians believed that pain served a useful purpose by preventing activity that could cause further tissue injury. The concern has also been expressed that the use of analgesia will mask signs of illness and result in inappropriate treatment. However, it is now accepted that pain rarely has any useful function and is more likely to be harmful to the animal. Physiologic changes seen in animals with untreated pain include increased fear and anxiety, decreased cardiovascular function, decreased appetite, slower wound healing, and greater risk of infection. Studies in seriously ill children show that survival rates are higher when pain is treated.

This is not to suggest that every patient must receive high doses of analgesic drugs. Overtreatment of postoperative pain can contribute to prolonged anesthetic recovery and may have significant side effects. In all cases, the need for analgesia must be weighed against the potential for serious side effects. Fortunately, many drugs are now available for pain control, and it is usually possible to select an analgesic that is safe for a given patient.

The goal of the anesthetist is to provide adequate analgesia and sedation to allow the patient to move, eat, and sleep without undue discomfort, particularly in the first 12 hours after surgery.

■ GENERAL PRINCIPLES OF ANALGESIA
Physiology of Pain

In recent years, significant progress has been made in understanding the physiology of pain. Pain results when nerve cells in the skin or deep tissues (called nociceptors) detect a noxious stimulus. Examples of noxious stimuli include heat, ischemia, distention or stretching, mechanical injury (such as a scalpel incision), or chemicals released by inflammation or tissue damage (including prostaglandins, leukotrienes, bradykinin, proteolytic enzymes, histamine, potassium ions, and serotonin).

Pain receptors convert the chemical, thermal, or mechanical stimuli into nerve impulses. There are two types of sensory neurons that transmit the majority of pain signals to the spinal cord and brain. A delta fibers transmit sharp, discrete pain signals that allow the patient to localize the source of the pain to an exact site. These neurons are large and myelinated, and conduct signals rapidly. Smaller, non-myelinated C fibers transmit dull, aching, or throbbing pain sensations that cannot be exactly localized. It is thought that somatic pain (that is, arising from skin, subcutaneous tissue, muscle, bones, or joints) is transmitted by both A delta and C fibers, whereas visceral pain (arising from internal organs) is primarily transmitted by C fibers only. The information from nociceptors is conveyed to the dorsal horn of the spinal cord, where transmission of pain signals is suppressed or augmented by the affect of neural hormones such as substance P and cholecystokinin. The information is then transmitted to the thalamus and the sensory cortex of the cerebrum, where the perception of pain occurs.

Pain can be classified in several ways. The intensity of pain may be mild, moderate, or severe, and the duration may be acute or chronic. Because surgical pain has an abrupt onset and relatively short duration, it is classified as acute pain. Acute pain can usually be satisfactorily treated with analgesic drugs. In contrast, chronic pain (for example, pain associated with cancer or osteoarthritis) has a slow onset, a duration of several months or years, and may be unresponsive to drug therapy. Referred pain is a term used to describe pain that is felt in a body part other than that in which the cause is situated (for example, human patients suffering from a heart attack may feel referred pain in their upper arms rather than the heart itself).

Monitoring Signs of Pain

It is well recognized that the amount of pain suffered in the postoperative period will vary depending upon the surgical procedure (Table 8-1). Significant pain is most likely to arise after orthopedic procedures (especially amputations or surgery involving the cervical vertebrae, femur, or humerus). Surgery of the ears, eyes, mammary glands, or joints may also be associated with severe postoperative pain. Other surgical procedures may result in a lesser degree of pain that can be treated with lower doses or less powerful analgesics.

TABLE 8-1

Severity of Pain Associated with Medical and Surgical Procedures

Irritating or Mildly Painful	Mildly to Moderately Painful	Moderately to Severely Painful	Severely Painful
Urine scald	Endoscopy with biopsy	Localized burns	Extensive burns
Clipper burns	Dental extraction	Corneal ulcerations	Pancreatitis
Intravenous	Arterial catheterization	Enucleation	Total hip replacement
catheterization	Aural hematoma	Thoracic or lumbar	Cervical disc surgery
Distended	Stabilized radial or tib-	disk surgery	Forelimb or hind
bladder	ial fracture	Onychectomy	limb amputation
Superficial	Castration	Stabilized femoral or	Ear ablation
lacerations	Ovariohysterectomy	humeral fracture	Thoracotomy (espe-
Eyelid		Pelvic fracture	cially sternal split)
procedures		Mastectomy	
		Cranial abdominal	
		surgery	

Modified from Carroll GL, *Small animal pain management*, Lakewood, Colo, 1998, AAHA Press.

The anesthetist must also recognize that there is considerable variation among patients in the amount of analgesic required to control pain. It has been documented in human patients that there is a fivefold variation in the amount of narcotic medication needed to control pain after a standardized surgical procedure. Observation of the patient is the only reliable means of determining whether sufficient analgesia has been provided. Because pain control is most critical in the first 24 hours after trauma or surgery, the patient should be repeatedly evaluated throughout this period to ensure that pain and discomfort are controlled as much as possible. If a patient has been treated with an analgesic but still appears uncomfortable, the veterinarian should be informed because it may be necessary to administer an additional dose of analgesic or to change the type of analgesic used.

It is sometimes difficult to judge when a patient no longer requires analgesic drugs. In human medicine, patients with severe postoperative pain are usually treated for 2 to 5 days with injectable analgesics before switching to oral analgesics. In the case of animals, 3 days of analgesia is often adequate; but after discontinuing the drug, the patient should be closely monitored for signs of discomfort that would indicate a need for further analgesia.

Detection of pain in a veterinary patient may be difficult, especially if the observer is not familiar with the animal's normal behavior. Some animals show no obvious signs of pain (particularly when interacting with people), or may demonstrate only subtle changes in their behavior. In the natural world, animals that show pain or distress are more likely to become prey than are healthy animals, and evolution has therefore ensured that animals have become expert at hiding signs of pain. Many hospitalized patients have been given sedatives, which may alter the behavioral response to pain (although not the perception of pain by the patient). For these reasons, the technician must be alert to even minor changes in normal behavior that may indicate that pain is present (Table 8-2).

TABLE 8-2

Behavioral Responses to Pain

Behavioral Response	Dogs	Cats
VOCALIZATION	Groan, whine, whimper, growl	Groan, growl, purr
FACIAL EXPRESSION	Fixed stare, glazed appearance, ears back	Furrowed brow, squinted eyes
BODY POSTURE	Hunched or laterally recumbent	Sternal recumbency
GUARDING/SELF-MUTILATION	Protects wound, limps, licks and chews wound and surgical site	Protects wound, limps, licks and chews wound and surgical site
ACTIVITY	Restless or restricted movement, trembling	Restricted movement, may see stereotyped movements such as circling
ATTITUDE	Increased aggression or fearfulness	Comfort seeking or hiding, may be aggressive
APPETITE	Decreased	Decreased
URINARY AND BOWEL HABITS	Increased urination, failure in house training, urinary retention	Failure to use litter box
GROOMING	Loss of sheen in hair coat	Failure to groom, unkempt appearance
RESPONSE TO PALPATION	Protecting, biting, vocalizing, withdrawing	Protecting, biting, scratching, vocalizing, withdrawing, attempts to escape

Modified from Carroll GL, *Small animal pain management,* Lakewood, Colo, 1998, AAHA Press

Animal caregivers who take the time to observe animals after painful surgical procedures will soon realize that there is considerable variation among patients in their reactions to pain. The age, breed, and sex of the patient will influence its reaction to pain, as will the patient's background, environment, and training. Some animals become agitated or restless, and may vocalize (for example, whimpering, groaning, barking, growling, and crying), whereas others appear quiet, depressed, and inactive. Some dogs and cats frown or squint, and lay their ears back. Some animals may become aggressive and resist handling, whereas others may seek contact with their caregivers. Other signs of pain may include panting, failure to sleep, and lack of appetite. Patients may lick, bite, or scratch the source of the pain sensation. Often, the patient will show stiff body movements and a reluctance to move. Often cats with severe pain are silent, assume a hunched position in sternal recumbency, and fail to groom themselves. Some dogs and cats may "stare into space," seemingly oblivious to their environment.

With close observation, it is sometimes possible to determine the location of the pain. For example, animals with ear pain commonly shake their heads and scratch the affected ear. Dental pain may cause salivation and a reluctance to eat or drink.

Animals with neck pain usually hold their neck straight and rigidly maintain that position. Patients with thoracic pain often have shallow abdominal respiratory movements and tend to sit in sternal recumbency, reluctant to move. Animals with abdominal pain may have tense abdominal muscles (*splinting*) and assume an abnormal sitting posture.

Pain may also cause changes in physiologic parameters, leading to increased blood pressure and heart rate,* increased respiration rate and decreased tidal volume, salivation, dilated pupils, pale mucous membranes, and prolonged capillary refill. Many of these changes arise from activation of the sympathetic nervous system. Laboratory findings may include neutrophilia and lymphocytosis, hyperglycemia, and elevated levels of cortisol, epinephrine, and other hormones. Patients that receive appropriate analgesia should show improvement in behavioral signs and physiologic parameters, including a reduction in heart rate and respiratory rate.

Recently, an attempt has been made to quantify the amount of pain experienced by an animal, based on the animal's behavior and physiologic parameters (Box 8-1). This assessment scale is only a guide, and individual patients may differ significantly from the normal pattern. Behavioral characteristics are a continuum, and a given patient may show some signs that indicate moderate pain and other signs that indicate severe pain.

Methods of Pain Control

Endorphins.   Given that pain may be harmful to an animal, it is not surprising that the body has an internal mechanism to control pain. Within the central nervous system, chemicals similar to morphine (for example, beta endorphin, leu-enkephalin and dynorphin) are released by neurons when the body is traumatized or under stress. These chemicals bind to opioid receptors and provide some analgesia. Acupuncture and transcutaneous electric nerve stimulation may effectively treat pain by stimulating the release of endorphins and other chemical mediators.

Nonpharmacologic pain control.   There are many approaches to pain control, not all of which involve the use of drugs. Patient discomfort can be reduced through conscientious nursing care, including keeping the animal clean and dry, affording ample opportunity for defecation and urination (including bladder expression or catheterization if necessary), providing comfortable bedding and quiet surroundings, and gentle reassurance of the patient. The patient should be positioned so that it does not lie on the surgery site, and some patients benefit from being turned every 2 to 3 hours. Treatments and monitoring should be scheduled such that the patient is not disturbed unnecessarily. Other nonpharmacologic methods of pain control that may be effective in some situations include massage therapy, application of cold (for acute injuries) or heat (for chronic injuries), physiotherapy, magnetic therapy, and homeopathic or herbal remedies.

---

*Although heart rate may be helpful in determining if pain is present, it is not always a reliable indicator of pain. Tachycardia may be mild or absent in painful animals, especially those that have received opioids. Also, tachycardia may be present in nonpainful animals as a result of excitement or other causes.

Box 8-1 Recognition and Treatment of Postoperative Pain

This is a guide for pain assessment in veterinary patients. Pain can be graded on a scale of 0 (no pain) to 9 (severe to excruciating pain).

0 No pain. Patient is running, playing, eating, jumping, and sitting or walking normally. Sleeping comfortably with dreaming. Normal, affectionate response to caregiver. Heart rate should be normal, but if elevated it is the result of excitement. Cats will rub their face on the attendant's hand or the cage, may roll over and purr. Cats and dogs will groom themselves. Appetite is normal. Behavior different from this, not associated with pain, may be associated with apprehension or anxiety in the hospitalized patient. *No treatment necessary.*

1 Probably no pain. Patient appears to be normal, but condition is not as clear-cut as above. Heart rate should be normal, or slightly increased as a result of excitement. Cats may still purr. *No treatment necessary.*

2 Mild discomfort. Patient will still eat or sleep but may not dream. May limp slightly or resist palpation of a surgical wound, but shows no other signs of discomfort. Not depressed. There may be a slight increase in respiratory rate and heart rate. Dogs may continue to wag their tail and cats may still purr. *Reassess within the hour, then give analgesic if condition appears worse.*

3 Mild pain or discomfort. Patient will limp or guard a surgical incision. The abdomen may be slightly tucked up if abdominal surgery was performed. Looks a little depressed. Cannot get comfortable. May tremble or shake. Appears to be interested in food and may still eat a little but somewhat picky. Respiratory rate may be increased and a little shallow. Heart rate may be increased or normal, depending upon whether an opioid was given previously. Cats may continue to purr and dogs may wag their tail, even when they are in pain; therefore, disregard these behavioral patterns as indicators of comfort. This stage may be a transition from 2 above because the animal changes from being comfortable to becoming restless as analgesia is wearing off. *Needs analgesia. The analgesic selected will depend on whether it is a repeat in patient with moderate to severe pain, or the patient has a problem resulting in mild to moderate pain. If the patient has been previously treated with an analgesic, continue with morphine IM or SC (dogs 0.3 to 0.5 mg/kg, cats 0.05 to 0.1 mg/kg), oxymorphone (0.05 to 0.1 mg/kg IV or IM), hydromorphone IV (0.1 mg/kg) or injectable NSAID if patient status allows. If patient has not been previously treated and this is a mild to moderate pain situation, oxymorphone or hydromorphone or morphine is not necessary because the patient may become dysphoric. Instead, administer butorphanol (0.2 to 0.4 mg/kg) or NSAID where appropriate.*

4 Mild to moderate pain. The patient resists touching of the operative site, injured area, painful abdomen, or neck, etc. If there is abdominal pain, guards or splints the abdominal muscles or stretches all four legs out. May lick or chew at the painful area. The patient may sit or lie in an abnormal position and is not curled up or relaxed. May remain recumbent, without moving, for several hours (because movement causes pain). May tremble or shake. May or may not appear interested in food. May start to eat and then stop after one or two bites. Respiratory rate may be increased or shallow. Heart rate may be increased or normal. Pupils may be dilated. May whimper (dogs) or cry (cats) occasionally, be slow to rise, and hang tail down. There may be no weight bearing or only a toe touch on an injured limb. Will be somewhat depressed. Cats may lie quietly and not move for prolonged periods. *Administer butorphanol 0.4 mg/kg every 2 to 4 hours for soft tissue injury or surgery, or pancreatitis. For orthopedic or soft tissue injury, administer an opioid every 3 to 6 hours: oxymorphone (0.05 mg/kg) or hydromorphone (0.1 mg/kg) or morphine IM or SC (dogs 0.3 mg/kg, cats 0.1 mg/kg). Consider NSAIDs for orthopedic procedures or soft tissue injury or surgery where there are no concerns for hemorrhage, renal insufficiency, or gastric ulceration. If the patient has already received an opioid, consider an NSAID as an adjunct to opioid.*

Continued

Box 8-1 Recognition and Treatment of Postoperative Pain—cont'd

5 **Moderate pain.** Patient reluctant to move, depressed, and inappetant. May vocalize, bite, or attempt to bite when the caregiver approaches the painful area. Trembling or shaking with head down, depressed. There is definite splinting of the abdomen if affected (as in peritonitis, pancreatitis, hepatitis, and incision). Patient is unable to bear weight on an injured or operative limb. The ears may be pulled back. The heart and respiratory rates may be increased. Pupils may be dilated. The patient is not interested in food, will lie down but does not really sleep, and may stand in the "prayer position" (tail and pelvis in the air, front legs extended and head close to ground) if there is abdominal pain. Cats may lie quietly and not move. *Treatment as for 4.*

6 **Moderate pain.** As in 5 but patient may vocalize or whine frequently, without provocation and when attempting to move. Heart rate may be increased or may be within normal limits if an opioid was administered previously. Respiratory rate may be increased with an abdominal lift. Pupils may be dilated. *Treatment with oxymorphone (0.1 to 0.2 mg/kg), hydromorphone (0.1 to 0.2 mg/kg), or morphine IM or SC (dogs 0.4 mg/kg, cats 0.2 mg/kg) every 3 to 6 hours, or morphine or fentanyl in IV fluids. (See p. 288.) If butorphanol was given within the last 20 minutes and the condition is still painful, a higher dose of morphine or oxymorphone is usually required because of the antagonistic effects of butorphanol; or may give injectable NSAID, especially if orthopedic pain and patient status permits.*

7 **Moderate to severe pain.** Includes signs from 5 and 6, and patient appears very depressed and is not concerned with its surroundings. The patient will urinate and defecate without attempting to move. Will cry out when moved or will spontaneously or continually whimper. Occasionally an animal doesn't vocalize. Heart and respiratory rates may be increased. Hypertension may be present, pupils may be dilated. *Patient requires a higher dose of morphine, fentanyl, oxymorphone, hydromorphone, or NSAID (if orthopedic pain) or combination of NSAID and opioid.*

8 **Severe pain.** Signs as in 7. Vocalizing may be more of a feature, or patient may be so consumed with pain that it does not notice your presence and lies quiet and unresponsive. The patient may thrash around in the cage intermittently. If it is traumatic or neurological pain, the patient may scream when approached (especially cats). Tachycardia and increased respiratory rate with increased abdominal effort and hypertension are usually present even if an opioid was previously given. *Treat with high dose oxymorphone, hydromorphone, or morphine IM, SC, or in IV fluids to effect (dogs) or with fentanyl (dogs and cats). Add an injectable NSAID if orthopedic pain and patient status permits.*

9 **Severe to excruciating pain.** As in 8 but patient is hyperesthetic. The patient will tremble involuntarily when any part of the body in close proximity to wound or injury is touched. Neurologic pain (entrapped nerve or inflammation around the nerve) or extensive inflammation (peritonitis, pleuritis, myositis, or pancreatitis) usually present. *Requires high-dose oxymorphone, hydromorphone, or morphine IM, SC, or in IV fluids given to effect (dogs), or fentanyl (cats and dogs), plus NSAIDs where not contraindicated. Consider combining analgesics with epidurally placed opioids or local analgesic block. Inciting cause must be found and removed.*

Modified from Mathews KA: Nonsteroidal antiinflammatory analgesics in pain management in dogs and cats, *Can Vet J* 37(9):539-545, 1996.

■ PHARMACOLOGIC ANALGESIA

There are many situations in which nursing care is clearly inadequate to prevent or treat pain, and the use of analgesic drugs is indicated. These drugs prevent pain perception by several mechanisms. Nonsteroidal antiinflammatory drugs (NSAIDs) such as aspirin or carprofen prevent the production of chemicals such as prostaglandins that mediate inflammation and pain. Local analgesics such as lidocaine block transmission of pain impulses by sensory nerves. Opioids such as morphine appear to affect multiple sites in the brain and spinal cord to diminish the perception of pain.

Because there are many pathways and mechanisms that lead to the perception of pain, it is unlikely that any one agent can effectively treat all patients for all kinds of pain. The nature of pain varies depending upon the surgical procedure and the patient, and the optimal analgesic treatment will therefore vary between cases. The anesthetist should have a good knowledge of several agents and techniques that can be used, and consult with the veterinarian on which drug or combination of drugs is most appropriate for a particular patient.

Whatever the type of analgesia chosen, there is considerable variation among patients in the amount of analgesic they require and the duration of its effect. Whether a patient receives injectable butorphanol, epidural morphine, a fentanyl patch, or an NSAID such as ketoprofen, the aim is the same: the patient should be able to sleep comfortably and move freely when awake. If this aim is not achieved after administration of an analgesic, the patient should be reassessed and further treatment given as necessary.

Delivery of Analgesic Drugs

The veterinarian has many options in choosing the method of delivering analgesic drugs. The first choice is the agent to be used, which may be an opioid, NSAID, local analgesic, or combination of these. The choice of analgesic is governed by the severity and type of pain and the animal's general condition. The veterinarian also selects the route of delivery, which may include injection (for example, subcutaneous, intramuscular, intravenous, intraarticular, epidural, or nerve infiltration), oral administration, rectal suppository, or transdermal patch. Finally, the veterinarian must decide whether the analgesic should be given before the surgery, during the surgery, in the postoperative period, or any combination of these.

Whatever the method selected, it is often advantageous to administer analgesics before the animal has an awareness of pain (for example, before or during surgery, rather than after surgery). This fundamental principle of analgesia is called *preemptive use*. A common example of this phenomena occurs in animals that are given preanesthetic cocktails containing butorphanol or meperidine before surgery. These animals are less likely to show signs of a painful recovery compared with an animal that has not received analgesics in the preanesthetic period. Because the effect of meperidine is short in dogs (1 hour or less), it is unlikely that the drug is still active in the body by the time the patient wakes up from anesthesia. Why then does the animal appear to have a less painful recovery then expected? It is thought that meperidine and other preanesthetic analgesics act during the surgical period itself to prevent the build-up of chemical mediators that intensify the pain response. In contrast, an animal that has not been treated with analgesics during the preanesthetic period will experience the build-up of these mediators within the spinal cord in response to surgical manipulation (a phenomenon called *windup*). Although the animal will not be aware of pain during the surgical period itself, it is likely to be painful when it regains consciousness in the immediate postoperative period. This results in the need for greater amounts of postoperative analgesic in these patients, compared with those that received preemptive analgesics.

In addition to providing effective pain relief in the recovering patient, preemptive use of analgesics also allows the anesthetist to reduce the amount of general anesthetic needed during the surgery itself. For example, a patient that has been given intramuscular morphine immediately before a surgery may require considerably less halothane for maintenance of anesthesia than an unmedicated patient.

The recommendation for preemptive use of analgesics applies best to opioid agents (such as butorphanol, meperidine, and morphine) and local analgesics (such as bupivacaine and lidocaine). In the case of nonsteroidal antiinflammatory agents such as ketoprofen, preemptive use may not be advisable because it may increase the incidence of adverse effects such as decreased blood flow to the kidney during anesthesia and hemorrhage at the surgery site. (See the section on NSAIDs later in this chapter.)

Classes of Analgesic Drugs

Pharmacologic analgesia can be achieved through a variety of agents, including opioids, nonsteroidal antiinflammatory drugs (NSAIDs), and local analgesics (also discussed in Chapter 7). Because these agents differ in their mechanisms of action, it is possible to combine two agents (such as an opioid and an NSAID, or an opioid and a local analgesic) to achieve more effective analgesia. This type of combination therapy is termed *balanced* or *multimodal analgesia.*

Opioid Agents

As outlined in Chapter 1 (See pages 35-41), opioids have many uses in veterinary anesthesia, including the following:

- Opioids are commonly included in injectable premedications, usually in combination with an anticholinergic and acepromazine (for example, Premix, BAA, and BAG). Although these premedications help prevent windup they do not eliminate the need for additional analgesics after surgery. The analgesic effect of these preanesthetic mixtures is generally gone by 2 hours after administration and may be inadequate to prevent or control even moderate postoperative pain.
- Opioids can be used on their own or in combination with other agents (for example, NSAIDs and local analgesics) to provide postoperative pain control. A discussion follows of the use of opioids in the postoperative period by injectable, epidural, transdermal, and other routes. Doses, routes, and side effects of opioids used for postoperative analgesia are given in Table 8-3.
- At higher doses, opioids can be used in combination with tranquilizers to induce a state of potent sedation (neuroleptanalgesia) that offers considerable analgesia throughout the surgical period and for some time after surgery. (See the discussion on neuroleptanalgesia on pages 37-38.)

Individual opioids vary in their potency, duration, and side effects. As a group, opioids can be divided into those agents that are potent enough to treat severe pain (pure agonists such as morphine, oxymorphone, and fentanyl) and those that are less effective (such as meperidine and mixed agonist/antagonists such as butorphanol*). Opioid agonists produce dose-dependent analgesia, and the dose required will therefore vary according to the level of pain present and the potential

---

*See page 36 for a discussion of opioid agonists and mixed agonist/antagonists.

TABLE 8-3

Dosages of Opioids Used for Postoperative Analgesia (Dosages are approximate and patient should be monitored for efficacy and duration.)

Drug	Species	Dosage	Duration
MORPHINE	Dog	Loading dose is 0.1 mg/kg slowly IV every 3-5 minutes until desired effect achieved. Add same dose to IV fluids and administer over next 4 hours. Maintenance dose is 0.2-1 mg/kg IM or SC, or 0.2 mg/kg/hr constant IV infusion. Oral dose 1-3 mg/kg every 4-8 hours orally (2 mg/kg every 12 hours for sustained release tablets)	3-4 hours for injection, 4-12 hours orally
	Cat	0.05-0.1 mg/kg SC	
OXYMORPHONE	Dog	0.03-0.2 mg/kg IM, SC, IV	3-4 hours
	Cat	0.03-0.05 mg/kg IM, SC	
HYDROMORPHONE	Dog and cat	0.1-0.3 mg/kg IV, IM, SC	4 hours
MEPERIDINE	Dog and cat	2-10 mg/kg IM, SC	Less than 1 hour
BUTORPHANOL	Dog and cat	0.2-0.8 mg/kg IM, SC, IV	1-2 hours for injection in dogs, 4 hours in cats
		0.5-1 mg/kg oral	6-12 hours orally
BUPRENORPHINE	Dog and cat	0.01-0.02 mg/kg IM or IV	6-12 hours

Modified from *Veterinary teaching hospital undergraduate manual,* Guelph, Ontario, Canada, 1992, Ontario Veterinary College

for side effects. Mixed agonist/antagonists are less potent than opioid agonists, and higher doses do not necessarily provide greater analgesia. These agents should therefore be reserved for use in preanesthetic mixtures or for treatment of mild to moderate postsurgical pain.

Opioids are metabolized in the liver and excreted in the urine. Animals with liver disease may have decreased hepatic metabolism and should be given reduced dosages.

The opioid agonists most commonly used in veterinary medicine are morphine, meperidine, oxymorphone, hydromorphone, and fentanyl. The mixed agonists/antagonists in most common use are butorphanol and buprenorphine.

Opioid agonists

Morphine (morphine sulfate, Duramorph, Astromorpho/PF). Morphine was the original opioid agent used in human and veterinary medicine, and is still extensively used in veterinary practice as a preanesthetic and analgesic. It is a pure agonist with affinity for both mu and kappa opioid receptors. (See Chapter 1.) Morphine can be used in both dogs and cats; however, the canine dosage may cause excitement in cats and a much lower dosage is recommended in this species. Restlessness is also seen in some dogs shortly after morphine administration, especially in the absence of pain.

Morphine is an inexpensive and effective analgesic for treatment of moderate to severe pain in most patients. It is effective in treating both visceral and somatic pain and can be given by several routes, including slow IV (dogs only), IM, SC, intraarticular, epidural, or spinal injection. A sustained release oral form is also available. Efficacy of morphine varies considerably among patients.

When giving morphine intravenously to dogs, care should be taken to avoid too rapid injection. One safe technique is to draw up a loading dose of 0.1 mg/kg, which is given slowly IV (over 3 to 5 minutes) and repeated until the patient appears free of pain. The same total dose is then added to the intravenous fluids and administered over the next 4 hours. Morphine can also be administered intravenously by constant rate infusion. In this technique, morphine contained in a syringe is slowly administered through an intravenous catheter by means of a syringe pump.

Administration of morphine (and oxymorphone or hydromorphone) by the IM route gives a slightly longer duration of action than IV administration and avoids the risk of hypotension. A 23- or 25-gauge needle should be used to reduce patient discomfort. Morphine can also be administered to cats by the IM route, but the SC route is preferred in this species because there is less vomiting and dysphoria. Cats should not receive morphine by the IV route.

Morphine has several undesirable side effects, including gastrointestinal stimulation, which may cause vomiting, salivation, and defecation in dogs (although not in cats) shortly after administration. Vomiting can be prevented by pretreatment with acepromazine (0.02 mg/kg IM, 10 minutes before the morphine is given). Morphine also has the potential to cause severe respiratory depression, although this is less common in animals than in human patients. Some animals experience histamine release (characterized by hypotension, red skin, and pruritus) when given morphine rapidly IV. Bradycardia (which is responsive to atropine), increased intraocular pressure, increased intracranial pressure, urinary retention, miosis (in dogs), mydriasis (in cats), and hypothermia are also encountered in some patients after morphine administration. Fortunately, these side effects are seldom a significant problem in patients treated with analgesic dosages.

Morphine has a strong tendency to cause physical dependence (addiction) in humans. It is therefore classified as a Schedule II drug in the United States* and is designated as a narcotic in Canada.

Meperidine/Pethidine (Demerol).   A synthetic opioid, meperidine has been extensively used in veterinary medicine as an analgesic and preanesthetic agent. Subcutaneous injection is preferred because IM injection may be painful and rapid IV injection may cause severe hypotension.

Meperidine has a wide safety margin and causes less respiratory depression and gastrointestinal stimulation than morphine. It may cause histamine release in some patients, and pretreatment with histamine blockers may be advisable before IV injection.

---

*In the United States, prescription drugs are listed in five schedules. Schedule I drugs have a high abuse potential and are not used in veterinary practice. Schedule II drugs have a high abuse potential and may produce psychic and physical dependence in humans. Schedule III drugs have moderate to low abuse potential, and Schedule IV and Schedule V drugs have low abuse potential. In Canada, drugs with high to moderate abuse potential are classified as narcotics, and drugs with less potential for abuse are classified as controlled drugs.

In the past, meperidine was commonly used on its own as a postoperative analgesic, at a dose rate of 2 to 5 mg/kg IM or SC. Unfortunately, its analgesic effect is weak and of short duration, particularly in cats. For this reason it is not considered to be an ideal postoperative analgesic, and in recent years it has been superseded by other opioids, particularly butorphanol.

Despite this fact, meperidine is still a useful drug for veterinary anesthesia and analgesia. Meperidine is commonly used to formulate preanesthetic cocktails in combination with atropine and low doses of acepromazine. (See box on pages 38-39.) When administered with a tranquilizer (usually diazepam or acepromazine), meperidine also provides effective neuroleptanalgesia in puppies. Meperidine is also used in conjunction with injectable NSAIDs such as ketoprofen because it confers analgesia during the 30 to 60 minutes before the NSAID takes effect.

Meperidine is a Schedule II drug in the United States and is classified as a narcotic in Canada.

Oxymorphone (Numorphan).   Oxymorphone is a pure agonist opioid with a greater analgesic potency than morphine, fewer side effects, and a longer duration of analgesia (4 to 6 hours). Despite these advantages, use of oxymorphone in veterinary practice is somewhat limited by its high cost.

Unlike morphine, oxymorphone does not stimulate vomiting or histamine release. It may cause respiratory depression in some animals, but paradoxically it also induces panting in many patients. Oxymorphone causes some animals to become hyperresponsive to sound, and affected animals are easily startled by sudden noises. Bradycardia is also a potential side effect of this drug.

Oxymorphone may be given IV to dogs, but intravenous administration may cause excitement in cats (a tranquilizer such as xylazine, acepromazine, or diazepam may be used concurrently if sedation is required). It can also be administered IM, SC, or epidurally. Oxymorphone mixed with sterile saline and administered by IV drip is a safe analgesic agent in very sick or debilitated animals.

Oxymorphone is classified as a Schedule II drug in the United States and as a narcotic in Canada.

Hydromorphone.   Hydromorphone is an opioid agonist with similar efficacy to oxymorphone and with a similar duration of effect. Hydromorphone is much less expensive than oxymorphone. It can be given IV, IM, or SC to both cats and dogs at a dose of 0.1 to 0.3 mg/kg. Unlike morphine, it is not associated with histamine release, and does not cause excitement in cats.

Fentanyl (Duragesic).   Among the most potent analgesics known, fentanyl has a short duration of effect in small animals (approximately 30 minutes after IM or IV injection). It is therefore most commonly administered by continuous IV drip or by means of a skin patch. (See page 293.) When given IV, the loading dose is 0.002 mg/kg in dogs (0.001 to 0.004 mg/kg in cats), followed by 0.001 to 0.004 mg/kg/hr in IV fluids. It can also be given by IM, SC, or epidural injection.

Fentanyl can induce profound sedation, bradycardia, and respiratory depression in humans, and like oxymorphone it may cause panting or increased sensitivity to sound. Side effects of fentanyl are further discussed in the section that follows on transdermal patches.

Fentanyl was formerly used in combination with droperidol in the injectable neuroleptanalgesic Innovar-vet; however this combination is no longer commercially available.

Fentanyl (including fentanyl patches) is a Schedule II drug in the United States, and is classified as a narcotic in Canada.

Opioid agonists/antagonists

Butorphanol (Torbutrol, Torbugesic, Stadol).   A synthetic opioid with both agonist and antagonist properties, butorphanol was first used in veterinary medicine as a cough suppressant. Butorphanol is widely used as a preanesthetic (at a dose of 0.5 mg/kg, or in mixtures with atropine and acepromazine) and is also an effective postoperative analgesic for mild to moderate pain.

Butorphanol is available in several concentrations, including 0.5 mg/ml, 2 mg/ml, and 10 mg/ml. Tablets are also available for long-term administration (at a dose of 0.4 to 1 mg/kg tid) and may be dispensed for postoperative pain. Injectable butorphanol may be given IV, IM, or SC. It is potentially toxic to the spinal cord, which limits its use for epidural injection.

The duration of analgesia provided by butorphanol may be short (as little as 1 hour in dogs after IM or SC injection). To avoid frequent redosing, butorphanol can be given as a constant rate infusion (in IV fluids or by syringe pump) at a dose of 0.1 to 0.2 mg/kg/hr, after a loading dose of 0.2 to 0.4 mg/kg.*

Butorphanol is a mixed agonist-antagonist agent in that it stimulates kappa receptors but not mu receptors. (See Chapter 1.) As such, it is not as effective as the pure agonists (for example, morphine, fentanyl, hydromorphone, and oxymorphone) for treating severe pain, especially orthopedic pain. Butorphanol is, however, an effective and safe treatment for mild to moderate visceral pain, especially cranial and abdominal pain, in both dogs and cats.

Butorphanol produces less sedation, dysphoria, and respiratory depression than most opioids. Although moderate doses of butorphanol may cause some respiratory depression, higher doses do not depress respiration further (a phenomenon known as the *ceiling effect*). Heart rate, blood pressure, and cardiac output may be decreased after the administration of butorphanol; however, the effect is less than that of morphine, and pretreatment with atropine is not usually required.

Butorphanol can be used as an antagonist to partially reverse respiratory depression and sedation induced by opioids such as morphine or fentanyl; however, it will also partially reverse the analgesic effect of these drugs. The dose used for reversal is 0.2 to 0.4 mg/kg, administered to effect as IV increments of 0.05 mg/kg. The antagonistic effect of butorphanol is less predictable and less potent than that of naloxone.

Since 1997, butorphanol has been classified as a Schedule IV drug in the United States. In Canada it is classified as a controlled drug.

Buprenorphine (Buprenex, Temgesic).   Buprenorphine is a mixed agonist/antagonist that can be given by the IV, IM, or epidural route. It has a delayed onset of action (15 minutes IV and 40 minutes IM) but provides a longer duration of analgesia than other opioids (authorities suggest as little as 6 hours or as long as 12

---

*The calculation of the butorphanol dose can be done as follows: suppose a 10 kg patient is receiving 100 ml of IV fluids per hour, and the dose of butorphanol selected is 0.2 mg/kg/hr. The patient should receive 2 mg butorphanol per hour (10 kg × 0.2 mg/kg/hr). Because the patient receives 100 ml of IV fluids per hour, 2 mg of butorphanol (0.2 ml of a 10 mg/ml solution) can be added to 100 ml of fluids in a burette. Or, one can add 10 × this amount (20 mg, or 2 ml of a 10 mg/ml solution) to a liter bag of fluids, and administer over the next 10 hours at a rate of 100 ml/hr.

hours). Like butorphanol, buprenorphine does not provide adequate analgesia for severe pain, but it is useful for mild to moderate pain. It is commonly used to provide analgesia for rodents and other species used in research, as well as postoperative analgesia for dogs and cats.

Like butorphanol, buprenorphine can be used to reverse the sedation and respiratory depression induced by other opioids while maintaining some analgesic effect. Its action as a reversing agent is not as dramatic as butorphanol because of the delay in its onset of action.

Buprenorphine at high doses may induce respiratory depression, which is difficult to reverse with naloxone. Analeptic agents such as doxapram may be effective in correcting buprenorphine-induced respiratory depression.

Although buprenorphine has little sedative effect on its own, it can prolong sleeping times with other agents.

Buprenorphine is a Schedule V drug in the United States and is not generally available in Canada.

Use of opioid injections to treat postoperative pain.   Opioids can be administered by a variety of routes for prevention or treatment of postoperative pain. In many practices, opioids are given by IM or SC injection, preferably before the animal regains consciousness from anesthesia. Injections may be repeated as necessary to prolong the analgesic effect. (See Table 8-3 for information on dosage and duration.)

From the standpoint of analgesia, one major disadvantage of opioid agents is their relatively short duration of effect when given SC or IM. Morphine offers 2 to 3 hours of analgesia for severe pain and 4 to 6 hours for moderate or mild pain; oxymorphone 1.5 to 5 hours; meperidine less than 1 hour; and butorphanol 1 to 2 hours in dogs and up to 4 hours in cats. Repeat injections can be used, but this tends to be expensive, requires hospitalization, and creates "peak-and-trough" blood levels instead of a constant, effective blood concentration.

A second disadvantage of opioid use is the potential for side effects such as respiratory depression, bradycardia, excitement (usually exhibited as apprehension, hypersalivation, and mydriasis), panting, auditory stimulation, urinary retention, and nausea. These side effects are seldom severe when analgesic dosages are used. However, it is probably advisable to avoid opioid use in high-risk patients such as those with hypotension, hepatic disease, preexisting respiratory difficulties, CNS disorders such as head injuries or increased intracranial pressure, or altered bowel motility.

Both disadvantages of opioids—their short duration and potential for side effects—may be partially overcome by giving these drugs by routes other than IM or SC injection. Alternative routes for opioid administration include epidural injection, transdermal patches, and intraarticular administration. When used by these alternative routes, opioids may produce effective, economical, and long-acting analgesia with minimal side effects. However, use of opioids by these routes constitutes off-label use in many animal species, and may require informed consent from the animal's owner.

Intraarticular use of opioids.   Opioids may be given by the intraarticular route, particularly after elbow or stifle surgery. In this technique, 0.1 mg/kg of morphine is diluted in 1 ml saline/10 kg body weight and instilled into the joint, using a sterile catheter, immediately after closure of the joint capsule. A tourniquet is applied to the limb for 10 to 15 minutes after opioid administration, and the animal should be placed in lateral recumbency (with the affected side down). This technique provides 8 to 12 hours of postoperative analgesia.

Epidural use of opioids.   By instilling a small dose of an opioid or other analgesic into the epidural space at the lumbosacral junction, it is possible to achieve excellent analgesia of the hind limbs, abdomen, caudal thorax, pelvis, and tail. At the present time, morphine is the drug most commonly used for epidural analgesia. Oxymorphone is more expensive, butorphanol is less effective and may have some spinal toxicity, and local analgesics such as lidocaine may impair movement, urination, defecation, and may cause a sympathetic blockade. (See Chapter 7.)

Morphine given by the epidural route offers more profound analgesia, and for a longer period, than morphine given by IM or SC injection. The analgesia is not sufficient for a surgical procedure unless supplemented with general anesthesia; however, it is an excellent means of securing postoperative pain relief. Epidural morphine has direct, long-lasting effect on the pain receptors in the spinal cord, but because it does not reach high concentrations in the bloodstream, side effects such as sedation (dogs), excitement (cats), respiratory depression, and nausea are rare.

To achieve preemptive analgesia for postoperative pain, epidural morphine is usually given after induction but before the surgical procedure. Epidural morphine is significantly less effective when administered in the postoperative period.

The technique for epidural morphine administration is similar to epidural administration of lidocaine. (See box on pages 258-260.) In very depressed animals that will lie in sternal recumbency, no sedation may be required. Otherwise, the animal must be anesthetized or deeply sedated and positioned in sternal recumbency with the head slightly elevated and the hind limbs pulled forward to open the lumbosacral space. An epidural puncture is performed. Once it is determined that the needle is in the epidural space, morphine is injected over 30 seconds. Currently, the recommended dosage for epidural morphine is 0.1 mg/kg in dogs, and 0.05 to 0.1 mg/kg in cats. Ideally, a single dose vial of formalin-free morphine should be used,* diluted with sterile saline to a volume of 0.3 ml/kg. The maximum volume that can be injected is 6 ml in a dog and 1.5 ml in a cat. Onset of analgesia is approximately 20 to 60 minutes after injection and lasts 6 to 24 hours.

Although epidural analgesia is regarded as a safe procedure, it should not be undertaken in animals with septicemia, local infections in the lumbosacral space, spinal trauma or neurologic disease of the spinal cord, or bleeding disorders. It should also be noted that it is relatively difficult to administer epidurals to obese animals. Epidural hematomas and abscesses may result from improper needle placement or unsterile technique. Urinary retention may occur in the first 24 hours after surgery and the bladder should be monitored closely in all patients that have received epidural analgesics. Urinary catheterization may be necessary in some patients. Pruritus, delayed respiratory depression, and nausea have been reported in human patients but are uncommon in dogs. These symptoms, if they occur, can be treated with naloxone hydrochloride (0.01 mg/kg).

---

*Solutions preserved with phenol or formaldehyde are potentially toxic when given by the epidural or spinal route. Methylparaben is considered to have minimal risk. Examples of solutions that are safe for epidural administration include Duramorph and Astromorpho/PF.

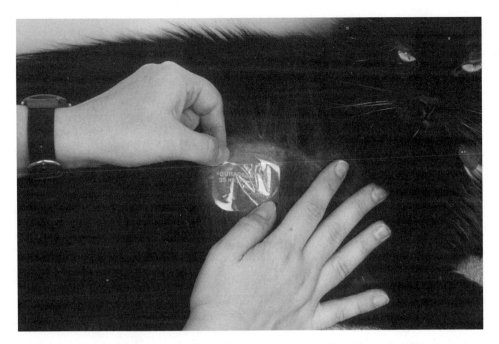

FIG. 8-1   Application of a fentanyl patch. (Photo courtesy of Dr. Margie Scherk)

Transdermal use of opioids.   Transdermal patches containing fentanyl are another convenient option for long-term opioid administration. Fentanyl patches (Duragesic patches) have been used for several years in the treatment of severe pain in humans. The analgesic effect of a fentanyl patch is thought to be comparable to IM oxymorphone, but the duration of analgesia is considerably longer.

A "patch" consists of a reservoir of 5 mg fentanyl enclosed in plastic. It can be applied to the clipped skin of a dog or cat and left in place for several days (Fig. 8-1). A 25-µg/hr patch is used in cats* and in dogs under 7 kg. A 50-µg/hr patch is used in dogs weighing 7 to 20 kg; a 75-µg/hr patch is used in 20 to 30 kg dogs; and dogs over 30 kg receive a 100-µg/hr patch. Patches should not be cut or trimmed because this will cause erratic drug release.

Because fentanyl is relatively slowly absorbed through the skin, there is a delay of 4 to 12 hours in cats and 12 to 24 hours in dogs before therapeutic blood levels are achieved. To achieve preemptive analgesia, the patch should therefore be applied at least 6 hours before the start of anesthesia in cats, and at least 12 hours before the start of surgery in dogs. If application of the patch is delayed until after surgery, it is necessary to bridge the patient with another opioid (for example, morphine or oxymorphone) or NSAID such as ketoprofen until the patch takes

*For cats weighing 6 kg or more, the entire patch is exposed by removing the protective liner. For cats weighing less than 6 kg, only one half to two thirds of the patch should be exposed, and the rest should remain covered by the protective liner. Some authorities suggest that fentanyl patches should not be used in cats weighing less than 3.5 kg.

▼ PROCEDURE 8-1
Applying a Fentanyl Patch

1. Various locations can be used for patch application, including the lateral thorax, dorsal neck, and the ventral abdomen.
2. The skin is clipped, taking care not to nick the skin (which may result in the fentanyl being absorbed too rapidly).
3. The patch is removed from its protective backing, and the adhesive side of the patch is held onto the skin for 1 to 2 minutes using hand pressure.
4. The patch should be handled by its edges, or gloves should be worn to avoid contact with the patch membrane.
5. Tissue adhesive should not be used to attach the patch to the patient because it alters the absorption of the fentanyl. If necessary, the patch may be covered using bandage material to prevent removal by the patient (particularly dogs*).
6. The patch remains in place for several days, during which time the fentanyl is gradually absorbed. Blood levels remain at therapeutic levels for approximately 5 days in cats and 3 days in dogs, although there is considerable variation in duration and effectiveness between patients.
7. At the end of this time the patch should be peeled off and disposed by flushing down the toilet. If the patient has been discharged in the interim, it should return to the clinic for patch removal and assessment.
8. If a longer duration of analgesia is required, a new patch can be applied at a separate, clipped site.

*Accidental ingestion of the patch produces no signs in dogs or cats if the patch reaches the stomach or intestines because any fentanyl absorbed is metabolized rapidly by the liver. However, overdose may occur after oral absorption (if, for example, a patch is chewed by the dog or cat).

effect. Mixed agonist/antagonists such as butorphanol should not be used because they may partially block the opioid receptors, reducing the fentanyl effect (Procedure 8-1).

There are many types of patients that benefit from a fentanyl patch, including postoperative patients (for example, after onychectomy, orthopedic procedures, or abdominal surgery) and those suffering from trauma, burns, painful abdominal conditions such as pancreatitis, and cancer.

Recent studies have shown considerable variation among animals in the concentration of fentanyl absorbed from a transdermal patch. One study showed that a 50-µg/hr patch in dogs delivered as little as 13.7 and as much as 49.8 µg/hr. Patients should be observed for signs of breakthrough pain (in cases of low fentanyl plasma concentrations) and supplemented with morphine, oxymorphone, hydromorphone, or ketoprofen as required.

Excessively high plasma fentanyl concentrations may develop in some patients. If this occurs, the most common signs are ataxia and sedation in dogs and dysphoria and disorientation in cats. Affected cats appear fearful or excited, hypersensitive to sound, and may have widely dilated pupils. Panting is also a problem in some animals. Treatment, if necessary, consists of removing the patch or giving a narcotic antagonist (for example, naloxone or butorphanol).

There have been some reports of death caused by respiratory failure when human patients self-administered more than one patch at a time, but respiratory depression is apparently uncommon in veterinary patients with fentanyl patches. Other side effects reported in human patients include constipation, physical dependence, muscle rigidity, miosis, mood changes, bradycardia, and bronchoconstriction. Use of fentanyl patches is not recommended in human patients with respiratory disease, increased intracranial pressure, impaired consciousness, bradycardia, pulmonary disease, hepatic or renal dysfunction, or brain tumors, and these recommendations may also hold true for animals. Some patients may exhibit a mild transient dermatitis at the patch site after removal.

Transdermal patches may release excessive amounts of fentanyl if they are heated, and fentanyl overdoses have been reported in humans who lie under electric blankets while wearing a patch. It is therefore suggested that fentanyl patches be avoided in cats with fevers and that patch contact with hot water bottles and other external sources of heat be avoided.

There is some concern regarding the potential for abuse or ingestion of the patch by a child. For this reason, the manufacturer does not support the use of fentanyl patches in animals. Some veterinarians address this concern by using the patch only on hospitalized animals, or by carefully selecting and educating owners before discharging an animal that is wearing a patch.

Nonsteroidal Antiinflammatory Drugs

Nonsteroidal antiinflammatory drugs (NSAIDs, also called nonsteroidal antiinflammatory analgesics or NSAAs) are a large group of agents that have been used for many years to control minor pain in humans and animals. The NSAIDs group includes such common drugs as acetylsalicylic acid (aspirin) and acetaminophen (Tylenol) and newer agents such as carprofen (Rimadyl) and ketoprofen (Anafen). Dose and toxicity information for NSAIDs is summarized in Table 8-4.

Traditionally, veterinarians have believed that NSAIDs are not powerful enough to treat anything other than mild postoperative pain. However, newer and more powerful NSAIDs such as ketoprofen, ketolorac, and carprofen are increasingly used for postoperative analgesia after procedures as diverse as ovariohysterectomy and fracture repair. In some cases (for example, degloving injuries and some orthopedic procedures) analgesia provided by injectable NSAIDs may be equal or superior to opioids. NSAIDs are also useful for treatment of dental pain, panosteitis, osteoarthritis, mastitis, and other painful medical conditions.

Mode of action.   NSAIDs have several useful effects on animal patients, including the following:

- All NSAIDs appear to be effective analgesics for somatic (musculoskeletal) pain. Some NSAIDs such as aspirin have little efficacy against visceral (for example, organ-related) pain, whereas others such as ketoprofen are potent analgesics for both somatic and visceral pain. All NSAIDs require approximately 30 to 60 minutes to achieve full analgesic effect, regardless of the route of administration.

TABLE 8-4

Dose and Toxicity of Nonsteroidal Antiinflammatory Drugs (NSAIDs)*

Agent	Dose	Comments
Aspirin (acetylsalicylic acid, ASA)	Dogs: 10-25 mg/kg p.o., every 12 hours Cats: 10 mg/kg p.o., every 48 hours	Gastric irritation. Enteric coated formulations decrease GI effects but unpredictable absorption. Increased bleeding time because of effect on platelets. Prolonged half-life in cats, neonates, and geriatrics.
Acetaminophen (Tylenol, Tempra)	Dogs: 10-15 mg/kg p.o. every 8 hours Cats: NONE!	Less potent than aspirin but less gastric irritation. Weak antiinflammatory effect. Very toxic to cats (hepatic necrosis, methemoglobinemia), hepatotoxic to dogs.
Ibuprofen (Advil, Motrin, Nuprin)	Dogs: 10 mg/kg p.o. every 24-48 hours but not recommended	Common cause of poisoning in small animals. Renal and gastric effects, severe gastric ulceration in some dogs. Gastrointestinal upset may occur at therapeutic doses. Narrow safety margin, especially for cats.
Flunixin (Banamine)	Dogs: 0.25-1 mg/kg IV, IM, or SC every 24 hours for three dose maximum. Cats: 0.25 mg/kg SC or IM, one dose only	Significant renal toxicity, especially in hypotensive patients. Risk of gastric ulceration. Use with ulcer prophylaxis, IV fluids. Do not use with methoxyflurane. Chief use is for ophthalmic surgery.
Ketoprofen (Anafen, Ketofen, Orudis, Oruvail)	Dogs and cats: 2 mg/kg first dose, give IV, SC or IM in dogs, SC in cats Maintenance dose 1 mg/kg p.o. every 24 hours	Potential for renal toxicity in hypotensive patients. Vomiting, abnormal stool, gastric irritation may occur at therapeutic doses. Potential for increased bleeding times. Potent analgesic, especially for orthopedics.
Ketorolac (Toradol)	Dogs: 0.3 mg/kg every 8-12 hours, IV or IM, one to three treatments only Cats: 0.25 mg/kg every 8-12 hours, one or two treatments only	Can cause gastric ulceration and renal insufficiency in geriatric or hypotensive patients. Use with misoprostol, sucralfate. Potent analgesic, comparable to morphine.

*Doses given are for healthy, young patients with normal renal function and no evidence of bleeding or gastrointestinal ulceration. For dose ranges, give lower doses IV and high doses IM or SC.
Adapted from Mathews KA: Nonsteroidal antiinflammatory analgesics in pain management in dogs and cats, *Can Vet J* 37(9):539-545, 1996.

Continued

- NSAIDs have antiinflammatory properties. This, combined with their analgesic effect, is the basis for the widespread use of drugs such as aspirin and carprofen in the treatment of osteoarthritis and muscular pain.
- NSAIDs are antipyretic (reduce fevers).

The clinical effects of NSAIDs stem chiefly from their inhibition of prostaglandin synthesis. Prostaglandins (often abbreviated PG) are a group of extremely potent chemicals that are normally present in all body tissues and are involved in the mediation of pain and inflammation after tissue injury. Most nonsteroidal antiinflammatory drugs prevent pain and inflammation by inactivating the enzyme *cyclooxygenase*

TABLE 8-4

Dose and Toxicity of Nonsteroidal Antiinflammatory Drugs (NSAIDs)* cont'd

Agent	Dose	Comments
Piroxicam (Feldene)	Dogs: 0-3 mg/kg p.o. every 24 hours	May cause vomiting, diarrhea, gastric ulceration. Use with misoprostol. Useful for urinary tract disease.
Carprofen (Rimadyl, Zenecarp)	Dogs: 2.2 mg/kg oral every 12 hours, 2-4 mg/kg IV, SC, IM, every 24 hours* Cats: same dose SC, one treatment only	Less potential for gastric ulceration than some NSAIDs. Renal toxicity seen in dogs and gastrointestinal ulceration in cats after chronic use. Hepatocellular toxicosis reported, especially Labrador retrievers.
Meloxicam (Metacam)	Dogs only: 0.1 mg/kg p.o. every 24 hours	Vomiting, diarrhea, inappetence may occur. Less potential for gastric ulceration and renal toxicity than some NSAIDs.
Tolfenamic acid (Tolfedine)	Dogs only: 4 mg/kg p.o. every 24 hours for 3 days May be approved for cats in future	Vomiting, diarrhea, inappetence may occur. Less potential for gastric ulceration and renal toxicity than some NSAIDs, but gastric erosions may occur after chronic use.
Meclofenamic acid (Arquel)	Dogs only: 1.1 mg/kg p.o. every 24 hours	Side effects include vomiting, diarrhea, and gastrointestinal ulceration.
Etodolac (EtoGesic)	Dogs only: 10-15 mg/kg p.o. every 24 hours	Difficult to accurately dose small dogs. Adverse reactions include vomiting, lethargy, diarrhea, and hypoproteinemia. Elevated doses may cause gastrointestinal ulceration and anemia because of fecal blood loss.
Naproxen (Naprosyn)	Dogs only: 3 mg/kg p.o. every 24-48 hours	Induces gastric ulceration; less toxic approved drugs are available.

*Injectable carprofen is not yet available in the United States.

(abbreviated COX), which catalyses one of the steps in the production of prostaglandins. There are actually two types of cyclooxygenase (abbreviated as COX 1 and COX 2). The relative effect of an NSAID on these enzymes will determine both the analgesic potency and the severity and type of adverse side effects after the administration of that particular drug. (See the separate section on side effects.)

Although most NSAIDs are active against prostaglandins in peripheral tissues only, some NSAIDs (for example, acetaminophen and ketorolac) exert their effects mainly upon prostaglandin synthesis in brain tissue, and are therefore said to be "central acting."

As a group, NSAIDs are well absorbed orally, and many are available in tablet or elixir form. Recently, potent injectable NSAIDs have also become available. Commonly, an injectable NSAID is given at the end of surgery to provide 24 hours of pain relief. If long-term analgesia is required, injections can be repeated in some cases, or tablets can be dispensed for oral administration.

All NSAIDs are eliminated by metabolism and conjugation within the liver, followed by renal elimination. For some drugs there is significant variation in duration of effect between species. For example, the plasma half-life of aspirin is 1 hour in the horse, 8 hours in the dog, and 38 hours in the cat. The prolonged half-life of aspirin in the cat is a result of the low levels of the enzyme glucuronyl transferase (one of the enzymes that metabolizes salicylate NSAIDs such as aspirin) in that species. There is also significant variation between species in the toxicity of particular NSAIDs. For example, ibuprofen is considered to be safe for use in humans but has significant toxicity in dogs. The safety of any NSAID in one species does not imply that it can be used with impunity in all species. (See Table 8-4 for dosages and cautions for specific agents.)

NSAIDs have some advantages over opioids: they are not subject to the storage, handling, and record keeping regulations that govern narcotics, they have little abuse potential, and they are effective when given orally. Unlike opioids, NSAIDs have negligible effect on the cardiovascular and respiratory systems. NSAIDs also do not depress the central nervous system and therefore lack the sedative effect of opioids.

Adverse side effects.   Unfortunately, NSAIDs have significant potential for toxicity in small animal patients. Most people who work in veterinary hospitals are aware of the toxicity of acetaminophen (Tylenol) in cats. A single 320-mg capsule may cause acute hepatotoxicosis within 4 hours of ingestion because of the formation of toxic metabolites within the liver. Fortunately, other NSAIDs are available that are relatively safe for use in both cats and dogs.

Many of the toxic effects of NSAIDs are attributable to the fact that they reduce not only the production of the prostaglandins that produce pain, inflammation, and fever, but also the production of beneficial prostaglandins. Pharmaceutical companies have attempted to formulate NSAIDs that will prevent the production of harmful prostaglandins while preserving the production of beneficial prostaglandins. This can be achieved if the NSAID inhibits the enzyme cyclooxygenase 2 (which is active in damaged or inflamed tissues and synthesizes the prostaglandins that cause pain) but does not affect cyclooxygenase 1 (which synthesizes the prostaglandins that help maintain normal physiologic functions such as protection of the gastric mucosa and modulation of blood flow to the kidney). In theory, it is possible to produce NSAIDs that have more than 1000-fold specificity for COX 2 over COX 1; however, the drugs currently available do not have this degree of specificity.

One example of a beneficial prostaglandin that is adversely affected by many NSAIDs is prostacyclin, which is normally present within the stomach mucosa and helps reduce gastric acid secretion and promote mucus production. When prostacyclin levels are reduced by the administration of an NSAID, gastric acid secretion increases and mucus production decreases, which sometimes leads to the production of stomach ulcers. Up to 50% of dogs treated with aspirin develop mild stomach ulceration, which may result in vomiting, gastrointestinal bleeding, and inappetence but more often is not clinically apparent. Occasionally, animals with gastrointestinal ulceration secondary to NSAID use may undergo a sudden episode of life-threatening hemorrhage.

In an effort to avoid gastrointestinal problems in animals receiving NSAIDs, pharmaceutical companies have prepared enteric-coated or buffered formulations. It is also helpful to administer oral NSAIDs with a meal to dilute the drug that is present in the stomach. In susceptible patients, it may be advisable to use gastrointestinal protectants such as sucralfate suspension (Sulcrate, at a dose of 0.25 to 0.5 gram p.o. tid in cats, 0.5 to 1 gram p.o. tid in dogs) in conjunction with an NSAID to prevent or treat gastrointestinal effects. Sucralfate forms a proteinaceous complex that adheres to damaged gastric mucosa, preventing further injury. Sucralfate should be administered on an empty stomach, 1 hour before meals.

Another helpful gastrointestinal protectant is the synthetic prostaglandin misoprostol (Cytotec), which is given orally at a dose of 2 to 4 μg/kg tid.* Histamine-blocking agents such as ranitidine are also helpful in treatment of stomach ulcers because they inhibit gastric acid secretion.

Another potential side effect of NSAID administration is renal toxicity. A beneficial prostaglandin, PGE_2, normally maintains adequate blood flow within the kidney. By blocking synthesis of PGE_2, NSAIDs have the potential to decrease renal blood flow, leading to renal hypoxia. This is a particular problem in anesthetized animals, which may already have decreased renal blood perfusion because of hypotension. One nephrotoxic NSAID, flunixin, is known to cause an elevation in blood urea nitrogen (BUN) in most human surgery patients for up to 30 hours after administration. To avoid the risk of renal damage in anesthetized patients, use of NSAIDs is usually postponed until after anesthesia, and preemptive or intraoperative use is not advised unless the patient is receiving intraoperative IV fluids and arterial blood pressure monitoring is available. Fortunately, NSAID-induced renal insufficiency is usually reversible (in young, healthy patients) with the administration of IV fluids.

Another potential side effect of NSAID administration is impaired platelet aggregation, which can lead to prolonged bleeding times. This effect may be beneficial in some circumstances (for example, by lowering the risk of stroke in human patients who regularly take aspirin). However, there is a potential for increased bleeding in patients that are given NSAIDs before or during surgery. This concern can be minimized by postponing the use of NSAID agents until after surgery is completed.

NSAIDs may antagonize the action of several drugs commonly prescribed for cardiac disease and hypertension, including ACE inhibitors (such as Fortekor and Enalapril), and some diuretics.

As with most drugs, there is great variation between individual patients in the potency, duration, and side effects produced by NSAIDs. Ideally, NSAIDs should only be used to treat postoperative pain in well-hydrated young to middle-aged dogs or cats, with normal renal and hemostatic function. The use of NSAIDs should be tempered with care or avoided entirely in dehydrated patients, geriatrics, and animals with liver or kidney dysfunction. Because of the potential for gastrointestinal ulceration, caution should be used when administering these agents to patients with gastrointestinal disorders or to patients that are receiving corticosteroids (which also contribute to ulcer formation). Animals that have hypotension, congestive heart failure, or hemostatic disorders such as thrombocytopenia are generally high-risk candidates for NSAID therapy. For some patients (for example, geriatrics and patients with renal disease) NSAIDs should only be used in conjunction with intravenous fluids and (if there is a potential for hypotension) blood pressure monitoring. Opioids may be a safer therapeutic option in some patients

---

*Misoprostol should not be given at the same time as sucralfate (ideally, it should be administered 1 hour before or 2 hours after). It should not be given to pregnant animals and should be used with caution in animals with a history of seizures.

Combination Therapy

Because there are several mechanisms by which pain is produced, it is sometimes helpful to use more than one type of analgesic to relieve pain. Combination therapy (for example, utilizing an opioid and an NSAID together) may be more successful than treatment with either agent on its own. For example, it has been shown in human patients that the use of piroxicam and buprenorphine together provides superior analgesia to use of either agent alone.

One familiar example of combination therapy is a mixture of acetaminophen and codeine (Tylenol 3, Tylenol 4), which is an effective oral treatment for moderate to severe pain in the dog. When given orally at a dose rate of 10 mg/kg acetaminophen and 0.5 to 1 mg/kg codeine every 6 to 12 hours, the combination is safe in healthy dogs for up to 5 days. If necessary, the codeine can be supplemented up to 4 mg/kg. Constipation and sedation are common side effects of this drug combination. Tylenol/codeine should not be given to cats or to dogs with hepatic disease.

Opioids and NSAIDs may also be given to the same patient at different times. For example, a dog undergoing orthopedic surgery can be premedicated with morphine (0.2 to 0.3 mg/kg IM) followed by administration of an injectable NSAID (such as ketoprofen or carprofen) at the end of surgery and then NSAIDs given orally for 3 days. This type of "balanced analgesia" allows the use of relatively modest doses of analgesics yet achieves effective pain relief in many patients.

Other Agents

Although opioids and NSAIDs are the mainstays of postoperative pain control, other agents may be useful in some circumstances. These include local analgesics, alpha-2 adrenergic agonists (for example, xylazine and medetomidine), and ketamine.

Local analgesics.   Local analgesic agents have long been used to allow surgical procedures in conscious animals, but their use in preventing or treating postoperative pain is relatively recent. (See Chapter 7.) As analgesics they have many advantages, including complete anesthesia of the affected area, low toxicity, and rapid onset of action. Unfortunately, the duration of action is relatively short, and the danger of CNS and cardiac toxicity prevents repeated use.

Of the various local analgesic agents available, lidocaine and bupivacaine are the most commonly used in veterinary medicine. Lidocaine is administered at a concentration of 0.5% to 2%, and bupivacaine as a 0.25% or 0.5% solution. Bupivacaine has a longer onset of effect (20 minutes) and a longer duration of effect (4 hours) than lidocaine (onset almost immediate, duration 1 to 2 hours). The dose of bupivacaine used should not exceed 2 mg/kg in dogs and 0.5 to 1 mg/kg in cats. Lidocaine is less toxic, with a maximum dose of 10 mg/kg SC or 2 mg/kg IV.

There are several ways in which local analgesics may be used to prevent or treat postoperative pain:

Infiltration of a surgery site before or during surgery.   In this technique (discussed in Procedure 7-1), lidocaine or bupivacaine may be administered by local infiltration, ring blocks, or splash blocks. Examples include infiltration of a nerve stump during amputation of a limb (by injection of 0.5% bupivacaine, 0.5 ml per nerve); interpleural or intercostal nerve blocks during thoracic surgery; and splash blocks after ear ablation. Bupivacaine can also be instilled through a chest tube placed at surgery. Specialty textbooks and journal articles provide complete descriptions of these techniques. Regardless of the technique employed, it is important to allow sufficient time for the tissues to absorb the anesthetic (15 to 20 minutes) before undertaking surgery. In the case of splash blocks this can be achieved by saturating a sterile gauze sponge with a mixture of the local analgesic and saline and laying the gauze on the site for 15 minutes before surgery.

Intraarticular administration. Bupivacaine has been shown to provide significant analgesia when injected into the stifle joint at the conclusion of cruciate surgery. A dosage rate of 0.4 ml/kg of 0.5% bupivacaine has been recommended. As with intraarticular use of morphine, the drug is injected immediately after the closure of the joint capsule.

Epidural administration. Local analgesics, like opioids, may be administered by the epidural route. Unlike opioids, however, lidocaine blocks not only sensory neurons (including those that transmit pain sensation) but also motor and sympathetic neurons. As a result, the patient is unable to walk and is at some risk of developing hypotension after epidural administration of lidocaine (and, to a lesser extent, bupivacaine). For this reason, opioids rather than local analgesics are the preferred drugs for postoperative pain control by the epidural route. Local analgesics given by the epidural route are most useful for preoperative use, to achieve patient immobilization and to provide analgesia during the surgical procedure itself.

Dental blocks. Although local analgesics are commonly used as the sole anesthetic agent in human patients undergoing dental procedures, their use in animals is limited by the fact that they do not immobilize the patient. General anesthesia is almost universally employed for small animal dentistry. Lidocaine and other local analgesics can be given after induction of anesthesia, however, and will provide long-lasting analgesia after the surgery. The infraorbital nerve can be blocked to provide pain control for the upper premolars, canines, and incisor teeth. The mental nerve can be blocked for procedures involving the mandibular canines and incisors, and mandibular or maxillary blocks are useful for procedures on the caudal teeth.

Topical use on skin. A topical cream containing 2.5% lidocaine and 2.5% prilocaine (EMLA cream) can be used to provide analgesia for superficial procedures such as arterial catheterization. The cream should be applied to intact, shaved skin and the area bandaged for 1 hour before attempting catheterization.

Alpha-2 adrenergic agonists. Although alpha-2 adrenergic agonists such as xylazine and medetomidine provide some analgesia, their use as analgesic agents is limited by three factors: (1) the short duration of their analgesic effect (in the case of xylazine, 30 minutes), (2) the profound sedative effect of these agents, and (3) the potential for serious cardiovascular side effects (respiratory depression, bradycardia, heart block, and hypotension, which may be exacerbated by opioids). These agents should only be used for young to middle-aged, healthy animals. However, when used in low doses (for example, xylazine at 0.1 to 1 mg/kg IV, IM, SC; and medetomidine at 0.001 to 0.01 mg/kg IV, IM, SC), these agents appear to potentiate the effect of opioids and may contribute to the quality of analgesia in the postoperative period. It is difficult to determine the quality or duration of analgesia in some patients because the sedative effect of these drugs remains even after the analgesic effect has worn off.

Recently, alpha-2 adrenergic agonists have been shown to give significant analgesia when administered by the epidural route (alone or in combination with opioids and other agents), but this is not yet a common procedure in clinical practice.

The analgesic effect of xylazine and medetomidine is antagonized by yohimbine and atipamezole.

Ketamine.   Ketamine is believed to be a good analgesic for superficial pain (such as that involving the skin and subcutaneous tissue) but a poor analgesic for muscle or visceral pain (such as pain originating in the abdominal and thoracic organs). The analgesic effect of ketamine is enhanced by concurrent administration of opioids such as butorphanol.

Ketamine can be used as an analgesic in two ways:

- Ketamine (5 mg/kg IM or SC) is sometimes used as a preanesthetic in cats, in combination with acepromazine and an anticholinergic.
- Ketamine at a dose rate of 1 to 2 mg/kg IV, 2 to 4 mg/kg IM or 10 mg/kg p.o. has been suggested as a means of controlling pain in dogs and cats, if opioids are not available. Duration of effect is 30 minutes. Catalepsy and unconsciousness are not seen at the lower dosages.

Ketamine should not be used in patients with hypertrophic cardiomyopathy or in cats with compromised renal function. Side effects of ketamine are dose-related and include tachycardia, increased blood pressure, increased intraocular and intracranial pressure, seizures and postoperative delirium, and salivation.

Tranquilizers.   Although acepromazine, diazepam, and other tranquilizers are not considered to be analgesics, they may potentiate the effect of opioids in some patients. Patients that have received adequate analgesia but are restless or dysphoric may become calmer after administration of acepromazine (0.01 to 0.05 mg/kg SC, IM, or IV) or diazepam (0.2 mg/kg IV). Because tranquilizers have no analgesic effect, they should not be used as a substitute for opioids or other analgesic agents.

✔   **KEY POINTS**

1. The veterinarian and veterinary technician have an obligation to provide analgesia for patients with painful medical disorders and for patients that undergo painful surgical procedures.
2. Pain has little, if any, beneficial effect and may decrease cardiovascular function, appetite, wound healing, and resistance to infection.
3. Pain is perceived when nociceptors are stimulated by mechanical injury, ischemia, heat, or chemicals such as prostaglandins. Pain is transmitted by several types of neurons, through spinal cord pathways to the brain.
4. Pain may be classified according to the location of origin (somatic or visceral pain), or duration (acute or chronic pain).
5. Animals vary in their behavioral response to pain, and close observation may be necessary to determine if a given patient is experiencing pain.
6. To some extent, pain may be quantified by observing behavior and physiologic parameters such as heart rate, respiration rate, pupil dilation, and hormone levels.

7. Patient discomfort should be addressed through nursing care, including the provision of comfortable bedding and allowing opportunity for urination and defecation.

8. Various classes of drugs can be used as analgesics. Classes vary in their site of action, potency, duration of effect, and expected side effects. If necessary, pain may be managed by administering more than one type of drug to a given patient.

9. Analgesics may be delivered by many routes, including injection (IV, SC, IM, epidural, intraarticular), transdermal patch, nerve infiltration, or oral or rectal administration.

10. Analgesic administration is most effective when used preemptively (that is, before the animal has an awareness of pain). This may not be possible in the case of nonsteroidal antiinflammatory drugs, which can interfere with blood clotting and may decrease renal perfusion during anesthesia.

11. Opioids may be used to provide analgesia during the preoperative, operative, or postoperative periods. Some opioids (for example, pure agonists) are potent enough to treat severe pain, whereas others (for example, agonist/antagonists and meperidine) are more suited to treatment of mild to moderate pain.

12. Side effects of opioid administration may include respiratory depression, bradycardia, and hypotension after IV administration, vomiting and defecation, urinary retention, increased intracranial and intraocular pressure, increased sensitivity to noise, and panting. Side effects are generally uncommon when analgesic doses are used.

13. The duration of effect of opioids may be extended if they are administered by the epidural, transdermal, or intraarticular routes.

14. Nonsteroidal antiinflammatory drugs (NSAIDs) have analgesic, antiinflammatory, and antipyretic properties. Their effects are mainly a result of inactivation of the enzyme cyclooxygenase, which catalyses the production of prostaglandins.

15. NSAIDs may cause gastrointestinal ulceration, platelet inhibition, and decreased renal perfusion during anesthesia. NSAID agents that preferentially inhibit the enzyme cyclooxygenase (COX) 2 have fewer adverse side effects than other NSAIDs. It is safest to reserve NSAID analgesia for young patients with normal renal, gastrointestinal, and hemostatic function. Patients receiving NSAIDs may benefit from IV fluids during surgery, and the use of sucralfate and other drugs.

16. Local analgesics such as lidocaine and bupivacaine may be used to prevent postoperative pain in patients undergoing surgery or dental procedures.

17. Alpha-2 adrenergic agonists and tranquilizers may be used to supplement the analgesic effect of opioids, but should not be used on their own to provide analgesia.

REVIEW QUESTIONS

1. Which of the following anesthetic agents provides some analgesia in the postoperative period?
   a. Isoflurane
   b. Halothane
   c. Thiopental
   d. Ketamine
2. Visceral pain arises from damage to:
   a. Muscle
   b. Skin
   c. Nerves
   d. Internal organs
3. Pain receptors are called:
   a. C fibers
   b. Nociceptors
   c. Prostaglandins
   d. Endorphins
4. If you wait until an animal shows signs of pain before treating with an analgesic, a higher dose will be required.
   True   False
5. Animals do not readily show pain compared with humans because:
   a. They do not feel as much pain
   b. Animals lack neurologic pathways for pain transmission
   c. Animals that appear stressed are more likely to become prey for other animals
   d. Animals release sufficient endorphins to alleviate pain
6. The dosage for morphine is greater for the dog than for the cat.
   True   False
7. Compared to butorphanol, meperidine has a _____ duration of effect.
   a. Shorter
   b. Similar
   c. Longer
8. Which of the following is an agonist/antagonist opioid?
   a. Oxymorphone
   b. Meperidine
   c. Butorphanol
   d. Fentanyl
9. When using fentanyl patches, one can expect a _____ onset of effect.
   a. Quick (less than 1 hour)
   b. Moderate (1 to 4 hours)
   c. Slow (more than 4 hours)
10. Increased amounts of fentanyl may be released from a patch if the patient has a fever or if heat is applied to the area where the patch is located.
   True   False

11. All of the following are characteristics of NSAIDs except:
    a. Decrease musculoskeletal pain
    b. Antipyretic
    c. Inhibit prostaglandin synthesis
    d. Reversed by naloxone or buprenorphine
12. Which of the following NSAIDs provides adequate analgesia for moderate orthopedic pain in the immediate postoperative period?
    a. Ketoprofen
    b. Ibuprofen
    c. Acetaminophen
    d. Aspirin
13. Opioids may interfere with the action of drugs used for treatment of cardiac disease.
    True   False
14. Lidocaine is less toxic than bupivacaine.
    True   False
15. Epidural lidocaine blocks motor, sensory, and sympathetic neurons, whereas epidural morphine only blocks sensory neurons.
    True   False
16. Which of the following can be used as a reversing agent for morphine?
    a. Oxymorphone
    b. Meperidine
    c. Butorphanol
    d. Fentanyl
17. Local analgesics provide pain control by:
    a. Preventing transmission of impulses through sensory neurons
    b. Decreasing perception of pain by the thalamus
    c. Decreasing the production of prostaglandins
    d. Interfering with synaptic transmission in the dorsal root ganglia
18. The potential side effects of opioids include all of the following except:
    a. Bradycardia
    b. Gastrointestinal bleeding
    c. Panting
    d. Increased sensitivity to noise
19. The potential side effects of NSAIDs include all of the following except:
    a. Platelet inhibition
    b. Decreased renal perfusion
    c. Respiratory depression
    d. Gastrointestinal ulceration
20. Tranquilizers such as acepromazine should be used instead of analgesics when treating painful, excited animals.
    True   False

Answers for Chapter 8

1. d   2. d   3. b   4. True   5. c   6. True   7. a   8. c
9. c   10. True   11. d   12. a   13. False   14. True   15. True
16. c   17. a   18. b   19. c   20. False

Selected Readings

CARROLL GC: How to manage perioperative pain, *Vet Med* 353-357, April 1996.

CARROLL GC: *Small animal pain management,* Lakewood, Colo., 1998, AAHA Press.

HANSEN BD: Analgesic therapy, *Compendium* 16(7):868-875, 1994.

HARDIER EM: Recognition and management of pain in small animals, *Small Anim Med Dig* 2(2):89-96, 1996.

HELLER PW, GAYNOR J: Acute post-surgical pain in dogs and cats: *Compendium* 20(2):140-153, 1998.

KO JCD, EATON-JONES TG: Epidural anesthesia in dogs and cats, *Vet Tech* 17(3):143-154, 1996.

KALES AE: Clinical pain management, *Perspectives,* March/April: 6-12, 1995.

KALES AE: Transdermal fentanyl, *Compendium* 20(6):721-726, 1998.

LEE VC, ROLLINGSTONE J: Preemptive analgesia: update on nonsteroidal antiinflammatory drugs in anesthesia, *Advances in Anesthesia 12,* Mosby Yearbook: 69-110, 1995.

MATHEWS KA: Nonsteroidal antiinflammatory analgesics in pain management in dogs and cats, *Can Vet J* 37(9):539-545, 1996.

QUANT. JE, RAILINGS CR: Reducing postoperative pain for dogs: local anesthetic and analgesic techniques, *Compendium* 18(2):101-111, 1996.

SOCMAN JE. Pain management. In McCurnin DM, editor: *Clinical textbook for veterinary technicians,* ed. 4, Philadelphia, 1997, WB Saunders.

SCHERK-NIXON M: A study of the use of a transdermal fentanyl patch in cats, *J Am Anim Hosp Assoc* 32(1):19-24, 1996.

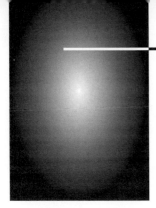

APPENDIX A

Standard Values and Equivalents

■ STANDARD VALUES
Metric Weights

1 gram (1 g) = Weight of 1 ml water at 4° C
1000 g = 1 kilogram (kg)
0.1 g = 1 decigram (dg)
0.01 g = 1 centigram (cg)
0.001 g = 1 milligram (mg)
0.001 mg = 1 microgram (μg)

Metric Volumes

1 liter (L) = 1000 milliliters (ml) or 1000 cubic centimeters (cc)
0.001 L = 1 ml
1 deciliter (dl) = 100 ml

Solution Equivalents

1 part in 10 = 10.00% (1 ml contains 100 mg)
1 part in 50 = 2.00% (1 ml contains 20 mg)
1 part in 100 = 1.00% (1 ml contains 10 mg)
1 part in 200 = 0.50% (1 ml contains 5 mg)
1 part in 500 = 0.20% (1 ml contains 2 mg)
1 part in 1000 = 0.10% (1 ml contains 1 mg) = 1000 μg per ml
1 part in 1500 = 0.066% (1 ml contains 0.66 mg)
1 part in 2600 = 0.038% (1 ml contains 0.38 mg)
1 part in 5000 = 0.02% (1 ml contains 0.20 mg)
1 part in 50,000 = 0.002% (1 ml contains 0.02 mg)
1 part in 200,000 = 0.0005% (1 ml contains 5 micrograms)

The number of milligrams in 1 ml of any solution of known percentage strength is obtained by moving the decimal one place to the right. For example, a 1% solution contains 10 mg/ml. By definition, a percent solution contains the specified weight (in grams) of the solute in 100 ml of total solution. For example, a 5% dextrose and water solution contains 5 g of dextrose dissolved in each 100 ml of water.

Approximate Equivalents

Weights

1 kg = 2.2 avoirdupois or imperial pounds
1 kg = 2.6 apothecary or troy pounds
1 oz = 30 g
(Avoirdupois or imperial = 28.350 g)
(Apothecary or troy = 31.1035 g)
1 lb = 453.6 g = 0.4536 kg = 16 oz

Volumes

1 liter = 10.6 U.S. quarts = 33.8 fluid ounces
1 U.S. pint = 473.2 ml
1 quart = 946.4 ml

Length

1 meter (m) = 39.37 inches (in)
1 in = $\frac{1}{12}$ ft = 2.54 centimeters (cm)

Pressure

1 lb per sq in (psi) = 0.070 kg/sq cm
= 51.7 mm of mercury (Hg)
= 70.3 cm of water (H_2O)
1 mm Hg = 1.36 cm H_2O
1 cm H_2O = 0.73 mm Hg
1 atmosphere = 760 mm Hg
= 14.7 lb/sq in
= 29.9 in Hg
= 1.03 kg/sq cm
= 33.9 ft H_2O
= 760 torr
= 1013.25 millibars
= 100 kilopascals (kPa)

■ EQUIVALENTS OF CENTIGRADE AND FAHRENHEIT THERMOMETRIC SCALES

Fahrenheit to Centigrade: $°C = (°F - 32) \times \frac{5}{9}$
Centigrade to Fahrenheit: $°F = (°C \times \frac{9}{5}) + 32$

Centigrade Degree	Fahrenheit Degree	Centigrade Degree	Fahrenheit Degree	Centigrade Degree	Fahrenheit Degree
−17	+ 1.4	5	41.0	27	80.6
−16	3.2	6	42.8	28	82.4
−15	5.0	7	44.6	29	84.2
−14	6.8	8	46.4	30	86.0
−13	8.6	9	48.2	31	87.8
−12	10.4	10	50.0	32	89.6
−11	12.2	11	51.8	33	91.4
−10	14.0	12	53.6	34	93.2
− 9	15.8	13	55.4	**35**	**95.0**
− 8	17.6	14	57.2	**36**	**96.8**
− 7	19.4	15	59.0	**37**	**98.6**
− 6	21.2	16	60.8	**38**	**100.4**
− 5	23.0	17	62.6	**39**	**102.2**
− 4	24.8	18	64.4	**40**	**104.0**
− 3	26.6	19	66.2	41	105.8
− 2	28.4	20	68.0	42	107.6
− 1	30.2	21	69.8	43	109.4
0	**32.0**	22	71.6	44	111.2
+ 1	33.8	23	73.4	45	113.0
2	35.6	24	75.2	·	
3	37.4	25	77.0	·	
4	39.2	26	78.8	100	212.0

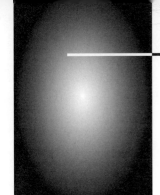

Catheter Comparison Scale

(For Comparison of Endotracheal Tube Sizes)

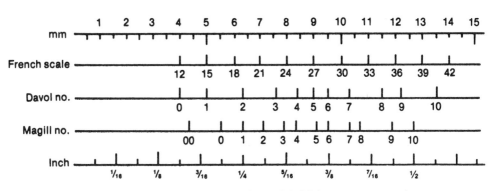

Modified from Lumb WV, Jones EW: *Veterinary anesthesia,* Philadelphia, 1973, Lea & Febiger.

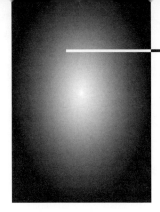

APPENDIX C

Equipment and Drugs for Use in an Emergency Crash Kit

The following list of equipment and supplies may be altered depending on the veterinarian's preference. Some supplies (for example, laryngoscope, Ambu bag, sterile fluids) that are easily accessible within the clinical setting may be omitted from the kit.

■ EQUIPMENT AND SUPPLIES

- **a.** Endotracheal tubes (various sizes)
- **b.** Penlight
- **c.** Adhesive tape (1-inch)
- **d.** Gauze roll (1- or 2-inch)
- **e.** Sterile gauze pads
- **f.** IV fluid administration set
- **g.** Burette for fluid administration
- **h.** Intravenous catheters (18-, 20-, and 22-gauge)
- **i.** Syringes (1-, 3-, 5-, 20-ml sizes)
- **j.** Needles (18-, 20-, 22-gauge)
- **k.** Alcohol swabs
- **l.** Sterile surgery instruments, including scalpel handle and blades, hemostats, thumb forceps, scissors, needle holder
- **m.** Sterile suture material (absorbable and nonabsorbable)
- **n.** Sterile saline for injection
- **o.** Sterile fluids (lactated Ringer's, saline, 5% dextrose)
- **p.** Vacutainer needles and tubes (lavender and red top)
- **q.** Stethoscope
- **r.** Sterile gloves
- **s.** Thermometer
- **t.** Sterile lubricant and lidocaine gel
- **u.** Ambu bag
- **v.** Laryngoscope

■ DRUGS

    a. Epinephrine (1 : 1000)—may be refrigerated
    b. Dopamine
    c. Sodium bicarbonate
    d. Atropine
    e. 10% calcium chloride or calcium gluconate
    f. 2% lidocaine without epinephrine
    g. Doxapram
    h. Dexamethasone
    i. Prednisolone sodium succinate
    j. Diazepam
    k. Naloxone
    l. Yohimbine
    m. Butorphanol
    n. Heparin
    o. Furosemide

NOTE: A list of emergency drug dosages should be posted or included in the kit.

INDEX

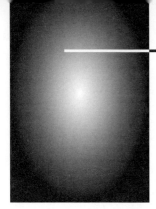

I N D E X

A

Abdomen
examination of, 10-11
splinting of, 284
Abdominal pain, 282
Abortion, spontaneous, and waste gas
exposure, 193, 194
Acepromazine, 302
benefits of, 24*t*
cyclohexamines used with, 121
dosages for, 22*t*
ketamine combined with, 124
meperidine used with, 289
opioids and, 286
as preanesthetic agent, 28-30, 38, 49
precautions for, 25*t*
Acetaminophen (Tylenol, Tempra)
dosages for, 296*t*
toxicity of, 298
Acetylsalicylic acid (aspirin), 296*t*
Activated charcoal canisters, 196, 199
Activity level, in physical examination, 6
Addiction, to opioid agents, 40
Advil (ibuprofen), 296*t*
Afghan hounds, in recovery period, 100;
see also Sighthounds
Age, in physical examination, 6; *see also*
Geriatric patients; Pediatric patients
Airway
in cardiac arrest, 237
obstruction of, 245
Alanine aminotransferase (ALT), 12
Alkaline phosphatase (AP), 12
Allergic reactions, with local analgesia, 262

Allergies, in patient history, 3
Alpha-2 adrenergic agonists, 301-302
Ambu bag, 232*f*; *see also* Bagging
American College of Veterinary
Anesthesiologists, 196
American Society of Anesthesiologists
(ASA), 14, 193
Anafen (ketoprofen), 296*t*; *see also*
Ketoprofen
Analeptic agents
defined, 140
in recovery period, 49
Analgesia
balanced, 300
in cesarean section, 221
choice of, 285
combination therapy for, 300
defined, 277
epidural, 202
with halothane, 136
long-term, 297
and nitrous oxide, 139, 140
pharmacologic, 284-302
principles of, 279-284
Analgesia, local
characteristics of, 253-254*t*
infiltration of, 255-256, 257*f*
mechanism of action of, 254-255
regional analgesia, 257-262
topical use, 255
toxicity associated with, 262-263
Analgesics, 284-285
alpha-2 adrenergic agonists, 301-302
classes of, 286

The letter *t* after page number indicates table.
The letter *f* after page number indicates figure.

Analgesics—Cont'd
  delivery of, 285-286
  ketamine, 302
  local, 300-301
  NSAIDs, 295-300
  opioids as, 37, 286-295
  postoperative, 103
  and propofol use, 127t
  tranquilizers, 302
Anaphylaxis, with local analgesia, 262
Anased (xylazine), 32-33
Anemia, as anesthetic risk, 17
Anesthesia
  balanced, 23, 47, 120, 216
  diagnostic tests for, 11-14
  dissociative, 120-121f
  early use of, 147-148
  fluids given during, 19
  hastening recovery from, 246
  for obese animals, 7
  and patient history, 3
  preanesthesia, 1
  preparation for, 2
Anesthesia, general, 46
  agents used in, 47f
  in cesarean section, 221-222
  classical stages and planes of, 50-54,
    52t-53t
  components of, 47-49
  definition of, 47
  induction in, 48
  maintenance of, 48, 71-100
  patient comfort during, 99-100
  recording information during, 95, 96f,
    97f, 98f, 99
  recovery from, 48-49, 100-104
  safety of, 49-50
Anesthetic agents
  cost of, 16
  orally-administered, 6
  for preanesthesia, 21-42
  spill procedures for, 203-204
Anesthetic chamber
  induction with, 6, 60, 61f
  waste gas control in, 201
Anesthetic depth
  indicators of, 88, 89t, 90f, 91f, 92f,
    93f, 94
  judging, 94, 95
  problems with, 226-229
  and response to surgical stimulation, 94

Anesthetic depth—Cont'd
  of stage III, 51-54
  treating excessive, 229
Anesthetic gas, waste; see Waste anesthetic
  gas
Anesthetic machines
  Bain system, 175f, 176f-177
  components of, 153f-165
  function of, 151-152f
  gas scavenging systems for, 196-199
  inhalation, 151-152, 153f, 154f
  leak testing for, 199-201
  misassembly of, 214
  with nonrebreathing systems, 173-177
  operation of, 172-173
  with rebreathing systems, 173
  schematic of, 155f
Anesthetic protocol, 47
  forms for, 96, 97f, 98f
  selection of, 14-16, 215
Antiarrhythmic effect, of phenothiazines,
  29; see also Arrhythmias
Antibiotics, in preanesthetic patient
  care, 21
Anticholinergics, 23
  action of, 24-25f, 26f
  effects of, 26f-27
  method of use for, 26
  opioids and, 37, 38t, 286
  toxicity associated with, 27–28
Anticonvulsants, in preanesthetic patient
  care, 21
Antiemetic effect, of phenothiazines, 29
Antihistamine effect, of phenothiazines, 29
Antisedan (atipamezole), 35
Antisialogogic activity, reduction of, 26-27
Apnea, and barbiturate use, 117
Appetite, in pain response, 281t
Appetite stimulants, 31
Arquel (meclofenamic acid), 297t
Arrhythmias, cardiac
  and barbiturate use, 117
  detection of, 234
  and oxygenation, 85
  treatment of, 235
ASA (aspirin), 296t
Aspiration, risk of, 124, 243
Aspirin (acetylsalicylic acid, ASA)
  action of, 284-285
  dosages for, 296t
Astromorpho/PF (morphine), 287-288

Ataxia, 125
Atelectasis
    cause of, 76
    prevention of, 162
Atipamezole (Antisedan), 302
    dosages for, 22t
    as medetomidine antagonist, 35
Atropine, 23
    action of, 24, 25f, 26f
    and anesthetic depth, 95
    in anesthetic emergencies, 240t
    benefits of, 24t
    dosages for, 22t
    effect on heart rate of, 93, 94
    effects of, 26f-27
    meperidine used with, 289
    and neuroleptanalgesia, 126
    for pediatric patients, 219
    in preanesthetic mixtures, 38
    precautions for, 25t
    to prevent unwanted effects, 22
    and pupil size, 93
    toxicity associated with, 27-28
Attitude, in response to pain, 281t
Auditory stimulation, opioid-induced, 291
Auscultation, of heart and lungs, 8
Autoclaving, 186
Autonomic nervous system, 24
Ayres T piece, 175
Azium (dexamethasone), 240t

B
Back pressure compensation
    and nonprecision vaporizers, 171
    of precision vaporizers, 169
Bagging, 54; see also Ventilation
    and atelectasis, 76, 232f
    reasons for, 162
Bain system, 175f, 176f-177
Balanced electrolyte solutions, in IV
    therapy, 19
Banamine (flunixin), 138, 296t
Barbiturates, 109
    adverse side effects of, 115-117
    and cardiac arrhythmias, 234
    classes of, 111
    commonly used, 117-120
    distribution of, 111-114
    effect on vital systems of, 114-115
    elimination of, 111-114
    in geriatric patients, 218

Barbiturates—Cont'd
    given "to effect," 119
    IV administration of, 55
    and medetomidine, 34-35
    and recovery period, 100
    short-acting, 111
    side effects of, 22
    tissue levels of, 113f
    ultrashort-acting, 111
    use in practice, 114
Benzodiazepines
    benefits of, 24t
    effects of, 30-31
    method of use for, 31
    as preanesthetic agents, 28
Bird Mark 7 Respirator, 268
Birds, preanesthesia for, 16
Bleeding, as anesthetic risk, 17
Bleeding times, NSAIDs and, 299
Blink reflex, assessment of, 89, 90f
Blood chemistry, 12
Blood clot formation, and IV therapy, 19
Blood clotting tests, 13
Blood gases
    determination of, 13
    during general anesthesia, 82
    monitoring of, 78
Blood loss
    and IV therapy, 18
    monitoring, 75-76
Blood pressure
    Doppler measurement of, 79-81
    monitoring of, 75, 78, 79-82
    during pain episodes, 282
    terminology, 79
Blood-to-gas solubility coefficient,
    133-134
Blood transfusions, 21
Blood urea nitrogen (BUN), 12
Blowpipe, for IM administration, 55
Body posture, as response to pain, 281t
Bolus induction, 56
Bordetella, preventing transmission of, 185
Boston terriers, 219
Bowel habits, and pain response, 281t
Boxers, sensitivity to phenothiazines of, 30
Brachial plexus block, 257
Brachycephalic animals, 6, 28, 33, 63
    and anesthetic emergencies, 211
    anesthetic risk in, 217t, 219-220
    dyspnea in, 245

Bradycardia
    on ECG, 87
    effect of halothane on, 135
    opioid-induced, 288, 291
    and oxygenation, 85
    in pediatric patients, 219
    and propofol use, 127
    treatment of, 234
Brain, anesthetic gas effects on, 192, 194
Breathing
    in cardiac arrest, 237
    monitoring, 76-77
Breed, identification of, 6
Brevital (methohexital), 111, 118*t*
Bronchodilation, promotion of, 27
Bulldogs, 6, 211, 219; *see also*
    Brachycephalic animals
BUN; *see* Blood urea nitrogen
Bupivacaine (Marcaine)
    as local analgesia, 253, 254*t*
    preemptive use of, 286
Buprenex (buprenorphine), 290-291
Buprenorphine (Buprenex, Temgesic)
    as analgesic, 290-291
    dosages for, 287*t*
Burette, in IV therapy, 19, 20*f*
Butorphanol (Torbutrol, Torbugesic,
    Stadol), 35, 290
    analgesic effect of, 278
    benefits of, 24*t*
    dosages for, 22*t*, 287*t*
    for pain, 283
    in preanesthetic mixtures, 38
    preemptive use of, 286
    in recovery period, 23
    in respiratory depression, 290

C
Calcium, in IV fluids, 21
Cancer, and waste gas exposure, 193
Capillary refill time (CRT), 8
    during induction period, 60
    monitoring of, 71, 74*f*
    during pain episodes, 282
    prolonged, 230, 231
Capnograph, 86*f*
Capnography, 78, 85, 86*f*, 87, 232
    in controlled ventilation, 268
    during general anesthesia, 84
Carbocaine (mepivacaine), 253, 254*t*,
    262

Carbon dioxide absorber canisters, 152*f*,
    153*f*, 154*f*, 155*f*, 164
    maintenance of, 185
    mechanics of, 164
Carbon dioxide absorber exhaustion,
    213
Carbon dioxide levels, during general
    anesthesia, 83-84
Carbon dioxide partial pressure (Paco$_2$),
    12*t*
Cardiac arrest
    during general anesthesia, 236-237
    incidence of, 211
Cardiac compressions, 237, 238*f*, 239
Cardiopulmonary resuscitation (CPR)
    aftercare, 242
    emergency drugs used in, 241*t*
    technique for, 237, 238*f*, 239
Cardiovascular disease
    and anesthetic risk, 217*t*, 223
    diagnosis of, 10
Cardiovascular function
    abnormalities of, 233-235
    during anesthesia, 52*t*, 54
    and cyclohexamines, 122
    effect of barbiturates on, 115
    effect of halothane on, 135
    with isoflurane, 137
    and methoxyflurane, 138
Carfentanyl, IM administration of, 55
Carprofen (Rimadyl, Zenecarp)
    dosages for, 297*t*
    mechanism of, 285
Carrier gas, flow rates for, 178-180, 181
Castration, anesthetics chosen for, 16
Catalepsy, 120-121*f*
Catheterization, intravenous, 17-21
Cats
    intubation of, 62*f*, 66-69
    mask induction of, 59*f*
    preanesthesia for, 16
CBC; *see* Complete blood count (CBC)
Central nervous system (CNS)
    cyclohexamines and, 120, 122
    effect of opioids on, 36-37
    waste gas effects on, 192, 194
Central venous pressure (CVP)
    measurement of, 82
    monitoring of, 78, 223
Cerebral spinal fluid (CSF), effect of
    cyclohexamines on, 122

Cesarean section, 216, 270
  as anesthetic risk, 217*t*, 221-222
  anesthetics for, 16
  barbiturates for, 115
  and IV therapy, 18
Cetacaine, 65
Chest, auscultation of, 8
Chlorofluorocarbons, 129
  desflurane, 139
  enflurane, 138
  halothane, 134-136
  isoflurane, 136-137
  methoxyflurane, 137-138
  pharmacologic properties of, 131*t*
  physical properties of, 130*t*
  sevoflurane, 139
Chloroform, 128
Chlorpromazine hydrochloride, as
  preanesthetic agent, 28-30
Circulating warm-water heating pad, 77, 78*f*
Circulation, in cardiac arrest, 237-238; *see
  also* Cardiovascular function
Closed systems, 173
CNS; *see* Central nervous system (CNS)
Coagulation disorders, 13
Colloid solutions, in IV therapy, 20*t*, 21
Combination therapy, to relieve pain, 300
Complete blood count (CBC), 11-12
Congenital abnormalities, and waste gas
  exposure, 193, 194
Consensual light reflex, 8, 9*f*
Consent forms, 4
Controlled Substances Act, 41
Corneal reflex, assessment of, 90
Corticosteroids
  for brachycephalic dogs, 220
  and neuromuscular blocking agents, 271
Cough reflex, during endotracheal
  intubation, 69
CPR.; *see* Cardiopulmonary resuscitation
Creatinine, 12
Crystalloid solutions, in IV therapy, 19
CSF; *see* Cerebral spinal fluid (CSF)
CVP; *see* Central venous pressure (CVP)
Cyanosis, 232-233
  during anesthesia, 74
  emergency care in, 230-231
  and nitrous oxide, 140
Cyclohexamines, 109
  action of, 120
  effect on vital systems of, 122

Cyclohexamines—Cont'd
  ketamine, 123
  tiletamine, 124-125
  use in practice of, 121-122
Cyclooxygenase (COX), 297, 298
Cytotec (misoprostol), 299

D

Data base, minimum patient, 2-14
Dehydration
  as anesthetic risk, 17
  clinical signs of, 7*t*
  indication of, 11
  IV therapy for, 18
Delta fibers, 279
Demerol (meperidine/pethidine), 288-289
Dental blocks, 301
Dental pain, 281
Depolarizing agents, 270, 271
Desflurane, 129, 139
Detector badges, 204
Detomidine (Dormosedan), 32
Dexamethasone (Azium), in anesthetic
  emergencies, 240*t*
Dextrose solutions, in IV therapy, 20*t*, 21
Diagnostic tests
  blood chemistry, 12
  for blood clotting, 13
  blood gases, 13
  CBC, 11-12
  ECG, 13
  radiography, 13
  urinalysis, 12
Diaphragmatic hernia, surgical repair of,
  224
Diastolic pressure; *see also* Blood pressure
  Doppler measurement of, 81
  normal, 79
Diazepam (Valium), 302
  and anesthetic depth, 95
  in anesthetic emergencies, 240*t*
  benefits of, 24*t*
  for brachycephalic dogs, 220
  in cesarean sections, 222
  cyclohexamines used with, 121
  dosages for, 22*t*
  effects of, 30
  in IV fluids, 21
  ketamine combined with, 124
  meperidine used with, 289
  method of use for, 31

Diazepam (Valium)—Cont'd
and muscle tone, 91
precautions for, 25t
Diethyl ether
characteristics of, 129
as inhalation anesthetic, 128
Differential count, in CBC, 12
"Diffusion hypoxia," 140
Digital display, for blood pressure, 80
Dilute concentrations, 115
Diprivan (propofol), 126-128
Disinfection, of anesthetic equipment,
185-186
Disposition, in physical examination, 6
Dissociative anesthesia, 120-121f
Divinyl ether, 128
DNA, and waste gas exposure, 193
Doberman pinscher, 13
Dobutamine (Dobutrex), 240t
Dobutrex (dobutamine), 240t
Dogs; see also Sighthounds
brachycephalic, 6, 28, 33, 63, 211,
217t, 219-220, 245
long-nosed breeds, 69
preanesthesia for, 16
Domitor (medetomidine), 32
Dopamine (Intropin), in anesthetic
emergencies, 240t
Doppler flow probe, 78, 79, 80f, 81
Dopram (doxapram), 140, 141, 240t
Dormosedan (detomidine), 32
Doxapram (Dopram), 140, 141
in anesthetic emergencies, 240t
in recovery period, 49
Drug reactions, in patient history, 3
Drugs; see Analgesics; Anesthetic agents;
Medications
Duragesic (fentanyl), 289
Duragesic patches (fentanyl patches),
293-295
Duramorph (morphine), 287-288
Dyspnea, 230-231, 232-233
in brachycephalic dogs, 220, 245
observation for, 10
in patient history, 3
during recovery period, 244-245

E
Ear flick reflex, 90
Ears
examination of, 8
pain in, 281

Electrocardiography (ECG), 78
during anesthesia, 72, 87-88f
uses of, 13
Electrolyte imbalances, and cardiac
arrhythmias, 235
Electrolytes, 12
Emergencies, anesthetic
anesthetic agents in, 215-216
cardiac abnormalities, 233-235
cyanosis, 230-231, 232-233
drugs used in, 240t
due to human error, 211-213
dyspnea, 230-231, 232-233
equipment failure and, 213-215
general approach to potential, 226, 227
pale mucous membranes in, 229-230
patient factors in, 216, 217t-218t,
219-225
prolonged capillary refill, 230, 231
response to, 225
shock, 230, 231
tachycardia, 233-234, 235
tachypnea, 231-233, 234
Emergency therapy, anesthesia in, 16
EMLA cream, 255
Endorphins, 282
Endotracheal intubation
advantages of, 61-62
anatomy of, 62f
excessive dead space in, 64f
problems associated with, 62-64
procedure for, 65, 66f, 67f, 68-70f
and vagus nerve, 26
Endotracheal tubes
for brachycephalic dogs, 220
classification of, 150t
correct placement of, 63f, 100
disinfection of, 70-71, 185-186
maintenance of, 203
and patient comfort, 99, 99f
pressure necrosis from, 64
problems with, 214-215
removal of, 102
securing in place, 70f
selecting, 151t
size of, 149-150
with stylet, 68f
types of, 148-149
and waste gas control, 201-202
End tidal carbon dioxide (ETCO_2),
85, 87
Enemas, during preanesthetic period, 17

Enflurane, 128, 129, 138
English bulldogs, 219
Epidural analgesia
    administration of, 301
    anatomic considerations for, 260-261f
    needle placement for, 259f
    procedure for, 258-260
    vs. spinal analgesia, 262
Epidural anesthesia, needle placement
    for, 261f
Epidural block, 257
Epinephrine
    added to local analgesics, 257
    in anesthetic emergencies, 240t
Equipment for anesthesia
    care and use of, 183-186
    disinfection of, 185-186
    endotracheal tubes, 148, 149f, 150f,
        151
    failure of, 213-215
    flowmeters, 153f, 155f, 159f, 160-161
    gas cylinders, 153, 154f, 155f, 156f,
        157f
    for IV induction, 148
    leak testing of, 199-201
    maintenance of, 183-186, 203
    operation of, 172-183
    setting up, 184
    vaporizers, 154f, 155f, 161, 165-172
Esophageal stethoscope, 73f, 185-186
Esophagus, accidental intubation of, 68
ETCO₂; see End tidal carbon dioxide
Ether
    diethyl, 128, 129
    flammability of, 205
Etodolac (EtoGesic), 297t
EtoGesic (etodolac), 297t
Etomidate, 109
    characteristics of, 128
    IV administration of, 55
Etorphine, IM administration of, 55
Evaluation, patient, 2
Excitement
    opioid-induced, 291
    postanesthesia, 243
"Excitement" stage
    barbiturates and, 116
    in general anesthesia, 51
Exhalation, defined, 264
Exhalation flutter valve, 163
Extubation, during recovery period, 102
Eyelid, third, 28f

Eye position
    during anesthesia, 53t, 54
    and anesthetic depth, 92-93f
    monitoring of, 72
Eyes
    corneal reflex, 90
    effect of cyclohexamines on, 122
    examination of, 8

F
Facial expression, as response to pain, 281t
F/air canister, 199
Fatigue, in patient history, 3
Fat solubility, with isoflurane, 137; see also
    Lipid solubility
Feldene (piroxicam), 297t
Femoral artery, palpation of, 10f
Fentanyl patches (Duragesic patches), 289
    application of, 293f, 294
    for preemptive anesthesia, 293-295
Fertility, waste gas effects on, 193
Fibrillation, on ECG, 87-88
Fibrosis, associated with local
    analgesia, 263
Fire safety precautions, 205
Flow compensation
    and nonprecision vaporizers, 171
    for vaporizers, 168
Flowmeters, 153f, 155f, 159f, 160-161
    checking, 213-214
    maintenance of, 183-184
    and waste gas control, 202
Flumazenil, 30
Flunixin (Banamine), 299
    dosages for, 296t
    nephrotoxicity of, 138
Flutter valves
    exhalation, 163
    inhalation, 163
    maintenance of, 185
Fresh gas inlet, 161

G
Gas, compressed, safe handling of, 205,
    206f
Gas cylinders, 153, 154f, 155f, 156f, 157f
    capacity of, 155t
    characteristics of, 158t
    labels for, 206f
    maintenance of, 183
    safe use and storage of, 205
    yoke for, 156, 157f, 158

Gastrointestinal problems, NSAIDs associated with, 298
Gastrointestinal tract, effect of opioids on, 40
Gauges, tank pressure, 158, 159f
Geriatric patients
    as anesthetic risk, 216, 217t, 218
    isoflurane for, 137
Gingivae
    assessing, 74f
    examination of, 8
Glucose, blood, 12
Glutaraldehyde solutions, 185-186
Glycopyrrolate (Robinul-V), 23
    benefits of, 24t
    dosages for, 22t
    effects of, 27
    and neuroleptanalgesia, 126
    as preanesthetic, 22
Greyhounds, recovery period for, 100; see also Sighthounds
Grooming, as response to pain, 281t
Guarding
    assessment of, 283
    as response to pain, 281t

H
Hair coat, condition of, 10
Hallucinations, cyclohexamine-induced, 122
Halothane, 109
    and anesthetic depth, 95
    and cardiac arrhythmias, 234
    contamination levels of, 195t-196
    effect on respiration of, 54
    hepatotoxicity of, 193-194
    leak testing for, 199-201
    MAC of, 166
    mask induction of, 215
    and neuromuscular blocking agents, 271
    NIOSH recommendations for, 195
    occupational exposure to, 191
    pharmacologic effects of, 135-136
    precision vaporizer used with, 15
    properties of, 130t, 131t, 134-135
    side effects of, 14, 22
    solubility coefficient of, 134
    toxicity of, 192
    vapor pressure of, 133, 166-167
"Halothane hepatitis," 194

Hazard Chemical Standard, OSHA's, 196
Head, examination of, 8
Heart, effect of local analgesics on, 263
Heart block, on ECG, 87
Heart rate
    during anesthesia, 54
    and anesthetic depth, 93, 94, 95
    for cats, 9
    for dogs, 8-9
    during induction period, 60
    monitoring of, 71, 72
    normal values for, 12t
    during pain episodes, 282
Heartworm test, 14
Hemoglobin (Hb)
    in CBC, 11
    normal values for, 12t
Hepatic disease, and anesthetic risk, 218t, 224
Hepatic necrosis, from waste gas exposure, 194
Herbal remedies, 282
Hernia, diaphragmatic, surgical repair of, 224
High pressure system tests, 200
Histamine release, morphine-induced, 288
History, patient, 2-4
    and anesthetic emergencies, 211
    prepared form for, 4
Homeopathic remedies, 282
Hydration status
    accidental overhydration, 18
    clinical signs of, 7t
    rapid rehydration, 19
Hydromorphone, 287t, 289
Hypercapnia
    and cardiac arrhythmias, 235
    determination of, 85-87
    and manual ventilation, 267
    in obese animals, 221
Hyperglycemia, transient, 33
Hyperkalemia, bradycardia in, 234
Hypertension, monitoring of, 75; see also Blood pressure
Hyperthermia, during general anesthesia, 78
Hyperventilation, during anesthesia, 76
Hypocapnia, determination of, 85-87
Hypoglycemia, prevention of, 218
Hypoproteinemia, indication of, 11

Hypotension
  diagnosis of, 10
  after epidural infusion, 263
  monitoring of, 75
  and oxygenation, 85
  and phenothiazines, 29
  and propofol use, 127
Hypothermia
  as anesthetic emergency, 229
  as anesthetic risk, 17
  bradycardia in, 234
  during general anesthesia, 50
  in geriatric patients, 218
  morphine-induced, 288
  in pediatric patients, 219
  prevention of, 77
  and recovery period, 100
Hypoventilation, 76
Hypoxia
  bradycardia in, 234
  determination of, 84-85
  diffusion, 140
  and nitrous oxide, 140
  and respiratory arrest, 235

I
Ibuprofen (Advil, Motrin, Nuprin),
  296t
Illnesses, in patient history, 4
Induction agents, 48
Induction period
  for brachycephalic dogs, 219-220
  monitoring during, 60-61
Induction process, 48
  dosages during, 50
  flow rates during, 178, 179
  with inhalation agents, 58-60
  with injectable agents, 55-56f, 57-58
Industrial hygienists, 204
Infiltration
  of local analgesia, 255-256, 257f
  of local anesthesia, 300-301
Inflammation, associated with local
  analgesia, 263
Inflated cuffs
  advantages of, 150-151
  endotracheal tube with, 62
  during intubation, 69
  and waste gas control, 201-202
Information recording, during general
  anesthesia, 95, 96f, 97f, 98f, 99

Informed consent, 4
Infrared spectrometer, 204
Inhalation, defined, 264
Inhalation agents, 109
  for brachycephalic dogs, 220
  disadvantages of, 110
  vs. injectable agents, 110
  and recovery period, 100
  in renal disease, 225
  and vagus nerve, 26
Inhalation anesthesia machine; see also
    Anesthetic machines
  with Ohio No. 8 vaporizer, 154f
  two-gas, 151-152, 153f
Inhalation anesthetics, 47
  characteristics of, 128-129, 130t-131t
  classes of, 129
  distribution and elimination of,
      132-134
  halothane, 134-136
  MAC of, 134
  mechanism of action of, 132
  nitrous oxide, 139-140
  properties of, 132-134
  solubility coefficient of, 133-134
  vapor pressure of, 133
Inhalation flutter valve, 163
Injectable anesthetic agents, 47, 109
  barbiturates, 111-120
  cyclohexamines, 120-125
  dosage ranges of, 112t
  etomidate, 128
  given "to effect," 50
  induction with, 55, 58, 56-57f
  neuroleptanalgesia, 125-126
  in pediatric patients, 219
  propofol, 126-128
  and recovery period, 100
Insecticides, in patient history, 3
Insulin injections, in preanesthetic patient
  care, 21
Intermittent positive pressure ventilation
  (IPPV), 62
International Association for Study of
  Pain, 277
Intraarticular administration, of local
  analgesia, 301
Intramuscular (IM) injection, induction
  by, 55-58
Intraperitoneal injection, of
  pentobarbital, 119

Intravenous (IV) catheterization
    fluid administration rates for, 19
    reasons for, 17-18
    risks of, 18-19
Intravenous (IV) fluids, 19-21
    for geriatric patients, 218
    for pediatric patients, 219
Intravenous (IV) infusion, of local
    analgesics, 262
Intravenous (IV) injection
    equipment for, 148
    during induction process, 55, 56-57*f*
Intravenous (IV) therapy, monitoring
    of, 72
Intropin (dopamine), 240*t*
Intubation, "blind," 63, 66; *see also*
    Endotracheal intubation
IPPV; *see* Intermittent positive pressure
    ventilation (IPPV)
Isoflurane, 109
    and anesthetic depth, 95
    leak testing for, 199-201
    MAC of, 166
    mask induction of, 58, 59*f*
    and neuromuscular blocking
        agents, 271
    NIOSH recommendations for, 195
    occupational exposure to, 191
    pharmacologic effects of, 136-137
    precision vaporizer used with, 15
    properties of, 130*t*, 131*t*, 136
    in renal disease, 225
    side effects of, 14, 22
    solubility coefficient of, 134
    toxicity of, 192
    vapor pressure of, 133, 166-167

J
Jack Russell terriers, 211
Jaw tone
    and anesthetic depth, 95
    monitoring of, 72

K
"Kennel cough," 70
Ketalean (ketamine), 123
Ketamine (Ketalean, Ketaset, Vetalar)
    administration of, 58
    as analgesic, 278, 302
    and anesthetic depth, 95
    for brachycephalic dogs, 220

Ketamine—Cont'd
    characteristics of, 123
    dosage ranges for, 112*t*
    effect on heart rate of, 93, 94
    IM administration of, 55-58
    IV administration of, 55
    and medetomidine, 34-35
    and muscle tone, 91
    side effects of, 22, 244
    tissue irritation caused by, 122
Ketamine/detomidine, 6
Ketamine/diazepam
    dosage ranges for, 112*t*
    IV induction with, 57
Ketamine/xylazine, 112*t*
Ketaset (ketamine), 123
Ketofen (ketoprofen), 296*t*
Ketorolac (Toradol), 296*t*
Ketoprofen (Anafen, Ketofen, Orudis,
        Oruvail)
    dosages for, 296*t*
    meperidine used with, 289
    preemptive use of, 286
Kidney, waste gas effects on, 194
Kittens; *see also* Pediatric patients
    delivered by cesarean, 222
    doxapram in, 141
    and injectable agents, 219
Kuhn circuit, 175

L
Lacrimation, and anesthetic depth, 93,
        94, 95
Lactated Ringer's solution, 19, 20*t*
Lameness, 11, 283
Laryngeal edema, 244-245
Laryngeal reflex, assessment of, 90
Laryngeal sprays, 65
Laryngoscopes, 63
    description of, 65
    disinfection of, 185-186
Laryngospasm
    during intubation, 63
    symptoms of, 244-245
Leukocytes, normal values for, 12*t; see also*
    White blood cells
Levallorphan tartrate, 40
Lidocaine (Xylocaine)
    in anesthetic emergencies, 240*t*
    epidural administration of, 292

Lidocaine—Cont'd
    for intubation, 65
    as local analgesia, 253, 254t
    preemptive use of, 286
Lidocaine gel, for endotracheal tube, 63
Limping, assessment of, 283
Line blocks, 256-257f
Lingual artery, palpation of, 74, 75f
Lipid solubility
    of barbiturate agents, 113
    of halothane, 135-136
    of inhalation agents, 132
    of propofol, 126-127
Liver, waste gas effects on, 193-194
Long-nosed breeds, intubation in, 69
Low pressure system tests, 200-201
Lubricant, for endotracheal tube, 63
Lymph nodes, palpation of, 11

M
MAC; see Minimum alveolar
    concentration (MAC)
Magill endotracheal tube, 149, 150t
Magnetic therapy, 282
Maintenance, of anesthetic equipment,
    183-186, 203
Maintenance period, in general
    anesthesia, 48
    anesthetic depth during, 71
    dosages during, 50
    flow rates in, 178-180
    monitoring during, 71-72
    muscle tone during, 91-92
    reflex activity in, 88-90
    vital signs during, 72-88
Mammary glands, observation of, 11
Mapleson A system, 175
Marcaine (bupivacaine), 253, 254t
Mask induction, 58, 59f, 60
    for brachycephalic dogs, 220
    halothane risk in, 215
Masks
    with activated charcoal, 199
    maintenance of, 203
    use of, 201
Massage therapy, 282
Meclofenamic acid (Arquel), 297t
Medetomidine (Domitor), 32, 33-35
    as analgesic agent, 301-302
    benefits of, 24t

Medetomidine—Cont'd
    dosages for, 22t, 34t
    precautions for, 25t
Medical procedures
    anesthetic requirements of, 16
    pain associated with, 280t
Medications; see also Analgesics;
        Anesthetic agents
    antiemetic properties of, 17
    in cardiac arrest, 239, 240t, 241t, 242
    incorrect administration of, 212
    in patient history, 3
    safety of, 49-50
Meloxicam (Metacam), 297t
Meperidine
    analgesic effect of, 278
    benefits of, 24t
    dosages for, 22t, 287t
    in preanesthetic mixtures, 38
    preemptive use of, 286
Meperidine/pethidine (Demerol),
    288-289
Mepivacaine (Carbocaine)
    as local analgesia, 253, 254t
    preference for, 262
Metabolic acidosis, effect of barbiturates
    on, 114, 116
Metabolites, toxic, 192
Metacam (meloxicam), 297t
Metacarpal artery, palpation of, 10f
Metatarsal artery, palpation of, 10f
Methohexital (Brevital), 111
    for brachycephalic dogs, 220
    characteristics of, 118t
    dosage ranges for, 112t
    lipid solubility of, 113
    pharmacology of, 119
Methoxyflurane, 109, 128, 129
    effect on respiration of, 54
    leak testing for, 199-201
    lipid solubility of, 132
    mask induction of, 58, 59f
    NIOSH recommendations for, 195
    occupational exposure to, 191
    pharmacological effects of, 138
    properties of, 130t, 131t, 137-138
    side effects of, 22
    toxicity of, 192, 194
    vapor pressure of, 133, 167
Methylated oxybarbiturates, 111

Midazolam
  benefits of, 24t
  dosages for, 22t
  effects of, 31
  ketamine combined with, 124
  method of use for, 31
Minimum alveolar concentration (MAC),
    133
  of halothane, 135, 166
  of inhalation anesthetics, 134
  of isoflurane, 136, 166
  of methoxyflurane, 137
  and nitrous oxide, 139
Minimum patient data base, 2-14
  classification of patient status in,
    14, 15t
  diagnostic tests in, 11-14
  history, 2-4
  physical examination in, 5-11
Miosis, 8
Misoprostol (Cytotec), 299
Monitoring
  importance of, 212
  instruments for, 78-88
  during maintenance period, 71
  with nonprecision vaporizer, 171
  pulse oximeter in, 84f
  during recovery period, 101
  of vital signs, 72-78
Morphine (Morphine sulfate, Duramorph,
    Astromorpho/PF), 287-288
  benefits of, 24t
  dosages for, 22t, 287t
  emetic properties of, 17
  epidural route for, 292
  preemptive use of, 286
Morphine sulfate (morphine),
    287-288
Mortality rate, associated with general
    anesthesia, 211
Motrin (ibuprofen), 296t
Mucous membranes
  during induction period, 60
  monitoring of, 72, 74, 74f
  during pain episodes, 282
  pale, 229-230
Murphy endotracheal tube, 149f, 150f
Muscarinic receptors, 24, 25f
Muscle-paralyzing agents, 270-271
Muscle relaxation
  effect of methoxyflurane on, 138

Muscle relaxation—Cont'd
  effect of nitrous oxide on, 139
  with halothane, 136
  with isoflurane, 137
Muscle tone
  during anesthesia, 53t, 54
  during general anesthesia, 91, 92f
Mydriasis, 8
  atropine-associated, 27
  morphine-induced, 288
Myelograms, 123

N
Nalbuphine (Nubaine), 40
Nalorphine hydrochloride, 40
Naloxone (Narcan)
  in anesthetic emergencies, 240t
  as narcotic antagonist, 40
Naproxen, 297t
Narcan (naloxone), 40, 240t
Narcotics, 35; see also Opioids
  for preanesthesia, 23
  side effects of, 22
National Institute for Occupational Safety
    and Health (NIOSH), 192, 195
Nausea
  opioid-induced, 291
  postanesthetic, 103
Neck pain, 108
Negative pressure relief valve,
    164-165, 199
Nembutal (pentobarbital), 111, 118t
Neonatal animals, isoflurane for, 137;
    see also Pediatric patients
Nerve blocks, 256
Neuroleptanalgesia, 37, 125-126, 286
  with meperidine, 289
  and propofol use, 127t
Neuroleptanalgesics, 109
  with local analgesia, 253
Neurologic disease, and waste gas
    exposure, 194
Neuromuscular blocking agents, 270-271
Neurons, anesthetic gas effects on,
    192, 194
Newborns, in cesarean section, 222
Nicotinic receptors, 24, 25f
Nictitating membrane, 28f
NIOSH; see National Institute for
    Occupational Safety and Health
    (NIOSH)

Nitrous oxide (N₂O), 109, 128, 129
in cesarean sections, 222
contamination levels of, 195
flammability of, 205
gas cylinders for, 156
in induction process, 58
leak testing for, 199-201
neurotoxicity of, 194
occupational exposure to, 191
properties of, 130*t*, 139
reproductive hazards of, 193
special precautions with, 140
stored in compressed air tanks,
158, 160
in total rebreathing system, 180-182
toxicity of, 192
Nitrous oxide tanks, maintenance of, 183
N₂O; *see* Nitrous oxide (N₂O)
Nondepolarizing agents, 271
Nonrebreathing systems
and carrier gas flow rates, 178-179
choosing, 177-178
vs. rebreathing systems, 174*t*
Nonsteroidal antiinflammatory drugs
(NSAIDs), 284-285
adverse side effects of, 298-299
benefits of, 24*t*
clinical effects of, 296-297
combination therapy with, 300
meperidine used with, 289
mode of action of, 295-298
for pain, 283
toxicity of, 298, 299
Norman mask elbow, 175
Nose, examination of, 8
Novocaine (procaine), as local analgesia,
253, 254*t*
NSAIDs; *see* Nonsteroidal
antiinflammatory drugs
Nubaine (nalbuphine), 40
Numorphan (oxymorphone), 289
Nuprin (ibuprofen), 296*t*
Nursing care, during recovery, 103, 104

O

Obesity
anesthetic risk in, 217*t*, 220-221
evaluation of, 7
Occupational Safety and Health
Administration (OSHA), 192, 195, 196
Ohio Metomatic, 268

Ohio No. 8 vaporizer, 154*f*, 169, 170*f*, 171
Ophthaine, as local analgesia, 253, 254*t*
Opiates
classification of, 35
IM administration of, 55
Opioids; *see also* Narcotics
action of, 35-36
adverse effects of, 38-40
agonists, 287-290
agonists/antagonists, 290-291
beneficial effects of, 24*t*, 36-37
in cesarean sections, 222
characteristics of, 286-287
disadvantages of, 291
dosages for, 287*t*
effect of, 36*t*
epidural use of, 292
intraarticular use of, 291-292
method of use for, 37-38
in neuroleptanalgesia, 125
for postoperative pain, 291
as preanesthetic agent, 49
precautions for, 25*t*
in recovery period, 23
regulatory considerations for, 41
reversibility of, 40-41
side effects of, 76
synthetic, 288-289
term for, 35
transdermal use of, 293-295
and vagus nerve, 26
Opisthotonus, side effects of, 244
Oral administration, induction by, 58
Oral cavity, examination of, 8
Organic compounds, halogenated; *see*
Chlorofluorocarbons
Oropharynx, visualization of, 63
Orudis (ketoprofen), 296*t*
Oruvail (ketoprofen), 296*t*
Oscillometer, blood pressure measured
with, 78, 80, 82
OSHA; *see* Occupational Safety and
Health Administration (OSHA)
Ovariohysterectomy, anesthetics chosen
for, 16
Overhydration, accidental, 18; *see also*
Hydration status
Oxybarbiturates, 111
Oxygen
flammability of, 205
during general anesthesia, 83

Oxygen—Cont'd
  leak testing for, 200
  during recovery period, 101-102
  stored in compressed air tanks, 158
  in total rebreathing system, 180-182
Oxygenation status, and respiratory arrest,
  235
Oxygen flow rate
  monitoring of, 72
  in nonrebreathing system, 176
Oxygen flush valve, 163
Oxygen partial pressure (PaO_2)
  measurement of, 83
  normal values for, 12t
Oxygen saturation (SaO_2)
  determination of, 84f, 84-85
  measurement of, 83
  monitoring of, 78
Oxygen tanks
  empty, 213-214
  maintenance of, 183
Oxymorphone (Numorphan), 289
  benefits of, 24t
  dosages for, 22t, 287t
  IV induction with, 55
  side effects of, 76
Oxymorphone/acepromazine, IV
  administration of, 55

P
Packed cell volume (PCV)
  in CBC, 11
  normal values for, 12t
PaCO_2; see Carbon dioxide partial pressure
  (PaCO_2)
Pain
  assessment of, 282-284
  behavioral responses to, 280, 281t-282
  detection of, 280
  monitoring signs of, 279-382
  perception of, 285
  physiology of, 279
  postoperative, 278-279, 291, 292
  referred, 279
  scale for, 283
  treatment of, 278-279
Pain control
  endorphins, 282
  nonpharmacologic, 282
  pharmacologic analgesia, 284-302
  postoperative, 286, 300

Palpebral reflex
  and anesthetic depth, 95
  assessment of, 89, 90f
Panting
  during anesthesia, 76
  opioid-induced, 291
PaO_2; see Oxygen partial pressure (PaO_2)
Parasitism, diagnosis of, 8
Parasympathetic nervous system, 25f, 26f
Parasympatholytics; see Anticholinergics
Paresthesia, with local analgesia, 262
Partial prothrombin time (PPT), 13
Partition coefficient, of inhalation
  anesthetics, 133-134
Patient care, preanesthetic, 16-21
Patients; see also Geriatric patients;
  Pediatric patients
  minimum data base for, 2-14
  positioning of, 99-100
  preventing self-injury of, 103-104
  during recovery period, 102-103
Patient status, classification of, 14, 15t
PCV; see Packed cell volume (PCV)
Pedal reflex, assessment of, 89-90, 91f
Pediatric patients
  anesthetic risk in, 217t, 218-219
  kittens, 141, 219, 222
  puppies, 141, 219, 222
Pekingese, 211, 219
Pentobarbital (Nembutal; Somnotol),
  6, 111
  in cesarean sections, 222
  characteristics of, 118t
  dosages for, 112t
  given "to effect," 119
  lipid solubility of, 113
  pharmacology of, 112, 119-120
  problems associated with, 120
Pentothal (thiopental sodium), 111, 118t
Peristaltic movement, and anesthetic
  agents, 27
Personality
  ketamine-induced changes in, 123
  and phenothiazines, 29
pH, blood
  effect of barbiturates on, 116
  measurement of, 83
  normal values for, 12t
Pharynx
  anatomy of, 67f
  examination of, 8

Phencyclidine, 120
Phenothiazines
    benefits of, 24t
    as preanesthetic agents, 28-30
Physical examination
    and anesthetic emergencies, 211
    importance of, 5
    organ systems in, 7-11
    signalment in, 5-6
Physiotherapy, 282
Physostigmine, for atropine overdose, 28
Pinna reflex, assessment of, 90
Piroxicam (Feldene), 297t
Plasma, in IV therapy, 20t, 21
Platelet counts, 13
Pneumothorax, 224
Pocket pets, preanesthesia for, 16
Pontocaine (tetracaine), as local analgesia,
    253, 254t
Pop-off valves, 154f, 155f, 163
    with active scavenging systems, 215
    problems with, 215
Positive pressure ventilation (PPV), 264
Postoperative pain
    opioid injections for, 291
    overtreatment of, 278-279
    preemptive analgesia for, 292
Potassium, tests for, 12
PPT; see Partial prothrombin time
    (PTT)
Preanesthesia, defined, 1
Preanesthetic agents
    anticholinergics, 23-28
    benefits of, 24t
    benzodiazepines, 30-35
    butorphanol as, 290
    dosages for, 21, 22t
    opioids, 35-41
    phenothiazines, 28-30
    precautions for, 23, 25t
    and propofol use, 127t
    reasons for, 21-23, 24t
    safety of, 49
    thiazine derivatives, 32-35
Preanesthetic period
    definition of, 48
    patient care during, 16-21
Precision vaporizers, 133
Prednisolone sodium succinate (Solu-
    Delta-Cortef), in anesthetic
    emergencies, 240t

Preemptive analgesia, 285-286
    of fentanyl patches, 293-294
    for postoperative pain, 292
Pregnancy, and waste gas exposure, 193
Pregnant animals, anesthesia for, 8
Premature ventricular contractions
    (PVCs)
    detection of, 234
    on ECG, 87
    during induction period, 115
Preoxygenation, in cesarean sections,
    222
Pressure manometer, 164, 165f
Procaine (Novocaine), as local analgesia,
    253, 254t
Proparacaine (Ophthaine), as local
    analgesia, 253
Propofol (Diprivan; Rapinovet), 109,
    126-128
    advantages of, 127
    for brachycephalic dogs, 220
    disadvantage of, 128
    dosages for, 112t
    IV administration of, 55
    IV induction with, 55
    and medetomidine, 34-35
    and preanesthetic agents, 127
Prostaglandins, 285, 297, 298
Protective equipment, for anesthetic
    exposure, 199, 203-204
Pugs, 219
Pulmonary edema, detection of, 223
Pulse
    during induction period, 60
    monitoring of, 72, 74-75f
    palpation of, 10
Pulse oximeters, 84
Pulse oximetry, 78
    during anesthesia, 84f, 83
    in controlled ventilation, 268
Pupillary light reflex, 8, 9f
Pupils
    during anesthesia, 53t, 54
    and anesthetic depth, 92-93f
    during pain episodes, 282
Puppies
    delivered by cesarean, 222
    doxapram in, 141
    and injectable agents, 219
PVCs; see Premature ventricular
    contractions (PVCs)

Q

Quill removal, under injectable anesthesia, 55

R

Rabies pole, for IM administration, 55
RAC; *see* Reticular activation center (RAC)
Radiography
  indications for, 13
  under injectable anesthesia, 55
Ranitidine, 299
Rapinovet (propofol), 126-128
Rebreathing systems
  and carrier gas flow rates, 179-180
  choosing, 177-178
  closed, 182, 183
  vs. nonrebreathing systems, 174*t*
  problems with, 213
  safety concerns with, 180-183
  total vs. partial, 173
  waste gas control in, 202
Recording, during general anesthesia, 95, 96*f*, 97*f*, 98*f*, 99
Records, anesthetic, 96*f*, 97*f*-98*f*
Recovery period, 48-49
  anesthetist's role in, 101-104
  dyspnea during, 244-245
  flow rates in, 180
  in geriatric patients, 218
  hastening, 245-246
  nursing care during, 103, 104
  problems during, 242-246
  prolonged, 245
  stages of, 101
Referred pain, 279
Reflexes
  corneal, 90
  cough, 69
  ear flick, 90
  during general anesthesia, 88-90
  monitoring of, 71-72
  palpebral, 95
  pedal, 89-90, 91*f*
  during stage III of anesthesia, 51-54
  swallowing, 89*t*
Regional analgesia
  epidural analgesia, 258
  technique, 257
Regurgitation, during anesthesia, 242

Renal disease
  and anesthetic risk, 218*t*, 224-225
  waste gas exposure and, 194
Renal failure, diagnosis of, 8
Renal function, effect of methoxyflurane on, 138
Renal toxicity, NSAIDs associated with, 299
Reproduction, waste gas effects on, 193
Reproductive status, in patient history, 4
Reservoir (rebreathing) bags, 161-163
  maintenance of, 203
  and waste gas control, 202
Respiration
  during anesthesia, 52*t*, 54
  apneustic, 122
  cessation of, 54
  effect of barbiturates on, 114-115
  effect of cyclohexamines on, 122
  effect of halothane on, 135
  effect of opioids on, 39-40
  with isoflurane, 137
  in obese animals, 221
  and propofol use, 127
Respiratory acidosis
  effect of barbiturates on, 116
  and manual ventilation, 267
Respiratory arrest
  during general anesthesia, 235-236
  treatment of, 236
Respiratory depression
  as anesthetic emergency, 213
  morphine-induced, 288
  with neuroleptanalgesia, 125
  opioid-induced, 291
Respiratory disease, and anesthetic risk, 217*t*, 223-224
Respiratory distress, as anesthetic risk, 17
Respiratory problems
  with fentanyl patches, 295
  treating, 232-233
Respiratory rate
  and anesthetic depth, 93, 94, 95
  defined, 265
  determination of, 10
  effect of methoxyflurane on, 138
  during induction period, 60
  monitoring of, 71, 76-77
  normal values for, 12*t*
  during pain episodes, 282
Reticular activation center (RAC), 102

Reversing agents
  defined, 140
  for thiazine derivatives, 35
Rimadyl (carprofen), 297t
Robinul-V (glycopyrrolate), 23
"Rocking boat" ventilatory pattern, 54
Romifidine, 32
Rompun (xylazine), 32-33
Rubber endotracheal tubes, 148-149
Rubber solubility, 132
  of halothane, 135
  of isoflurane, 136
  of methoxyflurane, 137-138
Russian wolfhounds, in recovery
  period, 100

S
Saline solutions, in IV therapy, 20, 20t
Salivation
  and anesthetic depth, 93, 94
  effect of cyclohexamines on, 122
  during pain episodes, 292
  reduction of, 26-27
Salukis, in recovery period, 100
SaO₂; see Oxygen saturation (SaO₂)
Scale, pain, 283-284
Scavenging systems, gas, 196-199
  active, 198f
  passive, 197f
Scottish terriers, 13
"Second gas effect," of nitrous oxide, 1
  39
Sedation, and phenothiazines, 29
Sedatives
  preanesthetic, 28, 49
  and propofol use, 127t
Seizure disorders, preanesthetic agents
  for, 30
Seizures
  and phenothiazines, 29
  postanesthesia, 244
Self-injury, preventing patient, 103-104
Self-mutilation, as response to pain, 281t
Semiclosed systems, 173; see also
  Rebreathing systems
Sensitivity, increased, 125
Sepsis, catheter-induced, 18-19
Sevoflurane, 129, 139
  pharmacologic properties of, 131t
  physical properties of, 130t
Shaking, assessment of, 284

Shock
  as anesthetic risk, 17
  and IV therapy, 18
Shock therapy, 19
Sighthounds
  anesthetic risk in, 217t, 220
  and barbiturate use, 117
  and propofol use, 127
  thiopental use in, 113
Signalment, 5-6
Signs and symptoms
  of hydration status, 7t
  in patient history, 3
Silicone rubber tubes, 149
Sinus arrhythmia, 9
Skin, examination of, 10
Small Animal Ventilator and Drager, 268
Sodium, tests for, 12
Sodium bicarbonate, in anesthetic
  emergencies, 240t
Solubility coefficient, 132
  of halothane, 135
  of inhalation anesthetics, 133-134
  of isoflurane, 136
  of methoxyflurane, 137
  of nitrous oxide, 139
Solu-Delta-Cortef (prednisolone sodium
  succinate), 240t
Somatic pain, 279
Somnotol (pentobarbital), 111, 118t
Species, identification of, 6
Sphygmomanometry, 79
Spinal (intrathecal) block, 257
"Sponge effect," 134
Squeeze cage, for IM administration, 57
Stadol (butorphanol), 290
Stephens Universal Vaporizer, 169
Stertor (snoring), 8
Stethoscope
  blood pressure monitoring with, 79
  esophageal, 73f, 185-186
Succinylcholine
  as depolarizing agent, 270
  and muscle tone, 91
Surgery
  pain associated with, 280t
  tables for, 100
Swallowing reflex, assessment of, 89t
Sympathetic blockade, 255
Systemic toxicity, with local
  analgesia, 262

Systolic pressure
    demonstration of, 80
    Doppler measurement of, 81
    normal, 79

T

Tachycardia
    as anesthetic risk, 233-234, 235
    on ECG, 87
    and propofol use, 127
Tachypnea, 231-233
    during anesthesia, 76
    treating, 234
Tear secretions, reduction of, 27; *see also*
    Lacrimation
Technician/anesthetist
    in emergency care, 225-226
    and patient history, 4
    role of, 2, 14
Telazol (tiletamine/zolazepam), 6, 55,
    124-125
Temgesic (buprenorphine), 290-291
Temperature, body
    monitoring of, 72, 77
    normal, 8, 12*t*
    and recovery period, 100
Temperature compensation
    and nonprecision vaporizers, 171
    of vaporizers, 168
Tempra (acetaminophen), 296*t*
Tetracaine (Pontocaine), as local analgesia,
    253, 254*t*
Thermoregulation
    with halothane, 136
    monitoring of, 77-78
Thiamylal, and anesthetic depth, 95
Thiazines, 32-35
    benefits of, 24*t*
    as preanesthetic agents, 28
    reversing agents for, 35
Thinness, evaluation of, 8
Thiobarbiturates, 111
    for anesthetic induction, 117
    in recovery period, 49
Thiopental sodium (Pentothal), 111
    administration of, 50
    characteristics of, 118*t*
    dosages for, 112*t*
    IV administration of, 55
    lipid solubility of, 113

Thiopental sodium—Cont'd
    pharmacology of, 111-112, 117
    tissue levels of, 113*f*
Thoracic pain, 108
Thoracotomy, mechanical ventilation
    for, 269
Tidal volume, 76
    defined, 265
    effect of methoxyflurane on, 138
    during pain episodes, 292
Tiletamine
    and muscle tone, 91
    tissue irritation caused by, 122
Tiletamine/zolazepam (Telazol), 6
    advantages of, 124-125
    IM administration of, 55
Titration process, 50
Toenail cuticle bleeding time, 13
Tolazoline, 35
Tolfedine (tolfenamic acid), 297*t*
Tolfenamic acid (Tolfedine), 297*t*
Topical use, of local analgesia, 301
Toradol (ketolorac), 296*t*
Torbugesic (butorphanol), 290
Torbutrol (butorphanol), 290
Total plasma protein (TPP)
    in CBC, 11
    normal values for, 12*t*
Toxicity
    atropine, 27-28
    of flunixin, 138
    of halothane, 193-194
    of local analgesia, 262-263
    nitrous oxide, 194
    of NSAIDs, 298, 299
    of waste anesthetic gas, 192-194
TPP; *see* Total plasma protein (TPP)
Tracheobronchitis, 70
Tranquilizers, 253
    cyclohexamines used with, 121-122
    ketamine in combination with, 123-124
    meperidine used with, 289
    opioids combined with, 37, 38*t*, 286, 302
    as preanesthetic agents, 23, 28
    and propofol use, 127*t*
    ventilation and, 265
Tranquilizing gun, for IM
    administration, 57
Trauma patients, anesthetic risk in, 217*t*,
    222-223

Trembling, assessment of, 284
Trichloroethylene, 128
Triflupromazine hydrochloride, as
  preanesthetic agent, 28-30
Tylenol (acetaminophen)
  dosages for, 296t
  toxicity of, 298

U
Urinalysis, 12
Urinary blockages, 225
Urinary habits, in response to pain, 281t
Urinary retention, opioid-induced, 291

V
Vaccinations, in patient history, 3
Vagal tone, effect of halothane on, 135
Valium (diazepam), 240t
Vaporizers, 154f, 155f, 161
  back pressure compensation for, 169
  in circle, 171, 172f
  flow compensation for, 168
  function of, 165-172
  maintenance of, 184-185, 203
  nonprecision, 169, 170f, 171
  out of circle, 171, 172f
  precision, 166, 167f-169
  precision vs. nonprecision, 166t
  problems with, 215
  temperature compensation for, 168
  waste gas contamination from, 196t
  and waste gas control, 202
Vapor pressure, 132
  of halothane, 135, 166-167
  of inhalation anesthetics, 133
  of isoflurane, 136, 166-167
  of methoxyflurane, 137, 167
Vasodilation
  effect of halothane on, 135
  and phenothiazines, 29
Ventilation, controlled
  in anesthetized animal, 265-266
  in awake animal, 264-265
  manual, 266 (see also Bagging)
  mechanical, 268-269
  risks of, 270
Ventilation assistance, 54
Ventilation systems, for waste gas control,
  202-203
Ventilator, 269f

Vetalar (ketamine), 123
VIC; see Vaporizers
Visceral pain, 279
Vital signs
  on anesthesia record, 98f, 99
  instruments for monitoring, 78-88
  monitoring, 71, 72-78
VOC; see Vaporizers
Vocalization
  assessment of, 284
  during endotracheal intubation, 69
  as response to pain, 281t
Vomiting
  during anesthesia, 242
  postanesthetic, 103, 242
  prevention of, 16-17
von Willebrand's disease, 13
Vulva, observation of, 11

W
Waste anesthetic gas
  contamination levels of, 195t-196
  control procedures for, 201-204
  defined, 191
  hazards of, 140
  leak testing for, 199-201
  long-term effects of, 192-194
  monitoring levels of, 204
  risk assessment of, 194-196
  scavenging systems for, 196-199
  short-term effects of, 192
  sources of, 196t
Weight, in physical examination, 6
Weimaraners, 211
Whippets, in recovery period, 100
White blood cells, in CBC, 12; see also
  Leukocytes
Windup phenomenon, 285, 286
Workup, for trauma patients, 223
Written consent, 4

X
Xylazine (Anased; Rompun), 32-33
  as analgesic agent, 301-302
  analgesic effect of, 278
  benefits of, 24t
  and cardiac arrhythmias, 234
  cyclohexamines used with, 121
  dosages for, 22t
  effects of, 32-33

Xylazine—Cont'd
  IM administration of, 57
  ketamine combined with, 124
  method of use for, 32
  and muscle tone, 91
  as preanesthetic agent, 49
  precautions for, 25*t*
  side effects of, 216
  and vagus nerve, 26
Xylocaine (lidocaine)
  for intubation, 65
  as local analgesia, 253, 254*t*

Y
Yobine (yohimbine), 35, 240*t*
Yohimbine (Yobine)
    in anesthetic emergencies, 240*t*
    as xylazine antagonist, 35, 302
Y piece, 163, 232, 233

Z
Zenecarp (carprofen), 297*t*
Zolazepam, combined with tiletamine,
    124-125